The
New
Psychiatry

The New Psychiatry

How Modern Psychiatrists Think About Their

Patients
Theories
Diagnoses
Drugs
Psychotherapies
Power
Training
Families
and
Private Lives

Jerrold S. Maxmen, M.D.

William Morrow and Company, Inc. New York

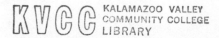

Copyright © 1985 by Jerrold S. Maxmen

I wish to express my gratitude to the authors, publishers, and copyright holders for permission to use the following material:

For a passage in Chapter 1, reproduced from Franz Alexander and Sheldon Selesnick (1966): *The History of Psychiatry*, Harper & Row, Publishers, Inc: New York, pp. 290–291

For a passage in Chapter 2, reproduced from Franz Alexander and Sheldon Selesnick (1966): *The History of Psychiatry*, Harper & Row Publishers, Inc: New York, p. 164

For two passages in Chapter 2, reproduced from American Psychiatric Association (1980): *Diagnostic and Statistical Manual of Mental Disorders*, Third Edition, APA:Washington, DC, pp. 222–223 and p. 6 (respectively)

For a passage in Chapter 2, reproduced from Donald Light (1980): *Becoming Psychiatrists*, W. W. Norton: New York, p. 19

For a passage in Chapter 6, reproduced from David Henderson and R. D. Gillespie (1952): *A Text-Book of Psychiatry*, Seventh Edition, Oxford University Press: London, p. 337

For Table 10–1 in Chapter 10, modified from Zebulon Taintor, Murray Morphy, Anne Seiden, and Eduardo Val (1983): "Psychiatric residency training: relationships and value development," *American Journal of Psychiatry*, 140(6): 778–780. Used with the permission of Dr. Taintor and the American Psychiatric Association.

Library of Congress Cataloging in Publication Data

Maxmen, Jerrold S.
The new psychiatry.

Bibliography: p.
Includes index.
1. Psychiatry—Methodology. 2. Psychiatrists—
Psychology. I. Title.
RC437.5.M39   1985   616.89   84-22798
ISBN 0-688-04242-2

Printed in the United States of America

First Edition

1 2 3 4 5 6 7 8 9 10

To Mimi

To guarantee confidentiality of patients, I have changed their names, ages, sex, religion, city, occupation, and marital status. Virtually all of the patients I describe are composites. At the same time, to convey psychiatric patients and practice as it occurs in fact and not fiction, these composites are of real people and events. Whenever I've altered the truth to protect a patient's confidentiality, I have kept the spirit of that truth. Because every patient mentioned here appears under a pseudonym, any resemblance to actual individuals with the same name is purely coincidental.

Acknowledgments

To portray how psychiatrists think, it is useful to know psychiatrists. In this respect, I have been most fortunate: Along the way, I've worked with many of our nation's finest psychiatrists at Wayne State University, Mount Zion Hospital (San Francisco), Yale University, Dartmouth College, The Albert Einstein College of Medicine (Bronx), and my current home, Columbia University's College of Physicians & Surgeons. These institutions—their faculties, students, and patients—have contributed to every page in this book.

Yet from among all these people, three psychiatrists stand out: Drs. Thomas Detre, Gary Tucker, and the late Edward Sachar. Their integrity, character, intelligence, and kindness have profoundly affected my career, and therefore this book. But more germane, each has helped to pioneer the revolution from psychoanalytic to scientific psychiatry that I'll describe.

Since people in every profession usually have firm ideas about what they do and why they do it, to characterize any profession is a delicate task. So, paraphrasing Montaigne's dictum that only a fool never suspects he could be foolishly mistaken, I sought, and received, much thoughtful advice from those who've read portions of this manuscript: Mary Rae Berman, James Berman, Philip Campanella, Stuart Colby, Dr. Francine Cournos, Diana Grant, Dr. Eric Marcus, Mimi Maxmen, Dr. Ronald Rieder, Dr. Steven Roose, Dr. James Ryan, Dr. Lawrence Sharpe, Dr. Michael Sheehy, Dr. Henry Spitz, and Dr. Gary Tucker. With such excellent help, whatever deficiencies and errors exist in this book are mine.

Finally, I would like to thank Carl Brandt, my agent, for his unfailing insights and support, as well as Nick Bakalar, my editor, for his patience and top-notch professionalism.

Contents

The
New
Psychiatry

ONE

Psychiatry's Second Revolution

This book describes the psychiatry of the 1980s. It shows how the old psychoanalytic psychiatry has been superseded by a new, and radically different, scientific psychiatry. It shows how a new psychiatric consensus has replaced the old "psychological versus biological" disputes. It portrays what modern psychiatrists do and why, what they think and how they think. It reveals what "professional" and "personal" thoughts run through the minds of psychiatrists when they see patients. It presents what people can expect, favorably or not, from scientific psychiatry and from contemporary psychiatrists. Although not a "how-to" book in the usual sense, it should help readers get the most from modern psychiatry.

The book also places psychiatrists on the couch. It analyzes what they are like as people—their motives, problems, and private lives. It depicts how modern psychiatrists view their theories, diagnoses, evaluations, drugs, psychotherapies, patients, images, friends, relatives, and themselves. In short, by describing the new scientific psychiatry, this book demonstrates how, in the 1980s, shrinks think.*

---

*Besides deriving from "headshrinker," the term "shrink" has an older and more favorable basis in the German *zurückschrecken*, "to shrink away"; unlike his

As a social history, this book is, to my knowledge, the first to present a panoramic view of this new scientific psychiatry, especially through the eyes of those who practice it. Until now, writers have discussed the components of this second revolution, such as the development of new drugs or the changing status of psychoanalysis, but they have not painted the larger picture of the revolution itself.

This book focuses on psychiatrists, because they wield more influence than all other mental health professionals. Although much of this material applies to other kinds of therapists, I felt best qualified to examine my own profession.

This will be neither an apology, nor a defense, nor an exposé of psychiatry. I don't care if you end up liking or disliking psychiatrists, wanting them as buddies, or seeking their counsel. This is not a book on what psychiatrists *should* think or on how they *should* behave, but rather on what they *do* think and on how they *do* behave. I want you to see psychiatry for what it is, understand psychiatrists for what they are, and recognize both for what they are not. If you do, I believe you can avoid the pitfalls of the new psychiatry, while capitalizing fully on what it offers.

Modern psychiatry is *not* what most people think it is. Despite popular belief, today's psychiatrists are not debating whether Freud is better than Jung; they are not preoccupied with discovering the meaning and purpose of life, or with providing mental health, or with exploring how psychoanalysis affects culture, or with fostering a sane society, or with interpreting dreams, or with curing a problem by simply unearthing its root, or with seeing how the unconscious causes symptoms. Historically, all these topics were key issues for psychiatrists, but no more.

There has been a revolution in psychiatry. In the 1980s, mainstream American psychiatry has switched from being primarily psychoanalytic to being primarily scientific. These radical changes, although well known to the profession, have largely escaped the public's attention. Consequently, never before has the public had such outdated views of what modern psychiatrists think and do.

When I trained as a psychiatrist from 1968 to 1971, there were two distinct camps within the profession arguing over whether the

---

colleagues, Freud was courageous in not "shrinking away" from the unknown and frightening.

cause and cure of mental illness lay with psychology or biology. Among psychiatrists this conflict no longer exists. Instead, because of this revolution there is now a consensus within the profession which values and integrates both psychology and biology.

Accustomed to the language of yesterday's paradigms, many psychiatrists still *say* the profession is split between biology and psychology; yet a simple look at what today's psychiatrists actually *do* quickly reveals that a consensus has replaced this split. Sure, some psychiatrists are more interested in psychology and others in biology, but in the office, most psychiatrists use both, each for its own purpose. Since recently most major advances have emerged from biological research, books for general audiences typically assert that the new psychiatrist is a biological psychiatrist. Untrue. Examine how modern psychiatrists are trained, what they are expected to know for board certification, what they read in the major psychiatric journals, and how they treat patients. Then it is clear that the new scientific psychiatrist practices an integrated biopsychosocial psychiatry.

American psychiatry's second revolution is as dramatic as its first—the Freudian revolution. Formerly, the center of psychiatric knowledge was psychoanalytic theory; other schools were of marginal or of secondary import. Today, psychoanalytic theory, along with psychosocial, biological, and moral-existential perspectives, is crucial to psychiatry, but the core of psychiatric knowledge derives from scientific evidence instead of psychoanalytic theory. This change is no fad; it represents a fundamentally different view of psychiatry, which involves far more than "drugs versus talk." This change has altered the psychiatrist's concepts of what is clinically true, how he defines the scope of his work, what he does with patients, and how he sees his role in society.

This revolution is of profound importance, since few professions exert as much power and influence as psychiatry. Although constituting less than 16 percent of all mental health personnel, 31,000 psychiatrists rule a mental health industry of over 200,000 professionals,* annually serving 8.2 million patients at an esti-

---

*In 1980, there were about 57,000 psychologists, 21,000 psychiatric social workers, and 100,000 psychiatric nurses, occupational and recreational therapists, and aides.

mated $50 billion a year. Because they are physicians, they can legally force drugs into the unwilling and hospitalize people against their will. By treating the emotionally vulnerable, psychiatrists profoundly affect patients and their families. Psychiatry has revolutionized nearly every American custom and institution, including marriage, sex, child-rearing, love, friendship, work, law, education, ethics, religion, language, entertainment, art, medicine, and death. How this new scientific psychiatry exercises its enormous authority will greatly affect our well-being, individually and collectively.

THE TYPICAL PSYCHIATRIST

There is no "typical" psychiatrist. Psychiatrists vary as much as members of any other profession. Yet given the limits of any generalization, I believe mine accurately reflect the profession. Some facts are beyond dispute.

Psychiatrists are physicians, that is, M.D.s who have completed, in sequence, four years of college, four years of medical school, one year of internship, and at least three years of formal psychiatric training called a residency. Legally, only physicians who have finished psychiatric residencies may call themselves psychiatrists. Since they are physicians, psychiatrists are the only mental health personnel who may give drugs and electroconvulsive (or "shock") treatments. Although roughly half of all psychiatrists obtain personal psychotherapy, it is not required.

In contrast, anyone, even without training, may legally call himself a psychoanalyst, though according to the American Psychoanalytic Association, 98 percent of all bona fide analysts have medical degrees.* Mostly after their psychiatric residencies, would-be analysts study five to ten years at a psychoanalytic institute; they spend three years in courses, five to ten years on the couch, and three to eight years receiving supervision on their conduct of two psychoanalyses. These requirements vary depending on the institute.

A psychotherapist can be, and in fact is, anyone who wants to

*In New York, if not elsewhere, many social workers and psychologists who have taken specialized training consider themselves psychoanalysts. Most psychiatrists find this presumptuous.

use this title. There are no legal or professional criteria for defining a psychotherapist. With no training and enough gall, anyone may claim he's a psychotherapist, hang up a shingle, talk to people, call it therapy, and charge for it.* Most psychotherapists, however, are psychiatrists, psychologists, or psychiatric social workers; some are psychiatric nurses or aides.

The "statistical" psychiatrist

Of the 31,000 American psychiatrists, statistically at least, the "typical" psychiatrist is forty-four years old, white (86 percent), male (82 percent), married (76 percent), Jewish (45 percent) or Protestant (30 percent), American-born (76 percent), and a graduate of an American medical school (75 percent). About 85 percent reside in metropolitan areas, usually on the East or West Coast, mainly in New York (17 percent), Los Angeles (6.5 percent), or San Francisco (5.3 percent).

Most psychiatrists conduct clinical practice (81 percent), though nearly a third teach for more than five hours a week. The primary work site for 56 percent of psychiatrists is their private office; their secondary work site is often a hospital (31 percent) or a medical school (25 percent). Since 1965, psychiatrists have moved away from working exclusively in private practice. In 1980, only 20 percent spent more than thirty-five hours per week in private practice, and the typical psychiatrist works in 2.3 settings. Roughly a quarter of American psychiatrists belong to the American Medical Association and 72 percent belong to the American Psychiatric Association.†

The "typical" psychiatrist is *not* a psychoanalyst; in fact, only

---

*That's almost exactly what Werner Erhard has done. Originally a businessman, he founded *est*—Erhard Seminars Training—a sixty-hour workshop held over two successive weekends, usually in a hotel, in which 250 people seek new outlooks on life. Although Erhard stresses that *est* is education and not psychotherapy, this distinction is more semantic than real. Charging $300 a clip, Erhard is sometimes accused of being a huckster who never left business, since he performs what amounts to psychotherapy without any formal training in it.

†Although the American Medical Association claims to speak for all American physicians, only 45 percent of them belong. This figure would be lower if membership in the AMA or one of its local chapters were not required in some areas to gain hospital staff privileges, malpractice insurance, or a license to practice by the state.

6 percent of American psychiatrists are psychoanalysts. Nonetheless, most psychiatrists still take for granted basic psychoanalytic concepts, such as the unconscious* and defense mechanisms, such as "denial" and "repression." Yet whereas psychiatrists once adhered to a single, usually psychoanalytic, approach, today they draw from *many* approaches. The "typical" psychiatrist prescribes medication, performs individual psychotherapy (89 percent), and treats families and couples (59 percent).

Stereotypes and realities

Psychiatrists are highly stereotyped. That is in part because of psychiatry's power, but also because people naturally feel queasy about doctors who can "read your mind" and "mess with your brain." The negative extreme of this stereotype is psychiatry's "3-D image": daffy, dumb, and dangerous; on the positive side is their "3-A image": altogether, all-knowing, and altruistic.

Even allowing for creative license, when movies like *One Flew Over the Cuckoo's Nest* and *Ordinary People* portray the profession's 3-D and 3-A images respectively, they reinforce the further misconception that psychiatrists are *extraordinary* people—either extraordinarily bad or good, but extraordinary nonetheless. Psychiatrists are *ordinary* people. They are neither sinners nor saints, villains nor heroes; they have all the virtues and frailties of the species.

What is extraordinary is not psychiatrists, but their *circumstances*. Indeed, how these ordinary people contend with these extraordinary circumstances reveals as much about human nature as it does about psychiatrists. When psychiatrists are mistaken for their circumstances, their 3-D and 3-A stereotypes cloud the understanding of what psychiatrists do and why.

THE BOUNDARIES OF PSYCHIATRIC EXPERTISE

Historically, another factor contributing to the wild stereotypes about the profession is that psychiatrists themselves had not

---

*A surefire clue that a person lacks psychiatric sophistication is when he says "subconscious" instead of "unconscious." Freud invoked the term "subconscious" in 1893 in *Studies on Hysteria* with Josef Breuer; yet by 1915 in *The Unconscious,* for largely semantic reasons, he had "outlawed" it; following suit, psychiatrists never use "subconscious" to mean "unconscious."

defined, or even clarified, their genuine areas of knowledge and skill. By claiming there were virtually no limits to psychiatric expertise, psychoanalytic psychiatrists led the public to overestimate the profession's abilities. Whereas this broader concept blurred the boundaries of psychiatric expertise, scientific psychiatrists have clarified these boundaries by drawing them more narrowly. To know what psychiatrists can do (and do well), it is crucial to understand these boundaries.

Mental illness: the sole consensus

Psychiatrists have always agreed their greatest expertise lies in diagnosing and treating patients with mental disorders.* Yet far more than psychoanalytic psychiatrists, scientific psychiatrists distinguish mental disorders from "problems in living." The failure to differentiate between them has created confusion over the boundaries of psychiatric expertise.

Although this distinction is explored in the next chapter, in brief, patients with mental disorders have *symptoms,* such as hallucinations, delusions, and constant sleep, mood, and appetite disturbances. Patients with problems in living are symptom-free; they come to therapy with *issues:* "I can't get along with authority figures," or "I can't find a woman and I'm bored with life." Patients with mental disorders have symptoms *and* issues, those with problems in living have issues only.

Among all mental health professionals, psychiatrists are the chief experts at caring for patients with mental disorders, but inherently no more (or less) expert at helping people with problems in living. Nowadays, many psychiatrists feel that during the psychoanalytic era the profession had lost sight of the fact that, first and foremost, psychiatrists are *physicians* who treat *patients*† with *illness.* Yet even the profession's expertise with mental disorders is questioned, since in comparison to other physicians, psychiatrists never seem to cure anyone.

It is generally unrecognized that psychiatrists are the *only*

---

*For literary convenience, unless specified otherwise, the terms "mental disorder," "mental illness," and "mental disease" will be used interchangeably.

†As do most psychiatrists, in this book I will use the term "patient" and not "client" to indicate anyone a psychiatrist treats, whether or not the person has a mental disorder.

medical specialists who treat disorders that, by definition, have no definitively known causes or cures. At the turn of the century, the most common mental illness was general paresis (i.e., syphilis of the brain). Other psychiatric patients had "myxedema madness" (a type of hypothyroidism), epilepsies, and psychoses caused by vitamin deficiencies and brain infections. Yet as soon as a definitive cause and cure was discovered for each of these conditions, the job of treating them shifted to physicians *other* than psychiatrists, such as internists and neurologists. Even today as the biological causes of and effective drug therapies for severe depression are surfacing, more depressed patients are being treated not by psychiatrists but by general practitioners and internists. Thus, although it's true that psychiatrists can't cure mental illness, that's less an indictment of psychiatrists than a reflection of how medicine assigns illness among its specialties.

During much of this century, because the psychiatrist didn't know the cause of mental illness (and since most biological research had been unproductive), his only option was to speculate, or to devise theories, to account for it. Because it's embarrassing to be "the expert" on the causes of illness when you don't know what they are, the all-too-human psychiatrist often treated his theories as if they were facts. For example, during the 1950s, he didn't speculate, but knew, that overbearing mothers caused schizophrenia. Meanwhile his colleague was equally certain that faulty parental communication caused schizophrenia. As psychoanalytic theories on the causes of mental disorders kept conflicting, psychiatrists' credibility as experts on mental disorders was undermined. So even in their chief area of expertise—diagnosing and treating mental disorders—psychiatrists have often been viewed as "nonexpert experts."

Because they perform psychotherapy for mental disorders and learn psychoanalytic theory, modern psychiatrists are also adept at treating patients with problems in living. Indeed, a large proportion of psychiatric patients have problems in living and not mental disorders. But without detracting from the psychiatrist's skills at helping patients with problems in living, I believe, unlike some of my colleagues, that psychiatrists are no better (or worse) at conducting psychotherapy for these patients than equally well-trained psychologists or psychiatric social workers.

The lurch into "mental health"

As experts on mental disease, psychiatrists are supposed to be experts on *all thinking, feeling, and behaving.* But since every human endeavor involves thinking, feeling, and behaving, psychiatrists are widely assumed to have *unique insights into absolutely everything*—the most obvious area being mental health. Because psychiatrists are the chief authorities on mental illness, they "should" be the chief authorities on mental health.

Yet what is "mental health"? Nobody knows, including psychiatrists. Is it merely the absence of mental illness, or is it more than that, like a heightened state of well-being? In and out of the profession, some claim that to "really" possess mental health, the person's life must have meaning and purpose. Many patients come to psychiatrists saying, "My life is meaningless; it lacks direction and purpose. I have no reason to live and I hope you can give me one." But if humanity's collective wisdom hasn't unearthed the meaning and purpose of life, how can the psychiatrist?

Freud suggested that mental health was the ability to love and to work, yet many people do both and are miserable. So even though nobody knows how to define mental health, how to recognize it, how to get it, and how to provide it, psychiatrists are supposed to be the experts in these imponderables.

Because mental health is often equated with happiness, people eagerly turn to psychiatrists as the "happiness experts." The public demands, and shrinks oblige. Admitting ignorance is no way to be an expert. As "experts" on mental health, many psychiatrists snow the public (and themselves) with flurries of speculations which are frequently conveyed and accepted as facts. Each flake of "fact" quickly melts or turns to slush. Psychiatrists tell us *the* proper way to raise children, even though *the* proper way keeps changing. In one breath psychiatrists encourage parents "to set limits on their kids," while in the next, "to facilitate their free expression." Being ordinary people, shrinks don't know anything more about finding happiness than anyone else; never once is the topic mentioned during their training. Still, psychiatrists are the "experts" at how to choose a mate, keep a mate, love a mate, divorce a mate, and live happily without a mate. Dr. Wayne Dyer writes *The Sky's the Limit,* and not only do shrinks claim they have the "sky" for sale, but plenty of folks buy it.

Nonexpert experts

Being "experts" on thinking, feeling, and behaving, psychiatrists are asked for insights not just on mental illness and health, but on every conceivable nonclinical topic. A business reporter from the *New York Times* contacted me to discover the "psychological reason" for the popularity of Izod-Lacoste shirts. I told her I hadn't the foggiest idea, and that psychiatrists don't have any special insights into such matters. My response didn't please her: She felt I was being coy and holding out on her. She demanded an explanation. The next day my joking with colleagues about this incident met with dismay: They insisted that psychiatrists *do* have unique insights into such matters. When I asked them to prove it by specifying why alligator shirts are the rage, one replied, "Well . . . I think it's due to conformity." Could be, but one hardly needs to be a psychiatrist to say so.

When, to their nation's disgrace, Team Canada lost 8–1 to the Russian hockey team, reporter Stan Fischler went straight to a shrink to understand why a team "chokes." He was told, "It is the inhibition of achievement-directed behavior when approaching success." I'm not sure what that explains. But no matter—there's nothing shrinks can't, don't, and aren't expected to explain.

There are books by psychoanalytic psychiatrists explaining just about everything. History is explained (e.g., *Young Man Luther*); religion is explained (e.g., *Moses and Monotheism*); student activism is explained (e.g., *Young Radicals*); fashion is explained (e.g., *The Psychology of Clothes*); racism is explained (e.g., *Children of Crisis*); nuclear war is explained (e.g., *Death in Life*); creativity is explained (e.g., *Art and Psychoanalysis*); films are explained (e.g., *The Movies on Your Mind*). Although these particular books provide interesting slants, their explanations are insightful only to the extent of the author's intuition, thoughtfulness, and scholarship; they are not derived from his experience as a psychiatrist, and for that matter, these books could have been written just as well by a psychoanalytically sophisticated layman.

Unlike the psychoanalytic psychiatrist, the scientific psychiatrist lays no special claim to nonclinical expertise. That one can see a psychiatrist on TV spouting "psychiatric" insights into terrorism or nuclear war only means that almost anybody can be enticed to say almost anything, if he can say it on TV. That psychiatric concepts are bandied about in respectable magazines as a way of explaining society merely demonstrates that people are free to misapply clinical concepts and write whatever they wish. Yet whenever this occurs, people are misled into believing the typical psychiatrist has expertise in understanding society.

Psychiatrists often reinforce this myth, and when the obvious limits of psychiatric knowledge are exposed, people wonder if psychiatrists know anything at all. Although contemporary psychiatrists are less apt to confuse political with clinical convictions, when they have, they look foolish. Psychiatrists can't diagnose politicians from afar. But to the profession's chagrin, in 1964 *Fact* magazine enticed almost 2,000 (out of 12,000) surveyed psychiatrists to judge whether then-candidate Barry Goldwater was mentally unfit to be president.* Psychiatrists can make an educated hunch about a celebrity's mental state, but unless they see the person clinically, it's no more than a hunch, and the shrink best serves everyone by keeping that hunch to himself.

Before the 1970s, a majority of psychiatrists assumed they had special abilities to understand and to improve society. This was more than a conviction, it was an obligation. Speaking for most of the profession, Dr. William Menninger, after proposing that psychiatrists had unique insights into practically every social ailment from unemployment to bigotry, concluded:

> Theoretically psychiatrists can limit themselves to diagnosis and treatment of patients in offices and hospitals. . . . [Yet] some of us would feel that we had at least accepted a responsibility in actively attacking these so-called social neuroses. . . .

By calling them "social neuroses," Menninger's semantic sleight of hand places social problems under psychiatry's purview. Although he never claims that psychiatrists can exactly solve these problems, he insists they can be of great help. So inspired, when Yale psychiatrists tried to "facilitate communication" between New Haven's police and blacks, a fight broke out. Each group discov-

---

*With clear political bias, 1,189 shrinks expressed doubts over Goldwater's fitness, 657 claimed he was fit, and 571 had enough sense (and taste) to admit they had insufficient information.

ered the value of poor communication and rediscovered what they already knew—they hated each other.

Today's psychiatrists rarely set such optimistic (or presumptuous) goals. Psychiatrists are not trained to "analyze a sick society"; they don't know what a "sick society" means, nor can they "heal" it. Psychiatrists are not oblivious to social conditions; they can't escape seeing poverty, racism, and sexism affect their patients. Yet knowing their time, energy, and skills are limited, most scientific psychiatrists restrict themselves to what they do best—diagnosing and treating mental disorders.

Despite the primary area of psychiatric expertise resting in clinical work, even here, the public isn't so convinced. With all the conflicting claims of nutritionists, sociologists, psychologists, and antipsychiatry groups (e.g., the Mental Patient's Liberation Front), whom can the public believe? In November 1982, 61 percent of voters in Berkeley, California, chose to abolish shock treatment. This was the first time a specific, well-established, and commonplace medical treatment was outlawed by popular election. The courts subsequently overturned the ban. But still, that this referendum passed at all, and that it was about a psychiatric and not a medical issue, indicates that the public doubts psychiatrists' clinical expertise far more than that of other physicians.

Psychiatrists are the only specialists in medical schools who are routinely asked by students, "Does psychiatry work?" Reflecting popular opinion, students will state, "I don't believe in psychiatry," as if psychiatry were a religion. They don't ask, "Does surgery work?" Nor would they say, "I don't believe in pediatrics."

Although many people claim they don't believe in psychiatry, what they mean is unclear. Are they suggesting that medications don't work, or that people don't have feelings, or that talking to people can't alter these feelings, or that psychotherapy can't influence behavior? Perhaps they mean that psychiatry is nothing more than glorified common sense—hardly something requiring experts.

Laymen reveal their view of the psychiatrist as nonexpert expert when saying, "I used psychology on him" (as if psychology were a commodity like hair spray or toothpaste), or "I'm a bit of a psychiatrist myself." Both statements have validity. Laymen are often quite adept at understanding and helping others with problems. Whereas few claim intimate, firsthand knowledge of and familiarity with, let's say, economics or surgery—would anyone say, "I'm a bit of a surgeon myself"?—everybody has direct experience with psychology and behavior. In contrast to economists and surgeons, psychiatrists are nonexpert experts because they have much less of a monopoly over what most people assume to be the field's wisdom—that is, anything to do with psychology.

In truth, psychiatrists are experts at only one area within psychology: that pertaining to mental illness.

Explaining versus understanding

A further source of confusion over the legitimate boundaries of psychiatric expertise stems from the public's, and worse yet, the profession's, incorrectly equating "explaining" with "understanding." Never once have I heard a therapist, teacher, or researcher even allude to this distinction; it appears in the psychiatric literature, but one must really dig for it. In this context, I'm not using "understanding" in the *explanatory* sense of "I understand *why* John hates his mother," but rather in the *descriptive* sense of "I understand *how* John hates his mother."

To explain is to view from the outside; to understand is to view from within. Explaining relies on logic and intellect, understanding on experience and empathy. Explanations try to be objective, whereas understandings can only be subjective. Psychiatric explanations invoke "madness" and "badness" to account for deviance; understanding never involves value judgments.

For different reasons, both explaining and understanding are crucial for clinical care. One is not better than the other; they're different. Explanations address the "why" of behavior, understanding the "what" of behavior.

By definition, psychiatric theories are explanations; they don't entail understanding. To theorize that someone's depression is caused by "repressed rage" or by "deficient biochemicals" might validly explain his unhappiness, but has nothing to do with understanding it.

Depending on how they're used, psychiatric diagnoses can help to explain or to understand. To say a person commits suicide because he has a mental illness called "depression" might be a valid explanation for suicide, but it doesn't enhance understanding of that person's suicide. In contrast, to say that people with the diagnosis of depression experience the world as bleak and hopeless conveys an understanding (and a description) of what it's like to have the illness of depression.

Psychiatrists often say they're "understanding" when they're actually "explaining." To show they "understand" a patient, a psychiatrist will say, "He is denying his anger." That might be so, but it's an explanation; by itself it doesn't reveal understanding. If the patient doesn't believe this explanation, he might respond, "You don't understand me." The psychiatrist then implies that he understands by claiming the patient's objection is a "resistance." This too might be so, but it too is another explanation.

Among themselves, psychiatrists say they talk *to* patients, never *with* patients. And no wonder. You explain things *to* people; you understand things *with* people.

It's not that psychiatrists never understand their patients; to different degrees, some do and some don't. Yet to the degree a psychiatrist does understand, it's more a product of his being a *person* than of his being a *psychiatrist*. Shrinks are no better or worse than anyone else at understanding people. A good novelist reveals a thorough understanding of a character's psychology without ever invoking a psychological term. To varying degrees, everyone understands behavior, because everyone experiences it firsthand.

Many would assume that just by spending so much time helping patients psychiatrists should be, and are, better able to understand people than are laymen. Yet there are different types of "understanding"; people understand in different ways and on different levels. Moreover, understanding of what? Of motivation? Of greed? Of patriotism? Of love? Does a psychiatrist who has never been in love understand more about love than a layman who has been? Does a heterosexual therapist understand more about homosexuality than a homosexual patient? Does a psychiatrist understand more about guilt than an actress who transforms herself nightly into a guilt-ridden Lady Macbeth?

By seeing so many people with mental illness, a psychiatrist does have unusual opportunities to understand what it is like to be mentally ill; but whether a psychiatrist understands more about *being* mentally ill than does the patient or the patient's spouse is questionable. When he sees a patient, a psychiatrist is concentrating almost exclusively on trying to explain the patient's psychology, or on reaching a correct diagnosis, or on deciding about medication; these are all worthy endeavors, but they are not understanding.

One might expect that psychiatrists are trained to understand. Not so. Explaining can be *formally* taught, understanding cannot. Although teaching clinicians to "empathize" more in order to understand more has been tried, it has flopped. Carl Rogers, the humanistic psychologist, had students act "empathetically" before a mirror. Self-consciously, the trainees muttered "ahas" and "uh-hums," practiced raising and lowering their eyebrows, polished their smiles, and rehearsed their "meaningful glances." All to no avail. To empathize, to experience as does another, to understand—these abilities are acquired in life and not in school. It can be no other way.

In contrast, by learning theory and diagnosis, psychiatrists are far more adept at explaining behavior. They can learn how the unconscious does this and how the id does that; they can learn how the brain's chemicals affect this and how the person's environment affects that.

Since "everybody" can understand, what distinguishes the psychiatrist is that he's better at explaining. Psychiatrists emphasize their explanatory skills, since one hardly demonstrates expertise by, or deserves a fee for, doing what everyone does.

Fellow professionals reward psychiatrists for the sophistication of their explanations, but not for the depth of their understanding. That's in part because when speaking with colleagues, it's easier to articulate explanations than to convey understanding. Explanations lend themselves to being displayed in public, understandings do not; they are best revealed in private, alone with a patient and away from colleagues. For all these reasons, psychiatrists overvalue explanations at the expense of understanding, and when psychiatrists fail to make this distinction, they can distance themselves from patients.

Karen, a psychiatric inpatient, was convinced she had no legs. When her psychiatrist went on vacation, she walked up to the staff and complained, more intensely than ever, of having no legs. Every time this occurred, a psychiatrist would reply, "You're walking, so that proves you have legs. But even so, you're obviously worried about having no legs because your doctor is on vacation." Karen was infuriated; she claimed the staff "doesn't understand me." The staff responded, "But we do understand: Your psychiatrist has gone away and you're understandably upset." Patient and staff talk past each other. The patient (accurately) feels she's being "explained away." The staff (mistakenly) thinks they're showing understanding, whereas in reality they're giving a (correct) explanation. A psychiatrist could demonstrate understanding by saying to her, "You must feel like a paraplegic. Of course you can walk, but the fact remains it's frightening to feel you have no control over your legs, or they don't work properly, or they don't belong to you. No wonder you're upset!" When a psychiatrist actually did tell her this, she felt somebody was finally on her "wavelength"; feeling understood, Karen was now ready to consider the explanation that her therapist's departure had upset her.

Advice versus therapy

Psychiatrists are experts at conducting therapy, but not at giving advice. Counselors, palm readers, and grandmothers are all experts at giving advice, and saying that psychiatrists have no particular talents in providing it in no way demeans it or psychiatrists. Except in dealing with mental disorders for which psychiatrists do have specialized knowledge, patients should not expect a psychiatrist to be more (or less) skilled than anybody else at giving advice on problems in living.

Freud knew this. He often stated that the analyst's skills were confined to making the unconscious conscious. That accomplished, he contended, the analyst has no extra skill at knowing how to cope with conscious material, which is giving advice; that's different from providing therapy, which involves examining the unconscious.

For example, a patient asks, "Doc, how can I get along with my husband?" The psychiatrist might well reply, "I don't give advice; that's not what I do. But your grandmother does, and probably good advice too. Ask her. Meanwhile, I wonder if your marital problems would occur no matter who your husband was. If you think they would, or say that such problems have arisen repeatedly in the past with other men, then I'll examine why these problems keep coming up. That's what I do."

THE NEW SCIENTIFIC PSYCHIATRY

Freud's first visit to the United States in 1909 so thoroughly revolutionized American psychiatry from the organic to the psychoanalytic that from the 1930s to the 1970s, psychoanalysis dominated American psychiatry to an extent that never occurred in Europe. Psychoanalytic insights were unique in being highly imaginative and scientifically based. Never before had science so illuminated the human condition. Psychoanalysis fascinated intellectuals and artists, while drawing psychiatrists who practiced it away from medicine.

During the 1960s and early part of the 1970s, psychiatrists developed other theories, in which parents, families, and society supposedly cause mental illness. Derived largely from psychoanalysis, these social theories, along with more traditional psychoanalytic theories, are the core of what I'm calling "psychoanalytic psychiatry."

The public still holds three fundamental beliefs that psychiatrists took for granted during the era of psychoanalytic psychiatry. First, that psychiatrists had to belong to one of two armed camps: psychological or biological. Second, that the core of psychiatry was psychoanalysis, and that everything else was at best second-rate. Third, that "good" psychiatrists used talking therapies, whereas "bad" psychiatrists drugged, shocked, and lobotomized people. Published in 1966, *The History of Psychiatry* reflected main-line psychiatric thought:

> There can be no question that the psychotropic drugs have great practical value. . . . However, psychological habituation to a chemically induced oblivion is an unrealistic solution and a basically unreliable crutch that only compounds the problems in day-to-day living. . . . In the final analysis, the situations that provoke emotional upsets and the subjective experience of psychic pain cannot be explained in terms of the nervous system but must be described in psychological language.

Psychoanalytic psychiatry insisted on a dichotomy between the biological and the psychological. Within the profession, psychiatrists who dared synthesize the two were deemed too wishy-washy to take a stand.

Today the polarization between psychological and biological psychiatry is still maintained by much of the public, even though most psychiatrists have discarded it. Inside the profession, the monopoly of psychoanalytic psychiatry crumbled during the mid-1970s, so that in 1980, when the American Psychiatric Association radically changed its official system for diagnosis (see Chapter 2), a revolution had occurred in American psychiatry: The central role of psychoanalytic psychiatry had been superseded by what I'm calling "scientific psychiatry."

As American psychiatry's second revolution, the conversion to scientific psychiatry extends far beyond the usual debates over "nature versus nurture," "talk versus drugs," and "psychology versus biology." This revolution doesn't involve a mere change of theories; it entails a fundamentally different *approach* to psychiatry: It has altered forever psychiatric views on mental illness, diagnosis, treatment, patients, the nature of clinical evidence, the profession's relationship to general medicine, and the boundaries of psychiatric expertise. Some psychiatrists regret this revolution, but none deny it has happened.

In describing these two psychiatries and the reasons for this revolution, this book emphasizes that today's scientific psychiatrist doesn't ignore psychoanalysis, but uses it differently. The old psychoanalytic psychiatrist virtually equated psychoanalysis and psychiatry, whereas today's psychiatrist employs scientific psychiatry first, and when its usefulness expires, he turns to other approaches.

In treating patients, modern psychiatrists apply, in sequence, three types of interventions. First, the psychiatrist prescribes medications to rectify *biological* abnormalities. Second, he performs psychotherapies to address *psychosocial* problems. Third, he uses the doctor-patient relationship to show that he values the patient as a person, the so-called *moral-existential* dimension of treatment. Throughout this book I'll detail how modern scientific psychiatrists employ this three-stage process. But for now, I merely wish to stress that although contemporary psychiatrists view science as the center of psychiatry, they believe that treating patients involves more than science.

The two psychiatries

Psychoanalytic psychiatry bases truth on authority; something is true because Freud said so. Scientific psychiatry bases truth on scientific experimentation; something is true because of the quality of the experiment and not because of who conducted it. The old psychiatry derives from theory, the new psychiatry from fact.

Psychoanalytic psychiatry emphasizes the abstract, scientific psychiatry the concrete. To the psychoanalytic psychiatrist, symptoms have meaning and are viewed as metaphors; to the scientific psychiatrist, symptoms are just symptoms. In psychoanalytic psychiatry, an explanation is true as long as it sounds right, whereas in scientific psychiatry, it must be proved right. During the 1960s, the following formulation was typical of those found in patients' charts:

> The patient has the fixed delusion that others (not near him) can smell his rectal gas and are terribly distressed by it. He tries to control his offensive anger by expelling his flatus in the bathroom, but not in the presence of people who could retaliate.*

The traditional psychiatrist used a single framework; the contemporary psychiatrist employs multiple frameworks. As a true believer, the psychoanalytic psychiatrist treated his theory as gospel and others as heresy. As an agnostic, the scientific psychiatrist uses, but doubts, every theory; although partial to "hard" science, he may overlook that science itself is also a system of belief.

To the psychoanalytic psychiatrist, madness is quantitative; we're all nuts, just some more than others. Under overwhelming stress any neurotic can become schizophrenic. To the scientific psychiatrist, madness is qualitative; one has it or doesn't have it. A few do, most don't. Under overwhelming stress and even if he tries, a neurotic cannot become a schizophrenic.

---

*As with this explanation, psychoanalytic explanations usually suffer from an overabundance of plausible yet ambiguous interpretations of the same information.

By dint of professional training and experience, the psychoanalytic psychiatrist feels uniquely qualified, if not obligated, to understand society and to correct its ills. The scientific psychiatrist restricts his expertise to the office. The psychoanalytic psychiatrist has universal theories of the mind which explain everyone's behavior—pathological or normal. The scientific psychiatrist's theories of the mind account only for psychopathology.

The psychoanalytic psychiatrist views himself as a psychiatrist first and a physician second; it's the reverse for scientific psychiatrists. The psychoanalytic psychiatrist avoids medicine, the scientific psychiatrist embraces it.

The psychoanalytic psychiatrist views psychotherapy more as an *artistic* endeavor, whereas the scientific psychiatrist believes psychotherapy should (and can) be as *scientific* as anything else in medicine.

Ideology primarily directs the psychoanalytic psychiatrist's choice of treatment, whereas pragmatism primarily directs that of the scientific psychiatrist. Although it gives lip service to biology, traditional psychiatry is a strictly psychological affair, which concentrates on the mind. The new psychiatry incorporates, but downplays, psychology; it emphasizes biology in general and the brain in particular.

Psychoanalytic psychiatrists focus on the *causes* of deviance, whether they stem from childhood experiences, family dynamics, social pressures, or universal symbols. Although scientific psychiatrists are also interested in the causes of deviance, they're mainly concerned with the *nature* of deviance. The *motivations* behind symptoms intrigue the psychoanalytic psychiatrist; their *descriptions* interest the scientific psychiatrist. The traditional psychiatrist asks, "Why?"; the contemporary psychiatrist asks, "What?"

Science and psychiatry

Most psychoanalysts claim their theory is a science, because it derives from systematic, objective, and repeated observations. Yet however "scientific" psychoanalysis may be and how intellectually disciplined an analyst might be, psychoanalytic theory and treatment are not "scientific" in the ways that other physicians use the term. Being so abstract, psychoanalytic concepts are virtually impossible to test scientifically.

Psychoanalytic findings lack "reliability," which refers to

whether observers can agree they are observing the same thing. When diagnosing a patient or indicating their chief psychological conflict, psychoanalytic psychiatrists usually give different answers; they display "low (interrater) reliability."

Research in scientific psychiatry shows much higher reliability largely because it's *quantified*. By investigating objective (and observable) phenomena, such as how long a patient slept or whether he hallucinated, numbers can be assigned. But even subjective judgments can be quantified, such as "On a scale from 1 to 10, how depressed are you?" "Numbers research"—as analysts call it disparagingly—allows for well-designed scientific studies, which use "double-blind" conditions, contrast experimental with matched control groups, and employ statistical methods to discover whether a finding is accidental or significant.

Statistical analysis can best produce scientifically valid results when there are large numbers of subjects. By its very nature, psychoanalytic research can only investigate very few subjects even though each patient is studied in depth. For instance, Freud's theory on hysteria derived from three cases, and his dictum that latent homosexuality caused paranoia was based on one patient (whom he never even met!). Thus, psychoanalytic psychiatry gave rise to relatively many theories based on relatively few observations, whereas in scientific psychiatry it is just the opposite.

The quality of this scientific research varies. Yet, as in every other medical specialty, the use of scientific experimentation in psychiatry means that modern psychiatrists can state facts and not just opinions.

When psychiatrists base their decisions on scientific studies instead of theoretical speculations, patients benefit. Diagnoses aren't just labels, but helpful guides for determining treatment. In scientific psychiatry, one can be relatively certain what various treatments can, or cannot, accomplish, and find out much earlier how they can harm. Today's psychiatrist can predict with far more accuracy the future course and outcome of a mental illness.

There are limits to scientific investigations. Rigorous experimentation might show whether psychotherapy helps anxious patients, but it doesn't illuminate what the psychiatrist should say to such patients. Studies might demonstrate whether losing a parent during childhood predisposes one to depression as an adult, but they will not reveal how an individual patient feels about losing his parent, nor what this loss symbolizes to him, nor how it will affect the rest of his life.

Today, many patients come to psychiatrists expecting the psychoanalytic psychiatry that has dominated the American scene for over half a century. But what they find is quite different, for psychiatry has undergone a revolution that's completely changed what psychiatrists do, how they think, and why.

TWO

How Psychiatrists Diagnose

On July 1, 1980, the ascendance of scientific psychiatry became official. For on this day, the American Psychiatric Association (APA) published a radically different system for psychiatric diagnosis called *The Diagnostic and Statistical Manual of Mental Disorders, Third Edition,* or more commonly, *DSM-III.* By adopting the scientifically based *DSM-III* as its official system for diagnosis, American psychiatrists broke with a fifty-year tradition of using psychoanalytically based diagnoses. Perhaps more than any other single event, the publication of *DSM-III* demonstrated that American psychiatry had indeed undergone a revolution.

With the emergence of *DSM-III* there has been a renaissance in psychiatric diagnosis. Before *DSM-III,* psychiatrists paid relatively little mind to diagnosis: Because a formal diagnosis was more important for insurance forms than for clinical care, psychiatrists rarely bothered to make a precise diagnosis. In contrast, with the development of *DSM-III,* psychiatrists have felt that diagnosis is essential for treating patients. Today's psychiatrists perform a careful diagnostic evaluation on *every* patient they see to determine if the patient has a mental disorder, and if so, what kind. (To spare patients from unnecessary or incorrect treatments, psychiatrists also want to know when patients do *not* have a mental disorder.)

Paradoxically, while psychiatric diagnosis was enjoying a revitalization within the profession, its reputation among intellectually sophisticated laymen was at an all-time low. The public widely concurred with America's best-known psychiatrist, Dr. Thomas Szasz, who claims, "The concept of mental illness is the pivotal mendacity of psychiatry." Szasz became famous by championing the view that psychiatric diagnosis is a cruel hoax psychiatrists perpetrate on nonconformists to deprive them of civil liberties, stigmatize them with meaningless labels, and undermine their self-confidence; psychiatrists diagnose just to inflate their egos, extend their power, and increase their incomes.

Is Szsaz correct? The question of how and why psychiatrists diagnose is crucial, because if Szasz is right, then not only are diagnoses meaningless, but *DSM-III*'s revitalization of psychiatric diagnosis will cause inordinate harm to patients.

THE PURPOSES OF PSYCHIATRIC DIAGNOSIS

A diagnosis should indicate the cause of a mental disorder, but as discussed later, since the etiologies of most mental disorders are unknown, current diagnostic systems can't reflect them. On the other hand, at present, psychiatric diagnosis can serve seven major purposes: (1) to determine whether a person's abnormal state is due to a mental disorder, (2) to guide treatment, (3) to predict outcome, (4) to illuminate if and how a mental disorder is inherited, (5) to facilitate intraprofessional communication, (6) to advance research, and (7) to uncover mental disorders.

Psychiatry, like other professions, has its own confusing jargon, yet a technical vocabulary does have a legitimate purpose: It affords professionals a convenient shorthand for conveying more complex information. But if technical terms mean different things to different people within the profession, a major reason to have a technical language is defeated.

During the era of psychoanalytic psychiatry, such "diagnostic anarchy" prevailed, with most psychiatrists having their own idiosyncratic notions of what constituted, for example, "schizophrenia" or "hysteria."* Yet by having an *external standard* which

---

*Of course, nobody "owns" a word or has "exclusive rights" to decide a word's "correct" meaning. Words are symbols; they're not what they describe. The word

defines diagnostic (and other technical) terms, as a dictionary defines words, psychiatrists can at least know what their colleagues mean by the term "schizophrenia" or "hysteria."

It's crucial to determine whether a patient has, or does not have, a mental disorder. For example, a patient can have insomnia, but if that insomnia is due to a mental disorder, it may well have long-term genetic, familial, behavioral, and therapeutic implications. On the other hand, if the insomnia is not due to a mental disorder, it may be a relatively minor matter. To make this distinction, diagnosis is essential.

If a patient does have a mental disorder, a patient's diagnosis should help to decide which specific biological and psychosocial treatments would be most therapeutic. An accurate psychiatric diagnosis should enable a psychiatrist to tell his patient how an illness is likely to affect his future. Will he improve, will he return to his normal level of functioning, and if so, will the illness recur? A useful diagnostic system should further indicate if and how a mental illness is genetically transmitted. Ideally, a diagnosis would show, for example, that if a parent is schizophrenic, the chance of his child's being schizophrenic is X percent.

A reliable diagnostic system is critical for effective clinical research. For instance, if one wishes to find out if drug A or B works better for the mental disorder of major depression, it is crucial to define "major depression." Whether the resultant definition is "right" or "wrong" is irrelevant; what's germane is that the researchers studied patients with similar clinical features and that readers understand what the researchers meant by "major depression."

As we'll see, another function of diagnosis is to reveal mental disorders that have been overlooked or confused with already-known disorders. Later I'll demonstrate how by paying close attention to diagnosis, psychiatrists "discovered," or more accurately uncovered, panic disorders. Instead of considering panic attacks as "just" another type of anxiety, psychiatrists found they

---

"chair" is not a chair; you may call it a "'penguin" or an "ishkabibble," but nobody would understand. A chair is only called a "chair" because it's a social convention for communication; dictionaries clarify and formalize these conventions. Each profession defines its own terms to convey specific meanings to fellow professionals, but when these terms are vague, they obfuscate.

were the cardinal symptom of a distinct disorder, which, among other things, required very different treatments.

Unlike that of the psychoanalytic era, today's diagnostic system affords psychiatrists these seven advantages, though how helpful they are varies greatly with the particular mental disorder. Understanding how psychiatric diagnosis came to its present state requires an understanding of a critical difference between psychoanalytic and scientific psychiatry.

TWO DIAGNOSTIC TRADITIONS

Except in America, psychiatric diagnosis has always been rooted in the older diagnostic tradition of "descriptive psychiatry." In America, however, psychiatric diagnosis was based on the psychoanalytic tradition, until scientific psychiatry resurrected the descriptive tradition.

Descriptive psychiatry is that aspect of psychiatry which describes the patient's symptoms, including his subjective experiences. Because descriptions should strive for accuracy, they're made at the lowest possible level of inference. The psychiatrist knows of these symptoms by direct observation (e.g., agitation, crying), or by indirect reports from the patient (e.g., sadness, hallucinations). In descriptive psychiatry, whether observed or reported, symptoms are delineated in detail; they are not interpreted.

Even though all psychiatrists use descriptive psychiatry, scientific psychiatrists rely on it far more than psychoanalytic psychiatrists. To scientific psychiatrists, symptoms are symptoms are symptoms, whereas in psychoanalytic psychiatry, symptoms are symptoms, but more significantly, they are symbols, important less for their existence and more for their meaning. In psychoanalytic thought, "symptoms" are based on theoretical concepts; they derive from relatively high levels of inference (e.g., "weak ego boundaries," "unconscious conflict").

Psychoanalytic psychiatry emphasizes the "why" of behavior, while descriptive psychiatry emphasizes the "what" of behavior. Although the differences between the why and the what are crucial, patients, and even medical students, rarely appreciate them.

In front of a group of first-year medical students I was interviewing a very bizarre patient who looked as if he hadn't washed for years. His scraggly beard was infested with lice and his hair caked with dandruff. His furtive glances avoided eye contact; nevertheless, they elicited sympathy as much as they threatened. His demeanor was kindly, his voice soft. His speech was mostly incomprehensible, but he managed to communicate the following: Having locked himself in his bedroom for the past seven months, he hadn't seen another person until the day before, when he was hospitalized. He was unhappy with life. He considered his parents "sinister" and "sadistic," since they "don't like how I live."

After the patient left the room, I asked these students for their assessment. They found nothing wrong with him. As one student explained, "With disapproving parents like his, no wonder he's unhappy. His problem is lousy parents, not mental illness."

Like most students, they were confusing the why with the what of behavior. Even if his parents were nasty and drove their son crazy, that's the why of behavior. That the son *is* crazy—or acts crazy, if you prefer—is still a fact; it is the what of behavior. Just because strange behavior seems "understandable" or we can guess why it occurs, that in no way alters the fact that it does occur.

In the descriptive tradition, diagnostic categories are defined exclusively by objective findings, such as symptoms, life course, and age of onset. In the analytic tradition, diagnostic categories are defined not only by objective findings, but also by subjective inferences about psychological mechanisms and forces.

The work of German psychiatrist Emil Kraepelin (1856–1926) best exemplifies the descriptive tradition. His fame was well deserved, for after describing the clinical features of thousands of very disturbed hospitalized patients, he created psychiatry's first major diagnostic system. He divided all the patients without obvious brain damage into two groups based primarily on prognosis and secondarily on age of onset. One group were patients whose delusions, hallucinations, and other bizarre traits initially appeared during their teens or twenties; despite transitory improvements throughout their lives and no matter how humane the treatment, these patients gradually and inevitably became worse. These unfortunates he diagnosed as having "dementia praecox," with "dementia" referring to the disorder's cardinal feature of a progressive downhill course* and "praecox" to its youthful onset. Since 1911, dementia praecox has been called "schizophrenia."

Kraepelin's second group of patients did not deteriorate, but typically returned to normal in between severe bouts of depression or mania. Although their depression or mania (or both) could arise at any age, patients with what Kraepelin called "maniacal depression" were usually not hospitalized until after the age of thirty.

Because during the depths of a patient's illness it can be hard to distinguish symptoms of manic-depression from those of dementia praecox (i.e., schizophrenia), symptoms could not always serve as the sole basis for diagnosis. Kraepelin showed that another criterion—the life course of an illness—could be used, and he was the first to build a psychiatric nomenclature using it.

Kraepelin's descriptive approach thrived in Europe, but fizzled in an America dazzled by psychoanalysis. From the 1930s to the 1970s, most American psychiatrists felt descriptive psychiatry was archaic, dehumanizing, vapid, and dumb. Published in 1966, the widely read book *The History of Psychiatry* reflected mainstream American psychiatry:

> What once in the past meant progress, when compared with subsequent [psychoanalytic] developments, often serves as a retarding influence . . . a rigid and sterile codifier of disease categories; even if these were valid, they contribute to neither understanding the causes of disease nor their prognosis. His [Kraepelin's] work is the culmination of that antipsychological era that . . . dominated the scene until Freud's motivational approach revived interest in the patient as a unique person with a unique history.

THE DEMISE OF ANALYTIC DIAGNOSES

The analytic tradition gave rise to the first two editions of America's official diagnostic system—*DSM-I* and *DSM-II*, published in 1952 and 1968 respectively. Yet, when *DSM-II* was re-

---

*Dementia praecox induced many patients to have terrible hygiene, frequently causing brain infections, which commonly produced a "true" dementia that hastened deterioration and death (often in their thirties).

leased, the analytic diagnostic tradition was already on the way out.

The transatlantic embarrassment

I doubt that any psychiatric research discredited the analytic method of diagnosis more than the US/UK Study, published in 1972. Indeed, just one part of this complex investigation can illustrate why the analytic approach was so unreliable as to be meaningless.

The researchers showed 250 British and 450 American psychiatrists videotapes of eight patients being interviewed by a psychiatrist. These experienced psychiatrists then were asked to diagnose each of the videotaped patients. Keep in mind that by looking at the identical videotapes, psychiatrists on both sides of the Atlantic saw the *same* patients presenting the *same* verbal and nonverbal information to the *same* psychiatrist. Nevertheless, most of the patients the British diagnosed as "depressed" the Americans diagnosed as "schizophrenic." The patients didn't change, nor did the data for diagnosing them; only the diagnosis changed. This finding did not address whether mental illness exists, nor did it tell whether the Americans or the British were correct. What it did show was that American and British psychiatrists used vastly different criteria for diagnosing mental illness.

A second finding was that with every patient, American psychiatrists "detected" many more symptoms, especially symptoms associated with schizophrenia. Following the dictum that even a trace of schizophrenia is schizophrenia, American psychiatrists had a much broader concept of schizophrenia and applied it more frequently.

Unlike British psychiatrists, who usually made the same diagnosis no matter where they lived, the diagnostic practices of American psychiatrists varied enormously depending on their city: Those residing in North Carolina and St. Louis diagnosed a bit more like the British, whereas those from New York, Boston, Baltimore, Topeka, and California diagnosed "American-style." As a result, the US/UK Study confirmed what the critics had charged all along: Psychiatric diagnosis was highly unreliable, and psychiatrists, especially Americans, couldn't agree on what constituted the major mental illnesses.

The study invalidated practically all research into mental disorders. When a researcher reported on a group of "schizophrenics," how could the reader know what kind of patients were being studied? American research was especially problematic. If a study claimed that drug X helped a hundred schizophrenics, the reader wouldn't know if drug X helped patients with depression, severe neuroses, mania, paranoia, schizophrenia, or something else.

The only way a reader could know what the researcher meant by a particular mental disorder was if the researcher explicitly listed his diagnostic criteria for that disorder. During the early 1970s, psychiatric researchers started doing so. The practice caught on; now it's virtually required in all scientific publications. More important, delineating specific diagnostic criteria, a practice which began strictly for research, resurrected the descriptive diagnostic tradition and became the cornerstone for *DSM-III*.

Is everyone crazy?

The descriptive tradition maintained by today's scientific psychiatrists holds that most people are *not* crazy. The analytic tradition holds that, as a price for civilization, to various degrees everyone is crazy. The descriptive tradition follows the medical model: Most people don't have disease, but when they do, they have distinct illnesses, such as asthma, diabetes, and angina. This "multiple qualitative" view differs from psychoanalytic psychiatry's "unitary quantitative" view. The analytic tradition implies there is but one mental illness, and its name is simply a relative matter, one of degree, not type—from the least severe to the most: "neuroses," "personality disorders," "manic-depression," and "schizophrenia."

That's why the psychoanalytically based and widely quoted Midtown Manhattan Study performed in 1954 and "reconfirmed" twenty years later arrived at the alarming conclusion that 80 percent of adults had symptoms of a mental illness. From a descriptive perspective, this conclusion is ridiculous.*

For example, in 1975, scientific psychiatrists from St. Louis published an article titled "Is Everyone Depressed?" Aware that

---

*When clearly defined diagnostic criteria were used in a survey of ten thousand adults—the largest psychiatric epidemiological study ever conducted—in 1984, the National Institute of Mental Health reported that 20 percent of Americans had a mental disorder (see Chapter 3).

many serious depressions are transmitted in part by genes, the researchers figured that if anyone should be depressed, it should be the blood relatives of depressed patients. Yet only 10 percent of this high-risk group had ever had a depressive illness, and only 26 percent could remember ever feeling severely depressed for more than several days. Their study concluded that although everyone gets moody, most people do *not* have a mental disorder—depression or anything else.

A major reason psychoanalytic psychiatrists overdiagnosed mental illness was that they focused often exclusively on the unconscious, which by definition is irrational. Consequently, psychoanalytic psychiatrists kept seeing people's craziness. Patients diagnosed as "neurotic" by analytic criteria would have "no mental disorder" by descriptive criteria. Psychoanalytic psychiatrists would often claim that as they "gained experience" they could detect "schizophrenia" in patients who otherwise appeared "neurotic." The notion that people were crazier than met the eye pleased the avant-garde, leading artists and psychoanalytic psychiatrists to reinforce each other's beliefs. The only thing missing was scientific evidence.

The excessive diagnosis of "schizophrenia" explained why many psychiatrists claimed to "cure" schizophrenia. Countless books like Mark Vonnegut's *The Eden Express* or Hannah Green's *I Never Promised You a Rose Garden* portrayed how ever-so-humane psychotherapy brought "schizophrenics" into "sanity." Yet by today's scientific criteria, these patients were never schizophrenic; in reality, they had mania, depression, or some other more benign mental disorder and eventually would have returned to normal without any psychological or biological treatments.

To assume that everybody is crazy is, in a sense, to believe that nobody is crazy. To consider everyone mentally ill, or everyone as being, to various extents, schizophrenic, defeats the main purpose of diagnosis, which is to identify meaningful categories of illness so that doctors know when to use, or not use, a particular treatment. Although the analytically oriented *DSM–II* never suggested that everyone was mentally ill, by not carefully defining the diagnostic criteria for each mental illness, *DSM–II* could not help psychiatrists determine treatment.

Further problems with DSM–II

Vagueness, more than anything else, undermined *DSM–II*. Although it never defined diagnostic categories, *DSM–II* did try to characterize them. Yet in "allowing for maximal clinical judgment," *DSM–II*'s diagnostic categories were so nonspecific they were meaningless.

Although *DSM–II*'s diagnostic descriptions included symptoms, they offered no guide as to how severe symptoms had to be, or how many symptoms had to exist before a particular condition qualified as a mental disorder. Moreover, *DSM–II*'s diagnostic descriptions did not show how one mental disorder differed specifically from another. (*DSM–III* answers these questions.) Yet to psychoanalytic psychiatrists, these deficiencies were minor, since *objective* descriptions were only a small part of diagnosis.

In their view, diagnoses should never be based on anything as "superficial" as objective features, but rather on the "deeper" matters of etiology and pathophysiology. This meant that most disorders sprang from unconscious mechanisms and came as "reactions" to something—real or imagined, past or present (e.g., an anniversary, a broken romance, a flunked exam). But even if these factors play the role they're supposed to—a dubious assumption—psychiatrists are unlikely to make the same diagnosis on a patient when their diagnosis depends primarily on such "deeper" matters. For what lies in the unconscious can't be proved or disproved, and events sufficiently stressful to trigger a "reaction" happen constantly. (Review your past week and you'll surely find some "stressful event" to justify your having a "psychotic reaction"). When a diagnostic system is based on factors that can't be defined, "facts" that can't be verified, and forces that can't be seen, its diagnostic criteria will be vague.

Psychoanalytic psychiatrists would claim to diagnose "by feel"; they'd say, "The patient must be schizophrenic, because he has that schizophrenic feel about him." By "that schizophrenic feel," psychiatrists usually meant the patient seemed remote, distant, and spaced-out, as if the patient were in a different room or someplace else. Other psychiatrists, however, would state that a patient "felt schizophrenic" because he seemed "empty inside." Diagnosis "by feel" was thoroughly subjective, idiosyncratic, imprecise, and widespread.

During my internship, when I asked a respected San Francisco psychoanalyst why he thought his patient was schizophrenic, he said, "Because she's a blob. Anybody who's that fat must have practically no ego boundaries." Noting my skepticism, he offered the definitive proof: "She's such an oral character, she has to be schizophrenic." However fatuous, this kind of diagnostic reasoning was common.

When the criteria for mental illness were vague, subjectively derived, and based more on inference and intuition, diagnosis was ripe for abuse. For instance, studies showed that blacks with the same clinical features as whites would more likely receive the bleaker and more damning diagnosis of schizophrenia. Without precise, objectified diagnostic criteria, if a psychiatrist did not like a patient, that patient was more likely to be labeled "schizophrenic." It is no wonder that patients often experienced diagnosis more as an accusation than as an assessment.

Since it served virtually no legitimate purpose for psychiatric diagnosis, *DSM–II* was hard to justify. Because psychiatrists were unable to demonstrate any usefulness for *DSM–II*, increasingly, artists, intellectuals, lawyers, patients, and the general public viewed diagnosis as nothing but "name-calling." By the late 1960s, a growing number of psychiatrists were agreeing, and by 1974, *DSM–II*'s diagnostic anarchy became so glaringly apparent that the American Psychiatric Association (APA) set to work on massively revising the profession's official nomenclature. In making this decision, the APA's leadership acknowledged the profession's need to become more scientific.

THE EMERGENCE OF *DSM–III*

Besides the mounting disenchantment with *DSM–II*, three developments in scientific psychiatry hastened the switch to *DSM–III*.

First, medications were discovered that worked specifically on different mental illnesses. Until the mid-1950s the only important treatments for mental illness were "talking" therapies, which patients received based more on their income than on their illness. Drug therapy was ancillary. The drugs were usually barbiturates, and their effects were nonspecific. These medications calmed everyone, "normals" as well as the mentally ill; they worked the same whether patients were depressed, schizophrenic, phobic, or anything else.

In contrast, the drugs of the new scientific psychiatry have no effect on "normals." Antidepressant medications (e.g., Elavil), for instance, do not make "normal" people happier, they only help patients with the mental disorder of depression return to normal. Moreover, these new drugs usually benefit a *specific* mental illness. In general, antipsychotic drugs (e.g., Thorazine) help schizophrenics, but not depressives; antidepressant drugs help only depressives.

But it was the introduction of lithium, which is specific for manic-depression, that truly revitalized American interest in diagnosis. Before lithium became available in the United States in 1971, whether patients were diagnosed "schizophrenic" or "manic" didn't matter; in either case they'd receive antipsychotic drugs. With lithium it became essential to distinguish between schizophrenia and mania, since that decision determined which drug was used.

Second, a scientific method that incorporated quantitative techniques was now being extensively used to study mental illness. Piece by piece, solid data accumulated showing which mental disorders ran in families, which were inherited, which had predictable life courses, which afflicted various demographic populations, which involved biological changes, which improved with one type of drug but not others, and so on.

These findings afforded psychiatrists many more objectifiable facts for making diagnoses. Because mental illnesses cause no gross physical changes, psychiatrists must rely on other criteria for diagnosis. The availability of all these new scientifically derived findings was making it possible to delineate meaningful diagnostic categories.

Third, researchers devised explicit, readily verifiable, and specific diagnostic criteria. *DSM–II* was never clear on how a mental disorder differed from normality or from other mental disorders. Professional papers in the psychoanalytic era typically read, "Patients were considered schizophrenic if two clinicians felt that was their diagnosis." Because these criteria were obviously too vague for decent scientific study, in 1972, psychiatric researchers from St. Louis published a landmark paper that defined each mental disorder by listing its exact type and quantity of pathological features. After some adjustment for clinical purposes, this research method for defining mental disorders became the basic approach of *DSM–III*.

Comparing DSM–II *and* DSM–III

To illustrate, let's see how *DSM–II* and *DSM–III* define a type of moderately severe depression, which the former calls a "depressive neurosis" and the latter a "dysthymic disorder." Please don't diagnose yourself. Just compare how each system characterizes the same disorder. My clarifications will be in brackets, *DSM*'s in parentheses.

DSM–II: DEPRESSIVE NEUROSIS

> This disorder is manifested by an excessive reaction of depression due to an internal conflict or to an identifiable event such as the loss of a love object [i.e., a person] or cherished possession.

DSM–III: DIAGNOSTIC CRITERIA FOR DYSTHYMIC DISORDER

[According to *DSM–III,* a patient has a mental disorder only if he satisfies *all* of the criteria—in this case, all six, from A through F.]

> **A.** During the past two years . . . the individual has been bothered most or all of the time by symptoms characteristic of the depressive syndrome but that are not of sufficient severity and duration to meet the criteria for a major depressive [i.e., very severe] episode [as defined elsewhere in *DSM–III*].
>
> **B.** The manifestations of the depressive syndrome may be relatively persistent or separated by periods of normal mood lasting a few days to a few weeks, but no more than a few months at a time.
>
> **C.** During the depressive periods there is either prominent depressed mood (e.g., sad, blue, down in the dumps, low) or marked loss of interest or pleasure in all, or almost all, usual activities and pastimes.

47

D. During the depressive periods at least three of the following symptoms are present:
1. insomnia or hypersomnia
2. low energy or chronic tiredness
3. feelings of inadequacy, loss of self-esteem, or self-deprecation
4. decreased effectiveness or productivity at school, work, or home
5. decreased attention, concentration, or ability to think clearly
6. social withdrawal
7. loss of interest in or enjoyment of pleasurable activities
8. irritability or excessive anger . . .
9. inability to respond with apparent pleasure to praise or rewards
10. less active or talkative than usual, or feels slowed down or restless
11. pessimistic attitude toward the future, brooding about past events, or feeling sorry for self
12. tearfulness or crying
13. recurrent thoughts of death or suicide

E. Absence of psychotic features, such as delusions, hallucinations, incoherence, or loosening of associations [i.e., speech in which thoughts seem unconnected].

F. If the disturbance is superimposed on a preexisting mental disorder, such as Obsessive Compulsive Disorder or Alcohol Dependence, the depressed mood, by virtue of its intensity or effect on functioning, can be clearly distinguished from the individual's usual mood.

The most striking difference between *DSM–II* and *DSM–III* is that the latter presents very specific diagnostic criteria, qualitatively and quantitatively. On the other hand, *DSM–II*'s description of depression merely indicates that depressed patients are depressed. By being so specific, *DSM–III*'s criteria for depression are more restrictive than those of *DSM–II*. In contrast to *DSM–III,* it's unclear in *DSM–II* if being sad (or depressed) for a week or even a day qualifies as a depressive neurosis. Whether *DSM–III* distinguishes a dysthymic disorder from normal human sadness in the best way is debatable, but in *DSM–III* the problem is acknowledged and a solution, which can be tested scientifically, is proposed, which is not so in *DSM-II*.

By making diagnostic criteria explicit, *DSM-III* establishes a standard for diagnosing a mental illness. In *DSM-II* there was no (external) standard; diagnostic criteria were idiosyncratic, based strictly on "clinical judgment." Just as physical disorders do not occur with identical symptoms in every case, so too with mental disorders. Yet unlike *DSM-II*, *DSM-III* recognizes this variability: As shown in criterion D, *DSM-III* has the psychiatrist pick from among several of a mental disorder's specific characteristics. Finally, *DSM-II*'s definition includes the disorder's (supposed) etiologies. *DSM-III* doesn't mention any etiologies.

HOW PSYCHIATRISTS MAKE DIAGNOSTIC CATEGORIES

Everyone "diagnoses," including you. We categorize people's madness by saying, "He's sick," "She's crazy," "He's neurotic," "She's a real hysteric," "I'm a superobsessive," "He's paranoid." These "diagnoses" are not baseless; they derive from very real observations of people. Psychiatrists also classify people's abnormal behavior—not people, but their behavior—but with more precision, information, and thoughtfulness. Therefore, diagnosis *per se* is no sin; we *all* do it. A greater concern should be if psychiatric diagnoses help anyone.

Are diagnoses random and capricious?

If you were a psychiatrist starting from scratch, how might you aid those people with highly atypical and distressing feelings, thoughts, perceptions, and behaviors—collectively called "symptoms"? Without knowing their cause, you might begin as doctors have always begun: by trying to identify, from among a vast array, those particular symptoms and features which cluster, which will follow predictable patterns in the future, and which are likely to respond to a specific treatment. What these categorizations should be, where the dividing lines should be drawn—that's what formulating a diagnostic nomenclature is all about.

Neither God nor nature draws these lines. Only men and women can, and do. Mortal psychiatrists huddle into committees, and after much research, discussion, and debate, decide by vote or by consensus on the best ways to do it.

Because they draw these lines so specifically—by claiming, for example, that a mental disorder has six rather than seven characteristics—*DSM–III*'s diagnostic criteria are accused of being random and capricious. In my view, *DSM–III*'s diagnostic criteria are indeed random, but not capricious; to miss this distinction is to misunderstand how all illnesses—physical and mental—are defined.

Why is hypertension defined as "blood pressure being over 120/80"? Why is the upper level (or systolic blood pressure) 120, and not 119 or 121? Why isn't the lower number (or diastolic blood pressure) 70 or 90 instead of 80? Who made these decisions? A committee. In selecting 120/80 and not some other numbers, this committee set boundaries, which, although random, were not capricious. For (I assume) studies showed that problems induced by hypertension escalated considerably when blood pressures exceeded 120/80 or thereabouts. Physicians realize that 120/80 is a man-made guideline for defining hypertension, not precise truths ingrained in stone and endowed by nature. Whether diagnostic criteria are defining diabetes, rheumatic heart disease, depression, or schizophrenia, they are inevitably random, but not capricious.

Although it's sometimes hard to determine if a single individual is mentally ill or "normal," that doesn't mean that mental illness and normality are fictions, or that there are no differences between them. At dawn and dusk I'm never sure if it's day or night, yet days and nights exist, and I usually have no trouble telling the difference. So too with mental illness and normality. That sometimes it's tough to separate the healthy from the psychotic doesn't change the fact that in most cases scientific psychiatrists have no problem determining whether people are or are not psychotic.

Similarly, that the line separating two mental illnesses might be vague or random doesn't argue against the existence of these two mental illnesses. Using *DSM-III,* the vast majority of scientific psychiatrists agree, for example, on who is manic and who is schizophrenic, even though at times the boundaries between them are murky.

In actual clinical practice, psychiatrists use *DSM-III*'s criteria as guides, not dogma. However precise, the diagnostic criteria in *DSM-III* require a psychiatrist's interpretation. For example, "social withdrawal" is one of *DSM-III*'s diagnostic criteria for dysthymic disorder. How socially withdrawn does a person have to be to meet this criterion? By dint of evaluating many, many patients, psychiatrists develop internalized norms of what is, or is not, social withdrawal. In part, psychiatrists base their assessment of a patient's social withdrawal on how actively the patient has been socially engaged during the rest of his life. Thus, psychiatrists employing *DSM-III* are not robots; they must consider each patient's particular circumstances.

Reliability and validity

In constructing *DSM-III*'s diagnostic criteria, psychiatrists tried using all the available scientific data to create categories with the utmost validity and reliability. The more "valid" a diagnostic category, the more it represents a genuine and meaningful disease entity. The more "reliable" a diagnostic category, the more psychiatrists will reach the same diagnosis when evaluating the same patient. The fundamental distinction between *DSM-III* and its predecessors was that the validity and reliability of its diagnostic categories were primarily based on scientific evidence instead of theoretical concepts.

To create valid diagnostic categories those formulating *DSM III* used only diagnostic criteria with relatively high degrees of reliability. Psychiatrists are far more likely to agree among themselves on, for example, the existence of symptoms (e.g., insomnia, slowed movements) and the duration of an illness than on "intact ego boundaries," "the quality of relatedness," or "repression."

The types of diagnostic criteria employed in *DSM-III* include symptoms, the patient's sex, age of onset, quality of onset (e.g., abrupt, gradual), life course (e.g., intermittent, continual), prognosis or long-term outcome, the family history of mental illness, genetic patterns, and how the patient and his mentally ill relatives have responded to psychotropic medications. The more all these factors cluster, the more valid the diagnostic category. The more valid the diagnostic category, the more the diagnosis can predict the disorder's future course, response to treatment, and patterns of inheritance.

Although the diagnostic categories in *DSM-III* have greater validity than those in previous *DSM*s, most psychiatrists believe the level of validity could be improved considerably by further research. On the other hand, an integral part of creating *DSM-III* involved testing the reliability of its diagnostic categories. When it was found that psychiatrists could not agree on whether patients had a particular diagnosis, the criteria for that diagnosis were changed. Thus, by the time they were published, *DSM-III*'s diagnostic criteria had demonstrated a high degree of reliability. Although psychiatrists are more satisfied with the reliability than with the validity of *DSM-III*'s diagnoses, they also realize that achieving high reliability is a prerequisite for obtaining greater validity. Therefore, *DSM-III*'s high reliability has made it possible to create more valid diagnoses in the future.

The personalities and politics of diagnosis

Being creatures of man, not God, diagnostic categories must evolve from personalities and politics as well as from science. "Politics" is not a dirty word; it simply refers to the acquisition and use of power to determine what happens. In formulating *DSM-III,* certain people exercised more influence than others. That should not be surprising, although how it occurs might be illuminating; neither is it scandalous, unless politics (and personalities) run roughshod over scientific evidence.

Although *DSM-III* drew substantially from scientific knowledge, because this knowledge was limited, personalities and politics did affect the formation of diagnostic categories. It had to be this way. How else could a psychiatric nomenclature be devised, given that many scientific questions had yet to be answered and many scientific studies had yielded conflicting results? A scientific finding gains credibility if replicated, so how much faith should one place in a topic that's been studied but once? In how many studies must a specific finding emerge before it's considered "true"? Complicating matters is that the method used in a scientific study is never "good" or "bad," but a *relative* matter requiring judgment. These types of problems arise in all the sciences, not just psychiatry, and when they do, human factors intrude.

So even though the use of objective, verifiable scientific findings was a leap forward from psychoanalytic psychiatry's use of theory as fact, still some truths were considered more significant than others. How the hazier areas of *DSM-III* ultimately turned out was influenced, at least in part, by the egos and pride of those who created it. People do what they do for many, often intertwined, reasons, and since every participant felt he was advancing arguments in good faith, it was hard to distinguish science from ego.

For example, if after a dozen years of accumulating data to show that catatonia isn't, as traditionally thought, a manifestation of schizophrenia but a symptom of manic-depression, how would you feel if those in charge of *DSM-III* did not think your findings were sufficiently compelling to be included? If your particular contributions to the scientific literature became enshrined in *DSM-III,* not only would your work be vindicated and your career advanced, but forever after your name would be remembered and inscribed in textbooks of psychiatry. Professional immortality was at stake.

When the "facts" were unclear, what finally made it into *DSM-III* depended in part on a psychiatrist's ability to muster scientific evidence and to present it persuasively. As *DSM-III*'s committees were trying to make good decisions, each member's status was never mentioned but always considered.

While the egos of scientific psychiatrists were being boosted or bruised, those of psychoanalytic psychiatrists were being brushed aside. Many psychoanalytic psychiatrists felt that when their approach to diagnosis was rejected, they themselves were rejected. Some felt time had passed them by, that they had been put out to pasture.

Psychoanalytic psychiatrists were also disappointed for many professional reasons. Even today, many of them feel that by not using psychological theories to link etiology with diagnosis, *DSM-III* is reductionistic and parochial; they argue that it is a grievous error to view, for instance, schizophrenia as a disease entity instead of a psychological reaction. Defenders of *DSM-III* countered that like most etiological formulations, whether schizophrenia is a psychological reaction is highly questionable, and that a diagnostic system should be based on scientific facts rather than on theoretical speculations.

For similar reasons, *DSM-III* does not consider homosexuality, by itself, a mental disorder. In doing so, *DSM-III* reconfirmed a decision voted on in 1973 by the membership of the American Psychiatric Association (APA). But once again, since standard psychoanalytic theory views homosexuality as a perversity, psychoanalytic psychiatrists (and many laymen) charged the APA had capitulated to gay-rights organizations. APA officials responded that the decision to delete homosexuality *per se* as a mental disorder was made for strictly scientific reasons, there being little or no objective evidence that in the absence of social prejudice, homosexuality causes disability or distress. Although the actual decision was scientifically based, psychiatrists acknowledge that gay groups had "forced" the profession to reexamine the scientific evidence for its position.* In this manner, gay-rights organizations were among the many pressure groups that indirectly influenced *DSM-III.*

Perhaps the most contentious issue involving psychoanalytic psychiatrists was that *DSM-III* discarded the diagnostic label of "neurosis." Despite the crucial position of the concept of "neurosis" in psychoanalytic theory, psychoanalytically oriented psychiatrists were unable to agree on how to define "neurosis." In response, psychoanalytic psychiatrists argued that even if the definition of "neurosis" is fuzzy, it is absurd to so cavalierly exclude such a highly familiar and time-tested term, while including such brand-new ones as "somatoform" and "schizotypal" disorders, which were known to few psychiatrists and would probably turn out to be fads. Whether the word "neurosis" was to appear in *DSM-III* developed into a battle royal between psychoanalytic and scientific psychiatrists. Just as the presses rolled, a patently political face-saving compromise was struck: When some disorders were introduced, the label "neurosis" would be placed in parentheses.

Writing *DSM-III* and using it clinically are different matters. Despite all the effort that went into *DSM-III,* what good is a diagnostic system if nobody uses it? There also was the question of whether American psychiatrists in 1980 were ready to switch from analytic to descriptive diagnoses. To find out, the prime movers of *DSM-III* had 550 psychiatrists not associated with it conduct "field trials." Never had a *DSM* been tested in "real" situations by masses of "real" psychiatrists *before* the final document was issued.† Overall, 12,667 patients in over 200 settings were evaluated. The field trials corrected practical problems, suggested that

---

*DSM-III has a diagnostic category called "ego-dystonic homosexuality," which refers to a patient's homosexual arousal being a persistent source of distress.
†More psychiatrists participated in these field trials than in any other single research project in psychiatric history.

most psychiatrists who were not in academia (e.g., were in private practice) would come to favor this new diagnostic approach, and that by using *DSM-III* psychiatrists would usually reach the same diagnosis with the same patient. The field trials were also good "public relations," since eventually the membership of the APA would have to vote for *DSM-III*. After much debate, it did.

WHAT IS A MENTAL DISORDER?

One of *DSM-III*'s major accomplishments is being the first official diagnostic system in America which strives to clarify what constitutes a mental disorder and to clear up many misconceptions about psychiatric diagnosis held inside, as well as outside, the profession.

DSM-III points out that to qualify as a mental disorder, a condition should produce either *distress* or a major *disability* (in one's personal, social, academic, or occupational life). Biological changes may or may not be involved. More specifically, *DSM-III* states:

> . . . a mental disorder is conceptualized as a clinically significant behavior or psychologic syndrome or pattern that occurs in an individual and that typically is associated with either a painful symptom (distress) or impairment in one or more important areas of functioning (disability). In addition, there is an inference that there is a behavioral, psychological, or biological dysfunction, and that the disturbance is not only in the relationship between the individual and society. (When the disturbance is *limited* to a conflict between an individual and society, this may represent social deviance, which may or may not be commendable, but is not by itself a mental disorder.)

DSM-III classifies *mental disorders* and not, as widely misperceived, *individuals* with mental disorders. That's why *DSM-III* goes out of its way to shun usages like "a schizophrenic" or "an alcoholic," but invokes clumsier constructions like "a patient with schizophrenia" or "a person with alcoholism."

A related misperception is that every person described as having the same mental disorder is alike in every important respect. The only similarity among ulcer patients is that they have symptoms of ulcers, and the only similarity among schizophrenics is that they have symptoms of schizophrenia. Illness—mental and physical—is a part of an individual's life, not its totality.

DSM-III insists that its diagnostic criteria are intended solely for clinical and research purposes. They are *not* designed to be used in court or for determining reimbursement from health insurance companies. Although *DSM-III* is to be employed for strictly professional reasons, many psychiatrists are afraid this principle will be violated.

PUBLIC CRITICISMS

Although the profession voted for *DSM-III,* the public, which over the years had become leery of psychiatric diagnosis, was surprised that psychiatrists were reemphasizing diagnosis. Indeed, many of the profession's critics were downright hostile toward *DSM-III.* Typical were the views of sociologist Donald Light, who in 1980 commented on the soon-to-be-released *DSM-III:*

> This expansion of diagnostic nomenclature is about to make a quantum leap with the publication of . . . *DSM-III.* It is an old technique for a profession to enlarge its clientele by expanding its criteria for treatment problems; this is how agencies serving the blind, for example, "made" more blind people. A review of the new manual concludes, *"DSM-III* widens the orbit of psychiatry, staking claims to a wide new territory of human problems." At the same time, it does so with much more precision by using explicit, descriptive criteria instead of theoretical concepts. Ironically, the effort to enhance psychiatry's professional stature by making diagnosis more scientific and precise may backfire. For in the process, the new diagnostic systems become less dependent on the clinical judgment or theoretical models of interpretation that distinguish the profession. . . . Yet the new diagnostic system is more organic, which favors physicians, and it is hard to imagine that clinical judgment or personal interpretation can be eliminated in any diagnostic approach to emotional problems.

Earlier in his book, Light scoffed at how the vagueness of *DSM-II*'s diagnostic categories led to the indiscriminate use of psychiatric diagnosis and how psychiatrists using *DSM-II* can't agree with each other on a diagnosis. Here he criticizes *DSM-III*'s diagnostic criteria for being precise and explicit.

The accusation that *DSM-III* expands the scope of mental illness to enhance psychiatrists' income is strange, because *DSM-III*'s very precision in diagnosis greatly *reduces* the number of people deemed mentally ill. During the psychoanalytic era, if a person weighed a ton, moved like a blob, or behaved like a jerk, he could be diagnosed as "schizophrenic." *DSM-III*'s very specificity established boundaries for what is (and is not) a mental disorder, thereby discouraging overdiagnosis. After considerable huffing and puffing, *DSM-III* did expand psychiatric turf in only one area; it made "tobacco dependence" a mental disorder. Otherwise, *DSM-III* greatly restricts the number of mentally ill.

Moreover, despite what Light claims, *DSM-III* will not recruit more patients for psychiatrists. Nobody sees a shrink because of the profession's current nomenclature. I'm sure that psychiatrists wish to expand business and that some will encourage people to obtain "treatment" when it's unnecessary; but the culprit here is the psychiatrist and not psychiatric diagnosis.

Contrary to what Light, and many psychoanalytic psychiatrists, charge, *DSM-III* is not "more organic." *DSM-III* appears this way because it is not based on a psychological theory. But then *DSM-III* is not based on *any* theory, not even biological ones.

Light claims that psychiatrists might not accept *DSM-III* because it obviates the need for "theoretical models of interpretation" or "clinical judgment," which, according to Light, "distinguish the profession." Although *DSM-III* is not based on theoretical models, it does require clinical judgment. Physicians in all specialties have been using specific and explicit diagnostic criteria without feeling any the less "professional." The same is true for psychiatrists using *DSM-III*. Indeed, because diagnosis is now based on a distinct body of knowledge and not on a theory open to countless interpretations, *DSM-III* has enhanced, quite justifiably, the psychiatrist's sense of professionalism.

If anything, *DSM-III* demands that psychiatrists have *more* professional skills and knowledge. By relying on a relatively fixed theory, psychoanalytic psychiatrists could (and did) use the same skills and knowledge they'd acquired years ago. Because scientific evidence continually expands, scientific psychiatrists must keep abreast of an ever-changing field.

By being so exacting, *DSM-III* shows how little psychiatrists actually know about mental disorders. Being vague, *DSM-II* could conceal the profession's ignorance. On the other hand, *DSM-III* specifies each mental disorder's major and associated features, age of onset, course, impairments, complications, predisposing factors, prevalence, sex ratio, familial patterns (of transmission), "differential diagnosis" (i.e., how it differs from similar-appearing mental disorders), and diagnostic criteria. Because solid data don't exist for so many of these topics, *DSM-III* spotlights the enormous gaps in factual information about mental disorders. From now on, a major goal of psychiatric research is to fill these gaps.

Psychiatrists are already looking forward to *DSM-IV*, not because *DSM-III* failed, but because it succeeded in making science, rather than theory, the basis for psychiatric diagnosis. Contrary to what Light predicted, *DSM-III* is being widely used by psychiatrists and by other mental health professionals. Every textbook of psychiatry and psychology employs *DSM-III* as the organizing principle for its table of contents. *DSM-III* is being translated into French, Chinese, and the Scandinavian languages. So when *DSM-IV* does appear—probably around 1990—it will vastly improve on *DSM-III,* not by abrogating, but by refining the scientific approach that made *DSM-III* the hallmark of psychiatry's second revolution.

THREE

Mental Disorders

What convinces the psychiatrist that mental illness is for real is his direct involvement with patients. While training, he sees hundreds of patients whose disturbances are not only far worse than everyday ups and downs, but also follow distinct and predictable patterns. During the first year of his residency, the psychiatrist usually treats inpatients, which means that on a typical day, the resident listens to a patient's fears of evaporating, a young man's hallucinations of skulls, and a depressed old man's obsessions over the color of his urine. He sees how as people each of these patients is unique, but he also recognizes that their "abnormalities" are not quirks but symptoms, not eccentricities but illness.

This early intense exposure to severely ill patients accounts in part for why most psychiatrists are appalled by the avant-garde notion that it's somehow good to be mentally ill. As tuberculosis had been romanticized as "glorious consumption," so have "antipsychiatrists," often inspired by R. D. Laing, viewed "mental illness" as a heightened state of awareness, a difficult yet ultimately rewarding journey.

When I started training in 1968, I was sympathetic to this perspective. Yet after a week of seeing real-life patients, I realized there was nothing glorious or romantic about mental illness; if being mentally ill is a rewarding journey, it's a trip that patients could do without. In a sense, their "problem" wasn't psychopathology, but that they didn't enjoy their psychopathology. Just as the only people who say "money isn't everything" are the people with money—the poor being more sensible—the only people who extol mental illness are those with "mental health"; the mentally ill know better. A twenty-year-old drug-taking schizophrenic puts it this way: "LSD and schizophrenia are totally different, because with LSD, no matter how bad the trip, you know the hallucinations will end. What I hate about my schizophrenia is that it never goes away."

MENTAL DISORDERS VERSUS PROBLEMS IN LIVING

Psychiatrists often hear people claim that what's called "mental illness" isn't really an illness, but a "problem in living." Sometimes the term "problems in living" is simply a euphemism for mental illness. To the psychiatrist, however, problems in living are of quite another order from mental disorders. To equate them is false and naive, and in my view, an inadvertent insult to the mentally ill.

"Problems in living" usually connotes things like dealing with a lousy boss, contending with a spineless husband, worrying about a sick daughter, fearing parental criticism, overcoming feelings of inferiority, keeping ahead of the bill collector, and being lonely. I don't wish to minimize the pain of such problems, but they are different in type and magnitude from mental illness.

Mental illness involves *symptoms;* problems in living don't. A mentally ill patient may be certain a television is zapping his spleen with x-rays or that skeletons are dancing in his closet; his dead grandmother's voice may be telling him to kill himself, or he may think he's Christ. These are delusions and hallucinations—symptoms—and to equate the diseases that provoke these symptoms with problems in living is to err in categorization and to trivialize the experience of the mentally ill.

Like everyone else, the mentally ill must contend with problems in living, but unlike everyone else, they must do so with the added burdens of psychiatric symptoms. Whether the patient is a schizophrenic who is convinced an electrode has been secretly implanted in his brain, a manic who has devised a foolproof plan for world peace, or a major depressive who is sure his innards are rotting with cancer, the patient must still contend with an irksome spouse, poor self-esteem, academic failures, occupational stresses, interpersonal rejections, and all the other problems inherent to the human condition.

On top of the extra hardship mental illness places on patients when they deal with problems in living, conducting the routine tasks we all take for granted becomes extremely difficult when the person has grossly distorted thoughts, feelings, and perceptions. It's hard enough to apply for a job, but try doing so while convinced that everybody is plotting against you. Writing a term paper may be stressful, but imagine doing so when your thoughts constantly race, or with no attention span, or with hallucinations that continually taunt you. Mental illness makes everything harder. Even simple chit-chat isn't so simple when you feel everyone is conspiring against you or that at any instant a bomb will explode in your stomach.

Given all their symptoms, what continually amazes me is not how poorly the mentally ill do, but how well. I find it insulting when "problems in living" are equated with "mental illness," because such an equation dismisses the very real pain and hardship of being mentally ill.

Can one fake mental illness?

In one of the most talked-about studies in the 1970s, psychologist D. L. Rosenhan had eight healthy students go to a state mental hospital with the single complaint of hearing voices. They all gained admission, and once hospitalized, ceased to report any symptoms. These "pseudopatients" were diagnosed schizophrenic and discharged in about a week. Rosenhan's central conclusions were that since mental illness can be faked, mental illness does not exist and psychiatrists cannot distinguish the sane from the insane.

Much can be said about this study, but what Rosenhan's findings demonstrate is that people can fool their doctors by lying about having psychiatric symptoms. The same is true for medical illness. A person can swallow a pint of blood, walk into an emergency room, and vomit. The person will be instantly hospitalized in order to "rule out a bleeding ulcer." *Why* somebody would do this is another issue.* Less bizarrely, it's common for people to exaggerate or embellish medical (or psychiatric) symptoms to gain sympathy, avoid jury duty, and so on. That "pseudopatients" can fake mental illness does not mean that mental illness doesn't exist or that doctors can't tell the difference between sanity and insanity.

Although people can fake mental illness, they can't do it for long. When a patient's relative notices how the patient can be more "with it" or "out of it" depending on what's "convenient," the relative begins to wonder if the patient is faking his symptoms. He's not, at least not in the sense of a deliberate deception or an outright fraud. Actors can feign mental illness for three hours a day, seven days a week, and twice on Wednesdays and Saturdays, but they can't keep it up for much longer; it's too exhausting. Only the mentally ill have the "ability" to pace for hours, to hide in corners for days, and to think of nothing but bowels and blood and dirt. If you have any doubts, try it! You can't keep it up. Or, if you wish, try hallucinating. Unless you're on funny chemicals or in a sensory-isolation chamber, you can't.

Although people can't fake mental illness for long, they can, during a given period, modulate or control their symptoms. It's not that patients are either "responsible and manipulative" or "completely unresponsible and crazed." The truth lies in between and is more complex.

Imagine being drunk (or stoned) when your parents call. What do you do? You stop giggling, quickly pull yourself together, and sound as coherent and as normal as possible. Can you do it? Of course. It takes more effort and it's harder to sustain, but it can be done. You can exert a modicum of self-control even though you have what psychiatrists call an "organic brain syndrome." Depending on your degree of intoxication and on what the situation demands, you can modify your behavior appropriately. In this sense, being mentally ill is like being drunk: Although genuine impairments exist, the patient can temporarily adjust or reduce his symptoms and do what's required, even though it's harder to accomplish and to sustain.

---

*For many odd reasons, there are a few people who do little else but fake medical illness. Having what's called "Munchausen syndrome," they subsist from hospital to hospital, switching whenever their "scam" is discovered.

Criminal behavior and mental illness

People often believe that being mentally ill or taking a drug like LSD, PCP, or alcohol is somehow an "explanation," and therefore a "justification," for committing antisocial acts. One often hears statements such as "Ron beat up Larry because Ron was drunk," or "It was the PCP Mary took which made her drown her child." Similarly, "Henry's schizophrenia caused him to murder his boss." Implicit in all these sentiments is that the patient/criminal has nothing to do with the act, as if the drug or the mental illness *made* him do the crime. As a group, schizophrenics are no more, or less, violent than any other group, so being schizophrenic *per se* does not make one violent. (If anything, schizophrenics are more likely than nonschizophrenics to be the victims of violence.) Being acutely psychotic may diminish normal social restraints or may bring out the violent tendencies a person already has or accentuate Ron's hatred of Larry, but that's different from blaming the illness for the violence and from disassociating Ron from his crime.

Many, but not all, psychiatrists believe that the few mentally ill who do commit crimes should be treated as criminals *and* patients, not as one or the other. Psychiatrist Robert Marcus points out:

> The either/or concept in mental illness and criminal behavior is a legal fiction and violates all we know about mental illness. It is also an inappropriate way of expressing compassion for the mentally ill. . . . There is no major mental disorder where the capacity to control one's behavior is an important or central feature. . . . In fact, mental illness, whether schizophrenia or alcoholism, is untreatable until appropriate controls are established over the person's behavior. . . . A mentally ill person requires "blame and punishment" to the same extent that those not mentally ill do.

The insanity defense is too complex an issue to be fully discussed here, yet it is worth stressing that the mentally ill criminal is a person, not a robot. If an imaginary voice demands that he kill someone, it is still *his* voice. While this patient may be tipped over the edge by the extenuating factor of his "command hallucinations," others are tipped over the edge by extenuating factors of jealousy, betrayal, and revenge. The extenuating circumstance of mental illness should be given the same consideration that other extenuating circumstances would be given in any ordinary criminal proceeding.

PERSONALITY AND MENTAL ILLNESS

Because personality and mental illness manifest as feelings, thoughts, and behaviors, the two are often confused. Technically, psychiatrists use the terms "personality" and "character" synonymously. Both refer to a person's enduring, ingrained, and dominant traits. Compulsive personalities, for instance, are meticulous, careful, and orderly; they're always cleaning up, writing lists, and insisting on punctuality. Preoccupied with details, they miss "the big picture."

Compulsiveness, like other personality traits, can be adaptive or maladaptive, depending on whether it helps or harms. Being compulsive is highly adaptive for an accountant if it leads him to check out every detail on a tax form, but it is highly maladaptive if it gets him so mired in details that he can't complete the tax form on time.*

In the psychoanalytic view, mental illness is either a breakdown or an extension of the patient's personality; the same forces which shaped the patient's character also give rise to his mental illness. Two examples: When a man with a compulsive personality develops a severe depression, the psychoanalytic psychiatrist might say that the failure of his compulsive defenses caused his depression. A psychoanalytic colleague said of a patient, "Being so histrionic, the only way she could get attention was by becoming psychotic."

By linking personality and mental illness, the analytic tradition implies that the patient caused his mental illness. In essence, psychoanalytic psychiatrists say to the patient, "If you weren't such a perfectionist, you would not be depressed." As a result, the pa-

*Most psychiatrists will describe themselves as compulsive personalities, feeling that such a personality is highly adaptive for becoming a doctor and a psychiatrist; it makes it possible for them to remember millions of facts, to conduct scientific experiments with great precision, and to have disciplined study habits.

tient feels accused, as if lurking within his personality is some character flaw, some misguided values, or some unsound attitude that is responsible for his mental disorder. Conversely, it is implied that if the patient behaves properly, if he stops being so perfectionistic, he could get over his illness. Until then, the patient is "causing" his illness, and, although it is rarely expressed this way, "deserves what he gets."

In contrast, scientific psychiatrists view personality and mental illness as distinct matters, which may or may not be related. Mental illness tends to accentuate the patient's personality. For instance, consider a person who, when healthy, takes "forever" to make a decision. When he becomes depressed, among his symptoms will be a total paralysis of decision-making. A depressed patient who usually spends five minutes every morning deciding on what shirt to wear is now unable to choose any shirt. When seriously depressed, a normally suspicious man becomes downright paranoid. An individual's personality influences how a patient expresses and contends with his mental illness.

Modern psychiatrists now believe the forces that shape personality differ from those that cause mental illness. Yet because both involve behavior, a patient's mental illness and his usual personality may be confused even by psychiatrists. For a layman, the problem is still tougher. When a patient who's naturally a worry wart gets depressed and then recovers from his depression, it can be hard to know if his worrying is a remaining symptom from depression or simply his typical behavior. For a patient's relatives, this poses a special problem. When a habitually compulsive man recovers from a serious depression, his compulsiveness, to the disappointment of relatives, persists. By not distinguishing between personality and mental illness, relatives may feel (incorrectly) that treatment has been only partially successful. The relatives' expectations would be like expecting a compulsive man who recovers from a heart attack to stop being compulsive.

There's a distinction between *personality traits* and a *personality disorder;* the latter is diagnosed when a patient's personality traits are sufficiently inflexible and maladaptive to cause significant impairment or distress. Unlike previous editions, *DSM-III* lists specific diagnostic criteria for each of the personality disorders, such as histrionic, paranoid, narcissistic, dependent, compulsive, and borderline.

More important, a major innovation of *DSM-III* is its use of a "multiaxial" diagnostic system, whose chief purpose is to show that personality and mental illness are two distinct, though at times related, entities. In fact, a *DSM-III* diagnosis has five axes: Axis I is for mental illnesses; Axis II is for personality disorders (or developmental defects); Axis III is for physical disorders; Axis IV is for the severity of the psychosocial events that have recently stressed the patient; and Axis V is for the patient's highest level of functioning during the past twelve months.

Although psychiatrists routinely consider the information in Axes IV and V for planning treatment and for predicting outcome, when making formal diagnoses, they tend to ignore these axes. On the other hand, depending on the patient, psychiatrists will use one or more of Axes I-III. For example, a *DSM-III* diagnosis might read:

> Axis I: Major depression
> Axis II: Compulsive personality disorder
> Axis III: Arthritis

By using a different axis for mental and personality disorders, *DSM-III* encourages psychiatrists to view them separately and to abandon the old psychoanalytic notion that the two are somehow inextricably linked.

ILLNESS, DISEASE, AND DISORDER

During informal conversations most psychiatrists use the terms "mental illness," "mental disease," and "mental disorder" synonymously, though with slightly different connotations. Technically, however, throughout medicine the word "illness" encompasses the patient's experience of the condition as well as the sickness itself. The word "disease" is more limited, referring specifically to the actual sickness, the clearly identified pathophysiology. "Mental disorder" is a more general term which carries neither connotation. In all three *DSM*s, "mental disorders" and never "mental illness" or "mental disease" are used as diagnostic labels.

When speaking casually to each other, psychiatrists tend to invoke the terms "mental illness" and "mental disease" to mean a mental disorder which (a) is serious and (b) has a significant biological component. To psychiatrists a mental illness or disease is an entity like schizophrenia, mania, major depression, or a panic disorder; in this sense, a large percentage of the patients many psychiatrists see in private practice do *not* have a mental illness, but a mental disorder (e.g., a phobia) or problems in living. (For administrative purposes, *DSM-III* has an actual category called "no mental disorder," and another called "no personality disorder." I believe these "diagnoses" are still underutilized.)

Among themselves, psychiatrists reserve the term "crazy" to mean "psychotic." This means impaired reality testing, in which the patient blatantly misperceives the world, grossly misinterprets events, or incorrectly processes information, to produce symptoms such as incomprehensible speech, hallucinations, and delusions. Psychiatrists especially apply the word "crazy" to patients who are out of control, or whose delusions and hallucinations are unusually bizarre.

In the psychiatrist's mind, being crazy or having a genuine mental illness is not some undefined mass of weird behavior or some histrionic madness as performed at the Metropolitan Opera. (I recently saw an actress imitate madness by flailing her arms and screeching, two diagnostic criteria overlooked in *DSM-III*.) When psychiatrists see "madness," or more properly see "mental illness," they observe patterns of symptoms. That's because people go crazy in *specific* ways.

I will describe five of the 210 mental disorders listed in *DSM-III*. That doesn't sound like a lot, but these five are the ones psychiatrists research, read about, think about, and see the most.* In its own way, each of these illnesses reveals a good deal about the new scientific psychiatry.

*The prevalence of mental disorders is controversial, and depends on how disorders are defined and how surveys are conducted. For instance, the frequency that psychiatrists see patients with particular mental illnesses is *not* the same as the frequency of these illnesses in the general population. Only 20 percent of patients with mental disorders, as defined in *DSM-III*, seek treatment, and these patients are more likely to consult general practitioners than psychiatrists. In 1980, according to the American Psychiatric Association, of the patients making office visits to psychiatrists, 27.6 percent have affective disorders (e.g., major depression, manic-depression, dysthymic disorder), 18.5 percent have "neuroses other

Do me a favor: Don't diagnose yourself. I'm all too familiar with "medical student's disease," that eternal affliction of proto-physicians in which they "catch" every illness they study. The student will think, "That patient who bruises easily has hemophilia. I bruise easily. Therefore, I have hemophilia." When a medical student who happens to be overly attached to his mother first sees a schizophrenic who is also overly attached to his mother, the medical student thinks he's a schizophrenic.

To have a particular mental disorder, the patient must have a *specific constellation of numerous characteristics,* not just one or two of them. In sketching these constellations, I'm leaving aside many details that *must* be considered before an accurate diagnosis can be made. (However, if you're concerned that you or someone close to you may have one of these mental disorders, a psychiatric consultation might be helpful, if for no other reason than to put your mind at ease.)

All five of these disorders are "functional" as opposed to "organic." Since they are physicians, psychiatrists are taught to distinguish "organic mental disorders," which constitute clear-cut alterations of or damage to the brain, from "functional mental disorders," in which the brain is not grossly affected. Organic mental disorders include dementias (e.g., Alzheimer's disease),

---

than depressive," 15.3 percent have personality disorders, and 10.8 percent have schizophrenia.

These figures vary considerably from the prevalence of mental disorders in the general population. Using *DSM-III* diagnostic criteria, interviewing over ten thousand adults—the largest survey ever—and published in 1984, the National Institute of Mental Health (NIMH) examined the frequency of mental disorders that occur during a six-month period. The NIMH showed that anxiety disorders were most common, affecting 31.1 million, or 8.3 percent of adult Americans. Anxiety disorders included phobias (affecting 7 percent of all Americans), panic disorders (0.8 percent), and obsessive compulsive disorders (1.5 percent). Substance abuse disorders—with 80 percent involving alcohol and the remainder involving other drugs—were next at 6.4 percent. About 6 percent had affective disorders, 1 percent had schizophrenia, and another 1 percent had antisocial personality disorder.

This landmark investigation corrected the long-held notion that women have higher rates of mental disorders than men. Previous surveys concentrated on depression and phobias, which more often affect women. By including alcoholism and antisocial personality disorders, conditions more frequent among men, this survey showed the overall rates of mental disorders for men and women were equal.

deliriums, and drug intoxications. Many symptoms of organic mental disorders are similar or identical to those seen with functional disorders. When a psychiatrist evaluates a patient, he considers whether the patient has an organic mental disorder before he diagnoses a functional mental disorder.

Scientific psychiatrists generally feel that separating mental disorders into "organic" and "functional" is misleading and arbitrary. As research methods become more sophisticated, it is being demonstrated increasingly that in many functional disorders, such as schizophrenia, there are changes in the brain's chemistry, physiology, and even anatomy. Nonetheless, for reasons having more to do with convention and convenience than with science, modern psychiatrists still make this distinction.

SCHIZOPHRENIA

Schizophrenia is not a "split personality" as in *Three Faces of Eve*. (Eve had a "multiple personality.") Schizophrenia is not a "nervous breakdown" or "insanity"; neither term has psychiatric meaning, the first belonging to laymen, the second to lawyers. Schizophrenia is not one illness, but a series of illnesses—"the schizophrenias"—all having similar features, much as epilepsy is a name for many diseases having similar characteristics.

Over the years, psychiatrists have defined schizophrenia differently, starting with Kraepelin's "dementia praecox," which emphasized its early age of onset (viz., usually the teens and twenties) and the patient's gradual deterioration of behavior. Initially, friends and family will say the patient "doesn't act the same," "is more withdrawn," "doesn't wash," or "is getting worse grades." From the patient's perspective, the world seems more and more overwhelming, as if everything's going too fast; feeling bombarded with stimuli, he retreats from the world and into himself. At first schizophrenia may arise abruptly, but it usually emerges over months or years before its full-fledged manifestations appear.

When schizophrenia becomes flagrant it presents with *specific* kinds of delusions and hallucinations. By "delusion," psychiatrists mean a fixed, firm, and patently false belief which is not widely held in the patient's culture or subculture. That a man staunchly believes Nixon to be innocent of Watergate is not a delusion, since it's a tenable position to many; if he is convinced Nixon is a woman, that's a delusion. In certain subcultures people feel that God speaks personally to them; that's not so in mine, and if I were to insist that he did, I'd be delusional.

Schizophrenic delusions tend toward the bizarre; they present in the "Twilight Zone." With a deadpan face a woman told me that her TV was sending messages specifically to her to purchase Bab-O. (She bought 250 cans of Bab-O. Her house remained a mess.) A man becomes furious at the telephone company for inserting a listening device into his brain. A woman is convinced that her in-laws are conspiring with Dan Rather to kill her.

In schizophrenia, *auditory* hallucinations are the rule. Hallucinations are blatantly false perceptions not based on any external stimuli. When brain tumors, drugs, or other types of organically induced hallucinations occur, they're usually seen, smelled, and felt, but not heard. Although schizophrenics may have visual hallucinations, they're more likely to hear imaginary voices. Because many people incorrectly consider their private thoughts to be hallucinations, the psychiatrist may ask a patient if the voices come from "outside your head." In schizophrenia, these voices often comment on the patient's actions or tell him what to do, such as "That's fine, Joe, but now look under the bed." The hallucinations may be a few words, like "Skyscraper" or "Toby likes car, Toby likes car"; these words may be heard for hours or even days. Sometimes the voices are two or more people conducting a conversation with the patient. The voices may be accusatory or frightening; occasionally, they comfort.

Incoherence frequently characterizes schizophrenia. Schizophrenic speech is illogical, senseless, or meaningless. Sentences are hard to follow: "I'm going to the grocery store. Hey, don't you think they've taken the 'hot' out of the dog? Don't tell me that's a church!" This quote is nonsense; the thoughts are not connected in any coherent or reasonable fashion. Nevertheless, friends and relatives, trying hard to "communicate" with the patient, often feel guilty about not comprehending. Psychoanalytic psychiatrists prided themselves in supposedly being able to "understand the inner meaning" of what the patient says. Yet most of the time no two psychiatrists could agree on such inner meanings, because to make sense of them, one had to *read* into them. Try it with this quote, and compare your hunch with mine, which is: "I'm going to the grocery, but I don't expect to get hot dogs that were as good as they used to be, and that's a sin. That grocery store is no church." Schizophrenic speech is often laced with double entendres, puns, word salads, neologisms, and words that have awesome personal significance but mean little to anybody else.

As the schizophrenic is being understood by fewer and fewer people, increasingly he dwells on his own thoughts and becomes socially isolated. The patient doesn't quite grasp why people are ignoring him, and so he imputes hostile or persecutory motives to others. He doesn't get a job, his grades decline, a friend doesn't return a telephone call. On the same day he receives no mail and there's an electrical breakdown in the neighborhood. "There must be an explanation for all this," the patient thinks. He tries harder and harder to bring clarity out of chaos, and then he spots or thinks of something that suddenly and amazingly "explains" everything. "Everything crystallized when I realized that on two consecutive days, telephone repairmen visited my neighbors. 'Why were they there?' I thought. 'And why are they going into everyone's home but mine?' That's what tipped me off to AT&T's plot to dispose of me. With all their connections, it was AT&T who made sure I didn't get a job, who ruined my grades, and who prevented people from talking to me."

Other schizophrenics, especially those who don't have a sudden onset of symptoms, develop an abnormal *affect*. This term refers to a person's mood at the moment. The schizophrenic's affect may be "inappropriate," meaning it's out of sync with his thoughts. The patient, for example, keeps chuckling while describing his father's funeral. He's not laughing away the pain, nor sharing fond or funny memories. While it's not clear what the patient is communicating, the listener's skin crawls. In more severe and chronic cases, the patient may giggle for no apparent reason. Although he may be responding to some inner thought, to the outsider the patient seems pathetic. The schizophrenic often displays a "flat affect," an emotional lockjaw, a monotone. Patients may describe a calamitous event—a death in the family, a suicide—or even a joyous one—a wedding, a World Series victory—all with a deadpan expression, as if nothing of significance had happened.

As the patient reacts more to private thoughts than to external events, he appears more distant and remote to outsiders. The patient is losing interest in the real world, and so he responds with less emotion and an increasingly flat or inappropriate affect. Preoccupied with the inner world, he begins to hear voices telling him, for example, "AT&T is making people's bodies conform to the shape of their clothes. Because only you realize this, you alone know that your mother's chemise dress is hiding a rectangular body, and that your brother's bell-bottom pants are hiding his dual knife-edged ankles." Afforded these "insights," the patient thinks, "That's why I couldn't help but laugh when my mother said she was going shopping for clothes. She thinks she's doing so on her own volition. I know better."

With such strange thinking and odd behavior, schizophrenics tend to drift to lower social standings or to the fringes of society. According to psychiatric folklore—and that's all it is—the schizophrenic's classic job is working the night shift at the post office. With their short attention spans, their impaired reality testing, and their interpersonal difficulties, they can handle only jobs that are simple and temporary; more complex jobs overwhelm their circuits. This "downward drift," even more than the adverse effects of poverty, is often given as the chief reason schizophrenia occurs more often among the poor.

Many patients who suddenly become psychotic appear to have schizophrenia, but don't; for instance, they may turn out to have manic-depression, or their delusions and hallucinations may simply melt away and stay away. To reduce the overdiagnosis of schizophrenia and all its ominous implications, *DSM-III* indicates that a patient must be ill for at least six months before a diagnosis of schizophrenia is made.

Although *DSM-III* sets the age of onset before forty-five, it's usually before forty or even thirty-five. (One pleasure of turning forty is knowing you'll never be schizophrenic.) Sexes are affected equally. Regardless of social or political system, throughout the world, a constant 1 percent of the population has schizophrenia. Each year, about 1.1 million schizophrenics receive treatment in the United States, with 200,000 being hospitalized and 900,000 being outpatients; another 1 million schizophrenics may obtain no treatment at all.

The annual cost of schizophrenia to the nation has been estimated at $11.6 to $19.5 billion, with about two-thirds of this cost due to lost productivity and one-fifth due to treatment expenditures (in 1975 dollars). Schizophrenics occupy roughly half of all hospital beds for psychiatric (and retarded) patients, and about 25 percent of all (medical and psychiatric) hospital beds. Schizophrenia devastates as none other.

MAJOR DEPRESSION

To psychiatrists, the word "depression" refers to either a symptom or a syndrome. As a symptom, it's being sad, down in the dumps, listless, joyless, blue. As a syndrome, which is how psychiatrists generally employ the term, it means a particular constellation of symptoms, with the symptom of depression usually, but not always, being present and prominent. Although at some point everybody has the symptom of depression, only some people have the syndrome, and when they do, it's most often what *DSM-III* calls "major depression."

At thirty-seven and married a year, Diana was struck by breast cancer. After a mastectomy, her surgeon "certified" her as cancer-free. Six months passed, but she was not getting back into the swing of things. She had been a successful graphic artist, but since the operation she had no desire to work. Although she loved the theater, she stopped going. In fact, nothing interested her; everything depressed her. Increasingly, she became guilty about her inactivity and felt that she'd "pulled a *Love Story*" on Jim, her new husband. She insisted that Jim felt her mastectomy scar made her "a sexual turn-off." Jim didn't think so, but nothing he could say or do dissuaded her. Although he felt awful for Diana, he was at his wit's end. Whenever he'd be supportive, she'd respond, "You're so good, I don't deserve you." Diana, Jim, and their friends all "realized" that "it was perfectly natural to be unhappy after having breast cancer." They also assumed that lingering worries about the breast cancer "explained" why for three months she'd been awakening in the middle of the night.

"Depression" and "insomnia," which Diana and Jim mistook for isolated *symptoms,* were actually features of a *syndrome,* or mental illness, known as "major depression."* Yet because what triggered her symptoms was "understandable," it never occurred to them that she was suffering from another illness. Obviously,

---

*"Major depression" has also been called "endogenous depression," "unipolar depression," "melancholia," and "psychotic depression."

breast cancer is stressful, but she now had an *added* problem, major depression. As with most patients, her major depression went away after four to six weeks of treatment with antidepressant medication. After she recovered, she still worried about breast cancer—who wouldn't?—but she worried like a "normal" person, not like a depressed one. She was no longer obsessed with her ex-cancer, but now could get her mind off of it for long stretches. She started socializing. She returned to work and her usual theatergoing.

Major depressions often erupt for no apparent reason; they "come out of the blue." Others, like Diana's, seem to begin after a major environmental stress: a lost job, a divorce, a death. However, no matter how the disorder starts—with or without an environmental stress—once major depression gets going, a classical pattern of symptoms emerges. These symptoms involve biological changes, and so no matter how a depression may begin, once these symptoms occur, biological treatments will effectively treat the depression.

The most prominent feature of major depression is usually a severe, paralyzing, and unrelenting sadness. Some patients, however, don't feel sad at all, but rather lose all interest or pleasure in things that normally gratify them. A baseball freak ignores the World Series; a family man no longer plays with his kids; a civil-rights activist doesn't care anymore. Technically, this is called "anhedonia," and to have a major depression a patient must have either anhedonia or profound sadness.

On top of being sad or anhedonic, patients with major depression must have, according to *DSM-III,* at least four of the following: (a) poor appetite or significant, unplanned weight loss; (b) insomnia or excessive sleep; (c) agitated or retarded movements; (d) loss of energy; (e) feelings of worthlessness, self-reproach, or inappropriate guilt; (f) much slower or indecisive thinking, and (g) recurrent thoughts of death or suicide. Symptoms (a) through (d), plus constipation, decreased libido, and a "diurnal mood variation" (i.e., consistently feeling worse in the morning and better as the day goes on) are called "biological signs of depression."

In addition to having many biological signs of depression, Diana experienced severe helplessness and hopelessness—both typical features of major depression. On first entering my office, she appeared drained, sickly, and fidgety; although she had never been there before, she immediately apologized for not knowing where to sit. She was deferential to the point of being obsequious. Like most patients with major depression, she was irritable and prickly. She'd tense up and convey annoyance whenever I said "cancer"; she would never use the word and would refer to her breast cancer as "that episode."

Some patients with major depression have a "masked depression," characterized chiefly by hypochondriasis. Although they have many biological signs of depression, they don't complain of sadness, and for that matter, of any feeling. They don't (or can't) articulate emotions. Ask them, "How do you feel?" and they respond, "My back hurts." If the doctor persists—"How's your mood, I mean emotionally?"—these patients will say, "I don't know. You're the doctor. I feel terrible, what else? My back hurts." These patients often frustrate physicians, and not infrequently become addicted to Valium-like drugs. Although Valium doesn't alleviate their symptoms, very often antidepressant medications do.

Whereas psychoanalytic psychiatrists usually equated psychosis with schizophrenia, scientific psychiatrists have shown that patients other than schizophrenics often have hallucinations and delusions. About a quarter of patients with major depression hallucinate. They see dead relatives and scenes of damnation; less often they smell putrid or foul odors; most frequently, they hear voices. Whereas the schizophrenic's voices are bizarre and unrelated to his mood (e.g., "You're turning into a computer"), the depressed person's reflect his mood and one can far more readily empathize with them (e.g., "You're vile and disgusting"). The same distinction occurs with delusions.

Even when they're not strictly delusional, they see the world through depressed goggles, and patients with major depression are virtually convinced that everything has been, is, and will be terrible. A severely depressed middle-aged man begs: "Please give me shock treatment. It's the punishment I deserve for my sins. . . . Twenty years ago I cheated on my wife and had an affair. As a teenager I stole a football. I deserve to die. Look! I caused my dear, dear mother so much pain, it made her die of a heart attack. My wife, a wonderful woman, would be better off without me. I can't concentrate. I'm useless, I'm garbage, I'm disgusting inside—always have been, always will be. Please, put me out of my misery."

He wants "out," largely because patients with major depression can think of nothing but depression. This man would recite this litany of "sins" about fifty times a day, and each time his wife would reassure him, but to no avail. From the patient's view what's most painful is that there's no escape from major depression, save one: suicide.

Fifty to 70 percent of all suicides result from either major depression or manic-depression. Although schizophrenics commit suicide more than the general population, they do so less often than the severely depressed. ("Rational" suicide is rare; virtually all suicides occur during a mental illness.) Fifteen percent of people with major depression kill themselves—a rate twenty-five times that of the general population. Because suicide is the ninth leading cause of death and the second most common among youth, in my view everyone should learn to recognize suicidal behaviors, just as everyone should learn first aid (see page 97–98).

At some time during their lives, 18 to 23 percent of women and 8 to 11 percent of men will have a major depression. About a third will be hospitalized. Untreated biologically, the average major depression persists six to nine months. About half the people who have one major depression will never have another; of those who do, half will have a third episode. The more often major depressive episodes occur, the more likely another will occur. Although depression can arise at almost any age, including childhood, patients are usually most depressed and hospitalized between the ages of forty and sixty.

MANIC-DEPRESSION

Before 1971, for eighteen years Ethel's illness led to three serious suicide attempts, a nasty divorce, and her two children "disowning" her. As was frequent American practice during this period, she was repeatedly diagnosed as "schizophrenic," despite becoming dreadfully unhappy every fall and dangerously ecstatic every spring; on average, she was hospitalized semiannually; in all, she had thirty-six admissions. For these eighteen years, she'd been treated with antipsychotic medications (e.g., Thorazine), which, although helpful for schizophrenia, were virtually useless for Ethel. Why? Because Ethel had been misdiagnosed; she did not have schizophrenia, but manic-depression. Accordingly, instead of taking antipsychotics, she should improve on lithium. She did. Since 1971, Ethel has taken lithium prophylactically and has never again been hospitalized; she has worked steadily, remarried, and reconciled with her children. Lithium isn't a cure-all, but when it works, it can be astonishingly effective, and it works for manic-depression.

Lithium attenuates the excessive highs and lows of manic-depression. The lows are similar to those of major depression, yet by definition, what distinguishes manic-depression is that the patient has at least one manic episode during his life.*

Up to a point, being manic can be lots of fun. One's on top of the world, high as a kite, in love with humanity. The manic behaves as a fast-talking stand-up comic, a Henny Youngman, but funnier. People laugh *with* the manic, not *at* him. Bursting with energy, engaging, and confident, the manic makes a supersalesman. He's a Max Bialystock (Zero Mostel in *The Producers*). Uninvited, an encyclopedia salesman entered my home and almost sold me a $300 set of books to "benefit my children." I have no children. Yet like most manics, the salesman was quite convincing. Before he goes bonkers, the manic goes from being incredibly productive to doing "twenty things at once." Even patients who have been greatly helped by lithium will stop taking it just because they miss the manic euphoria, ecstasy, and productivity. Who can blame them? (The main reason they take lithium at all is to avoid the depressions.)

Unfortunately, this high gets out of control. The manic feels so great he begins to concoct grandiose schemes, spend money wildly, run up long-distance phone bills, and travel anywhere on a whim. An eighty-year-old woman flew into my office, gave me her Cadillac (with keys), and wrote me a check for $1 million. (Yes, she could afford it, and yes, on second thought, I returned her check.) A University of California undergraduate called the Kremlin to persuade Brezhnev to ban the bomb. The student didn't get Brezhnev, but he did reach a member of the Politburo. His friends were amused, but not his parents—they got stuck with the $850

---

*Because patients with manic-depression have highs as well as lows, their depressions are called "bipolar depressions." Because patients with major depression are never high but only low, their depressions are called "unipolar depressions."

telephone bill. Being so busy, manics aren't bothered by their insomnia and diminished appetite. It's like being on "speed."

Since he is so sure of being right about everything, the manic gets irritated at anyone who doubts him. He becomes edgy and provocative, flattering people one moment, insulting them the next. It's uncanny how manics can detect and hit a person's soft spots, as when a hospitalized manic introduced himself to another inpatient, a pudgy and insecure teenager, by saying, "You have a very nice face for someone so disgustingly fat." The manic constantly tests limits. He will evoke anger and then disavow his actions and their consequences, usually by blaming others. When a nurse criticized this manic for causing the insecure teenager to burst into tears, the manic replied, "It's not my fault; I was merely joking. If her doctor did his job properly, this girl wouldn't be so vulnerable." By habitually getting under people's skin and by overestimating their own combative abilities, manics frequently provoke fights only to get bashed up.

As the manic increasingly senses that people dislike his actions, he often begins to feel persecuted. Even when no disfavor is intended, the manic finds it: "Why didn't you compliment my new shirt?" Paranoids do have enemies, but that's mainly because they're paranoid. Paranoid people are very unpleasant. They get extremely suspicious, accusatory, and defensive. Sometimes they're violent. Yet unlike many paranoids who keep their ideas to themselves, manics act them out, and eventually suffer the consequences.

Manics develop grandiose delusions, such as "I'm the greatest poet-philosopher-scientist ever," or "I've devised a foolproof plan for preventing war." Another manic designed a ninety-story building that would stand on one square foot of land. He brought his family near bankruptcy in spending over $100,000 for architects, city planners, and attorneys, as well as for a guru, Bruce, who was to bless the edifice. Unlike schizophrenics, who are too disorganized, and depressives, who are too lethargic, manics are hyped with energy and driven by conviction, and so they act out their schemes and delusions.

If untreated with medication, mania typically lasts two to four weeks, while depression usually persists nine to twelve months. In contrast to the depressions of major depression, those of manic-depression are more likely to last longer, feel worse, affect the sexes equally, manifest earlier (e.g., age thirty instead of forty), prompt suicide, and run in families.

Relatives commonly refer to the patient as a "Jekyll and Hyde," who is normally an upstanding, likable high achiever, and then for distinct periods becomes outrageously manic or dreadfully depressed. Unlike schizophrenics, who rarely return to normal, patients with manic-depression usually function exceedingly well in between episodes, and if they have some brains or talent, they're often among society's most successful people. Nevertheless, the pain and carnage of the acute episodes severely scars the family. In one study, after manic-depressives and their spouses learned of the increased risk of familial inheritance and the long-term burdens of the illness, 5 percent of patients and about half of the spouses indicated that if given a second chance, they would not get married or have children.

BORDERLINE PERSONALITY DISORDER

Psychiatrists are usually gratified in treating the previous three disorders because there are relatively effective therapies available. Moreover, the patients' symptoms are so obvious, it's clear the patient is ill; they have Axis I mental disorders. For borderline patients it's different: Their symptoms are less blatant and more enduring; they have an Axis II personality disorder. Because effective treatments are still elusive and they become unrelentingly demanding and dependent, they drive psychiatrists buggy. At one moment the psychiatrist's heart goes out to these patients; at the next, he wants to strangle them. (Borderlines usually feel the same way toward their therapists.)

Everybody knows borderlines. They're chronically unhappy and demoralized. When coaxed into attending a party, they'll enjoy it; they won't, however, initiate a party or go on their own. Being "injustice collectors," they're always "cheated" by life. Whatever one does for them is never enough. Relationships, platonic and romantic, become all-or-nothing. They're in love with love, but not with people. On first meeting them, they seem perfectly normal, and often delightful. Yet they look better than they are. They are great starters and lousy finishers; they don't stick with anything for long.

Relations quickly become so intense and dependent that attempts to cool things infuriate them; they become demanding, vindictive, and abusive. They'll weep and scream and swear and carry on and insist they'll never see the person again. They are, as Dr. Donald Klein says, "rejection-sensitive." To them, minor slights become major catastrophes.

Many possess a slew of "neurotic" symptoms—phobias, anxiety, somatic complaints, roller-coaster mood swings. Unlike the mood changes in major depression and manic-depression, the borderline's rapidly alternating moods last for hours (not weeks) and are clearly triggered by environmental events. Under sufficient stress, borderline patients sometimes become *briefly* psychotic. When taking psychological tests that have definite answers, they respond rationally, but when taking psychological tests without correct answers (e.g., "inkblots"), they give off-the-wall responses. Indeed, the term "borderline" originated with the now widely doubted belief that these patients are "on the border" between schizophrenia and neurosis.

Most are women, and they often present as exaggerations of the worst female stereotypes—flamboyant, grasping, illogical, seductive, manipulative, fickle, narcissistic, egocentric, and vain. Female borderlines are constantly trying (and in their own minds, failing) to fulfill what they believe others expect of them.

Inside, these patients feel empty, bored, and evil. Privately, they believe they do not have the right stuff to make it in society, to establish enduring intimate relationships, and to be loved. Publicly, they continually bitch that others aren't sufficiently understanding, interesting, and kind. After a rocky year-long relationship, a borderline patient was met by her boyfriend at the O'Hare airport. Casually, the boyfriend said that a passerby was "attractive"; the patient became incensed, opened her suitcase, throwing clothes all over the place, spent thirty minutes cursing him as loudly as possible, and left the airport by herself. Although by evening she calmed down, for months she saw nothing wrong, or even excessive, about her behavior. She would pout, "The cluck knows I'm sensitive. Why couldn't he say something nice about *my* body?"

Feeling bored, they're addicted to excitement and novelty. Feeling empty, they expect others to fill their ever-drained gas tanks. Feeling worthless, they're driven to see if people love them enough to put up with their "garbage," which usually includes much self-destructiveness, such as repeated suicide attempts, alcoholism, drug abuse, pathological gambling, and promiscuity.

At other times, these patients are often engaging, clever, intelligent, talented, and kind. Perhaps most annoying is that despite their genuine capabilities, they almost inevitably let themselves and everyone else down, including their therapists.

Since these patients are so frustrating for therapists, the topic of "borderlines" has become one of modern psychiatry's hottest issues. That's partially because psychiatrists believe, rightly or not, that they're seeing more of these patients. While these patients have a *personality* disorder (Axis II), many of them also have severe demoralization and unhappiness, and therefore, a *mental* disorder (Axis I) called "atypical depression." In general, psychotherapy helps patients with borderline personality disorders, and medication helps those with atypical depressions.

THE "DISCOVERY" OF PANIC DISORDERS

Imagine walking into your corner bakery, and without warning or cause, you're suddenly terrified and struck mute. Imagine being in church, and pow!—you're paralyzed by fear, frightened you'll die right on the spot; your dread is senseless, yet all-consuming. Imagine entering your garage and, for no reason, you're overwhelmed by a sense of impending disaster, destruction, and doom. Technically, these episodes are called "panic attacks," and they afflict 1 to 2 percent of the population.

In general, panic attacks occur out of the blue. The victims are thoroughly overcome by fears of imminent doom or death, such as a global holocaust, a nuclear war, or a heart attack; sometimes they don't even know what frightens them, they're just frightened. Patients know their fear is irrational, and that scares them all the more. Their hearts pound and they breathe rapidly. Many feel choked and suffocated. Sometimes they faint. Their legs may feel rubbery. During panic attacks, victims sense the only immediate relief will come from going outside, leaving the bakery, church, or garage. Once outdoors, patients relax and return to normal.

Although at first these attacks are totally unexpected, in time many patients find they occur in only *one* location; the patient might have panic attacks solely in Whitney's drugstore. Yet as the symptoms of panic *attacks* evolve into a full-fledged panic *disorder,* patients go from avoiding Whitney's drugstore to fearing every store, to being scared of being outside, to feeling terrified of leaving home. Many psychiatrists claim that panic disorders occur in three stages: (1) the panic attack itself, (2) "anticipatory anxiety" over the attack happening again, and (3) phobias about going more and more places so that eventually the patient is terrified to leave home. These patients live in constant dread of having another panic attack.

Most patients are reluctant to tell family or friends about their attacks for fear of being dismissed as crazy. A concentration-camp survivor told me her panic attacks were more frightening than anything she remembered at Auschwitz. Until recently, most patients had never heard of panic attacks, and therefore thought they were losing their minds and that they were the only ones in the world with this affliction.

Yet despite the severity of this common disorder, not until the mid-1970s did psychiatrists realize that panic attacks existed, or that they were anything more than anxiety. The most popular comprehensive psychiatric textbook published in 1967 never mentions "panic disorders"; it briefly discusses "panic attacks," but simply as one, among many, symptoms of anxiety, such as palpitations and nervousness. *DSM–III* was the first official American diagnostic system to list panic disorders.

But given how much stark terror panic attacks produce, how could psychiatrists overlook it for so many years? There are many reasons, but among them was that in psychoanalytic psychiatry, what counted was not the overt symptom, but the unconscious. Psychiatrists did not view symptoms as anything worth treating in their own right. Symptoms were significant only to the extent they were symbols of unconscious conflicts; they needed not treatment, but understanding. Yet because these unconscious conflicts, like those over "castration anxiety," were not specific to panic attacks but existed in everyone, psychiatrists could not see that panic attacks (and disorders) were distinct entities. Psychiatrists were so busy looking at what (supposedly) was "below" (and by implication, meaningful), they didn't see what was "above"; that would be too superficial!

Patients were complaining of panic attacks, but shrinks weren't listening. Psychiatrists began to "discover" panic disorders when they stopped inferring what patients' complaints "meant" and started clarifying what the complaints actually were. It was only after they focused on *describing* complaints—what precisely happens, when it happens, what happens along with it—that psychiatrists "discovered" panic disorders.

One way to determine if, in this case, panic disorder was a genuinely distinct disorder was to see if these patients had a specific response to a specific medication. Although panic attacks are not helped by antipsychotic agents (e.g., Thorazine) or by sedatives (e.g., Valium), they are prevented by the antidepressant Tofranil.*

The "discovery" and diagnosis of panic disorders meant that laymen started hearing about them, which helped victims realize they were not alone and that effective treatment existed. All of these patients I've known have described their great relief on first hearing they had a genuine illness; they were not going nuts, they had a "real" problem. They do not feel the diagnosis stigmatized or demeaned them, but rather that it unburdened them of the implied (or stated) blame that somehow they "caused" their symptoms.

ILLNESS OR ALLNESS

Contemporary psychiatrists are convinced that with the possible exception of borderline personality disorders, the other four mental disorders are genuine illnesses that cause severe distress or disability, have consistent constellations of symptoms, and, as I'll show later, have specific genetic patterns, characteristic responses to drugs, and similar biological features. If so, what else can these disorders be called other than "illness"? Any other label seems euphemistic and absurd, resembling how the actor Frank Langella described Dracula—"a man with a problem."

Patients can sense the difference between a problem in living

---

*When these patients finally consult a psychiatrist, many have become so afraid of another panic attack that even though they know that Tofranil will prevent it, they are still severely incapacitated by the second and third stages of the disorder—"anticipatory anxiety" and "agoraphobia." Tofranil does *not* help these later symptoms, but other treatments do.

and an illness. When ill, patients feel their illness runs them; when well, patients feel they run themselves.

Yet even when a patient is ill, his personality doesn't disappear. He is still the same person. What has changed is that this "same person" must now contend with a mental illness. Just as no two patients with an ulcer act the same, so too with major depression and every other mental disorder.

To paraphrase Dr. John Dorsey, a favorite mentor for generations of medical students, "illness is not allness." That someone is mentally ill does not mean that everything the patient feels and does is without meaning or purpose. Each individual's response to his illness is unique. For example, depending on their life experiences, personalities, and unconscious concerns, two patients with major depressions will express the symptom of overwhelming hopelessness in different ways. One man with a "dependent" personality may cling to his wife and constantly beg for reassurance, whereas a reserved New England Yankee may sit alone in the corner of a room and refuse all help or even conversation. Both men have the symptom of hopelessness that is characteristic of depression, yet each man is an individual in how he manifests this hopelessness.

People do not go crazy in some randomly amorphous way, but in specific patterns. That's why when psychiatrists evaluate patients, among the first questions they ask themselves is whether a mental illness exists, and if so, which one.

FOUR

How Psychiatrists Evaluate Patients

The questions I'm most frequently asked by friends and acquaintances are "How should I choose a therapist?" and "Whom should I see?" That's not surprising, given all the conflicting advice people get about psychiatry and psychotherapy from friends, relatives, and the media.

In looking for a therapist, people frequently err by prematurely determining what kind of therapy they require without first obtaining a thorough evaluation. Although exceptions exist, such as the person seeking couples therapy for what's clearly a marital problem, most of the time, prospective patients are jumping the gun. For example, a chronically unhappy friend wanted the name of a good psychoanalyst. As I told him, I'd gladly give him some names, but I'd suggest he first receive an evaluation to assess the nature of his unhappiness and the best possible treatment. My friend was surprised, for like many people, he'd always assumed the only decent psychiatric treatment was psychoanalytic psychotherapy. In most cases, it's premature to decide on a therapy before having a formal evaluation.

A thorough assessment has become far more important with scientific psychiatry. During the psychoanalytic era there was only one basic treatment—psychoanalytic psychotherapy; the psychiatrist's evaluation merely aimed to determine how best to apply this therapy. In contrast, the scientific psychiatrist must figure out the best way to employ many different types of treatment.

SELECTING A PSYCHIATRIST

When friends and acquaintances ask me about finding a therapist, although my advice varies depending on the person, some considerations apply to everyone.

I first try to determine if the person wants help with *symptoms,* such as phobias, incapacitating depression, and insomnia, or if he seeks help only with *issues,* such as an unrewarding professional life, a low self-image, a lousy social life, or a precarious marriage. Everyone has issues; only some have symptoms.

If my friend has symptoms, I suggest that at least initially he should see a psychiatrist. If he does not have symptoms, if his concerns are limited to issues, then I'll recommend he consult a therapist of any discipline, especially psychiatry, psychology, or psychiatric social work. If I'm not sure if my friend has symptoms, I'll play it safe and suggest he first receive an evaluation from a psychiatrist.

When I believe the friend should receive an assessment from a psychiatrist, I'll suggest that he see a "generalist," somebody who is familiar with a large variety of treatments—drugs, individual psychotherapy (of all kinds), family and group therapies, behavior therapies, hypnosis, etc. Unlike the "specialist" who does, let's say, nothing but psychoanalysis or nothing but drug therapy, the generalist is not ideologically beholden to a particular brand of therapy nor restricted to viewing patients from only one theoretical perspective. That psychiatrists are increasingly being trained to be generalists is fortunate, since it is much easier for patients to go from a generalist to a specialist than the other way around.

Nobody *really* knows if a psychiatrist is good or bad with patients. Neither I nor any other shrink knows what Dr. X actually does in his office. I can tell if he sounds brilliant or stupid when talking with colleagues; I can have a sense of his personality. But I can't say how much this reveals about his work with patients. These reservations aside, psychiatrists can make fairly good predictions about which people will do well with which psychiatrists because they have an idea of a colleague's personality, knowledge, skills, and limitations.

As in choosing any physician, one receives the most dependable information about a good psychiatrist from residents-in-training. Being in training enables psychiatric residents, and to a lesser degree interns and advanced medical students, to have the best firsthand view of how psychiatrists work with patients and think about them. The next most dependable source is psychiatrists who are already in practice. After them, one may get some good names from other physicians or mental health professionals. And then, while asking friends and relatives for advice, one should also contact the department of psychiatry of a nearby university. After that, call the local branch of the American Psychiatric Association, and if there isn't any, try the local office of the American Medical Association.

Once the consultation has been set up, I remind friends that they will be evaluating the psychiatrist as much as the psychiatrist will be evaluating them. One should ask about where the psychiatrist trained, for how long, and if in any psychiatric subspecialties. Although it is no guarantee of excellence, a psychiatrist certified by the American Board of Psychiatry and Neurology is likely to be a "safe" psychiatrist, and probably much better than someone who isn't board-certified.

It's harder to determine if a psychiatrist is up-to-date. Nonetheless, patients can glean some idea by asking if all his therapy is based on one theory, or if he draws from many theories and pragmatically choses treatments from a variety of therapies. When asked about their professional orientation, psychoanalytic psychiatrists usually portray themselves as some type of "Freudian," whereas scientific psychiatrists will say they are "eclectic" or "general" psychiatrists. It will surprise the psychiatrist, but ask him what professional journals he reads. Most psychiatrists who keep abreast of current developments will mention (among others) the *Archives of General Psychiatry* and the *American Journal of Psychiatry.**

If the shrink gets defensive when you inquire about any of these matters, get another shrink. Note how the psychiatrist responds

---

*A journal the psychiatrist will not mention is the *Journal of Polymorphous Perversity.* Its first issue contained articles such as "Psychotherapy of the Dead" and "New Improved Delusions." Shrinks reading this satirical journal might not be better psychiatrists, but at least they would have a sense of humor.

when you doubt something he says. If the psychiatrist gets miffed, feels slighted, or insists you agree with him, be cautious.

The patient should ask about the psychiatrist's fees, and whether he charges for telephone calls and for missed sessions, especially when the patient has given advance notice. Also inquire if he's available by telephone in an emergency. The patient should not forget to ask if each session lasts forty-five, fifty, or sixty minutes.

In all these matters as throughout the consultation, the patient must decide whether he trusts the therapist, feels he's competent, and senses he can do the job. In selecting a psychiatrist, a patient should be far more concerned with whether the psychiatrist can help *him* in particular, and not with how good the psychiatrist might be in general. Whether the psychiatrist is a famous researcher, has published numerous professional papers, has written books for a general audience, or boasts a fancy academic title—these matters are of less importance than whether the patient feels comfortable with the psychiatrist. A psychiatrist may be great for some patients, but not for others.

THE PSYCHIATRIST'S PERSPECTIVE

First impressions always leave their mark, but so striking for the psychiatrist is that in just one hour, a total stranger reveals his biggest problems, deepest fears, greatest hopes, and darkest secrets; the patient divulges information he's never told a soul. Intimacies are normally reserved for intimates, but not here. That's why no matter how long a psychiatrist has practiced, he never tires of hearing a new patient unfold his story. For the psychiatrist it's like watching a live drama, but the script is real and so are the players.

Psychiatrists know that patients are evaluating them as much as they are evaluating patients. In assessing the psychiatrist's skills, knowledge, experience, and personality, a patient wants to see if the psychiatrist inspires confidence and hope; a patient wants to know if *this* psychiatrist can help him. In trying to fulfill these wishes, psychiatrists sometimes feel they must impress patients; at other times, they feel they are auditioning for patients. With every patient, fulfilling these wishes presents challenges.

At a first meeting, what exactly should one do to inspire confidence and to convey hope? Be honest and open? That sounds fine, but how honest and how open? Telling the patient that he's ugly may be honest; it's also stupid. Be oneself, act naturally? That sounds fine too, but I'd hope the psychiatrist doesn't behave toward his friends as he does with his patients.

In one sense, during this initial session, the psychiatrist puts on an act. I don't mean that he's phony, but that he tries to gauge what he thinks will make the patient comfortable, and then acts accordingly. If he isn't acting something of a role, he will not be doing his job. For example, those security-conscious patients who want their doctor to ooze confidence and to convey certainty are greatly relieved when a psychiatrist says, "Hey, don't worry! Everything's going to be okay." On the other hand, saying exactly the same thing to a suspicious patient courts disaster: The patient might think, "This shrink can't tell me not to worry when he doesn't even know me. What's this guy up to?" Some patients prefer a psychiatrist who listens a lot, others a psychiatrist who talks a lot. Within the boundaries of what the psychiatrist finds proper and comfortable, he always modifies his act to make the patient feel more at ease.

It's nice to make the patient feel comfortable and hopeful—that is, to be "supportive"—but that's quite different from conducting an assessment; doing both tasks is necessary for a successful first interview. Performing the assessment involves gathering a history, making a diagnosis, arriving at a formulation, and devising a treatment plan.

The initial meeting has a built-in tension between its "supportive" and "assessment" functions. The psychiatrist is frequently conflicted over how much time to devote to each. How he decides depends on the patient. If, for example, the patient keeps insisting he's scared of seeing a psychiatrist, the therapist will offer relatively more support. Most outpatients aren't as fragile. They want to know if the shrink knows his stuff, and for them it's most reassuring to see the psychiatrist conduct a skillful and sensitive assessment.

GOALS OF ASSESSMENT

At the initial consultation, many patients say they want "to *understand why* I'm depressed." What they actually want is quite different: They want to stop feeling depressed. Psychoanalytic psychiatry has indoctrinated the public to confuse means with ends. "Understanding why" is one among many means to reach the end, which in this case is to stop feeling depressed.

From the psychiatrist's perspective, the overall purpose of an evaluation is to determine what, if any, treatment program can best meet the patient's needs. To make this decision, the psychiatrist conducts the evaluation to answer, to his own satisfaction, the following ten questions:

1. Does the patient have a mental disorder as defined in *DSM-III,* and if so, which one(s)? If the patient has no mental disorder, what is the precise problem?

2. What psychological, social, and biological factors have initiated, sustained, or shaped the patient's disorder or problem?

3. Why is the patient coming *now?* The answer is obvious sometimes, but not always. When it's not, finding out "why now" often uncovers critical information. To illustrate: I saw a woman who said she had been unhappy for years; only after pursuing the answer to "why now?" did she reveal that she'd recently placed her mother in a nursing home and felt terribly guilty about doing so.

4. Is the patient suicidal or homicidal?

5. What is the patient's personality style and characteristic "defense mechanisms"*? The psychiatrist's conduct of psychotherapy is greatly influenced by whether, for example, the patient is habitually dependent or suspicious, or if he usually blames others or blames himself. The psychiatrist also needs this information when prescribing medication. For instance, a patient who uses a lot of denial is far more likely to stop medication prematurely, and therefore requires more careful monitoring.

6. What is the patient's current "mental status"? This phrase refers to an objective *description* of the patient's *present* mental functioning, such as how he speaks, feels, thinks, and perceives.

7. How "psychologically minded" is the patient? More psy-

---

*The psychoanalytic concept of "defense mechanisms" has been incorporated into mainstream modern psychiatry. Defense mechanisms are the psychological ways people protect themselves against unwanted feelings. In most situations, people use defense mechanisms unconsciously—that is, they're unaware of using them. Everyone employs defense mechanisms; they can be adaptive or harmful. "Denial," "projection," and "reaction formation" are commonly used defenses.

chologically minded people are especially curious about their own feelings and motives; they're relatively introspective; they're also more willing to examine themselves instead of blaming others. How the patient describes his history and problems conveys his degree of psychological-mindedness. In addition, several times during the interview the psychiatrist will either make or suggest an interpretation and see how the patient deals with it. A woman told me that three hours after her mother died, she decided to become a nun. When I asked her how the two events were related, she looked genuinely baffled: "What makes you think they're related?" Such virtual absence of psychological-mindedness dissuades the psychiatrist from recommending insight-oriented psychotherapy.

    8. What has been the patient's previous experience with psychiatric treatment? What has helped? What has failed?

    9. Do I want to treat this person? If so, why? If not, why?

    10. Can I help this person? If so, how? If not, who can?

CONDUCTING THE INTERVIEW

Every psychiatrist has his own particular way of eliciting the answers to these questions. Nonetheless, some generalizations can be made.

Most initial assessments take one to three hours, in one or more sessions.

Since there is limited time to achieve the "support" and "assessment" purposes of this initial interview, the psychiatrist often pursues both purposes simultaneously. For instance, when the psychiatrist shakes hands with a new patient, he's being cordial, but he's also collecting data: Does the patient have a limp or a crunching handshake? Does his palm sweat? Is his hand rough or smooth, that of a hard laborer, an office executive, or a prima donna?

How psychiatrists shape the interview

Psychiatrists direct the initial evaluation from the general to the specific. During the first half of the session, the psychiatrist is relatively quiet; occasionally he encourages the patient to speak, and offers support and, if needed, redirection. Otherwise, the psychiatrist listens, observes, introspects, and (mainly to himself) hypothesizes. During this period the psychiatrist wants to see the patient relate his story in *his* way. Because the psychiatrist is interested not only in *what* the patient says but also in *how* he says it, the psychiatrist gives the patient as much room as possible to reveal his personal style. Moreover, by being relatively silent, the psychiatrist hopes to be supportive by allowing the patient to "get things off his chest."

The psychiatrist devotes the latter half of the session to tying up loose ends, clarifying apparent contradictions, and answering the patient's questions. To gather these details, the psychiatrist speaks more and asks more specific questions.

The form of question asked by the psychiatrist varies as he goes from the general to the specific. During the first part, he uses relatively more "open-ended questions," whereas in the latter half he relies more on "closed-ended questions." In an open-ended question, such as "How do you feel about your wife?" the patient is given considerable latitude and can answer in a variety of ways. A closed-ended version of this question would be "Do you like your wife?" The form of this question restricts the patient's range of potential responses to yes or no. Open- and closed-ended questions each have their place.

Getting started

For all patients, but especially for those who've never before consulted a psychiatrist, this first hour can be quite stressful. Faced with squeezing all of one's problems and history into fifty minutes, patients are often surprised by their own anxiety and confusion. Normally articulate people are embarrassed by their disorganized presentation of their problems. Yet why should it be otherwise? Nobody I know is in the habit of presenting his problems and history in an orderly and succinct way; even if he were, the stakes for the patient are high and the pressures on him considerable. Anxiety is inevitable.

During the first hour, patients frequently apologize—"Everything is so confusing, I don't know where to begin." Psychiatrists hear this concern so often, they're used to replying, "Why don't you start by telling me what mainly worries you." Or "Don't worry about it; most people find it hard to know exactly where to start. Begin anywhere, and I'm sure you'll cover the important issues. If necessary, I'll step in and redirect you." In presenting their history, other patients will say, "I'm not doing well enough," or "I'm not doing it right," as if the consultation were a test, and as if there were a "right" and "wrong" way of outlining one's problems.

Despite patients' many concerns over leaving out significant details, and although some matters inevitably go uncovered, what's striking is the great amount of important information that does get conveyed to the psychiatrist. What is left out at the first meeting can always be brought up at the next one. Similarly, the patient who fears he's given the psychiatrist a false or misleading impression can always rectify matters later on.

When recounting distressing events, many patients are disturbed or surprised by becoming "too emotional"; they're worried about looking "foolish" in front of the shrink. Others, having spent weeks anticipating this session, expect a massive catharsis. When it doesn't occur, as is the usual case, they're disappointed. The psychiatrist is accustomed to these concerns, and if they arise, he will try to be reassuring.

To start the interview, the psychiatrist usually says, "Can you tell me what's been troubling you?" or "What brought you to consult me?" or "What do you think I should know?" Once the interview is launched, the psychiatrist primarily follows the patient's lead. This strategy differs from that used by many physicians, who conduct the interview by asking their own predetermined set of questions.

In following the patient's lead, the psychiatrist will intercede mainly to have the patient elaborate on a particular subject. If the patient says his father is overbearing, how does the psychiatrist know what the patient means by "overbearing"? Therefore, the psychiatrist might ask, "Can you say more about that?" or "Can you give me an example of how he's overbearing?" I cite this specific example because I recall a thirty-five-year-old patient who claimed his father was overbearing for not giving him a big enough allowance, and on the other hand a teenage girl who used the term "overbearing" to describe a father who had been sexually abusing her for nine years. "Overbearing" is hardly the word I'd use to describe either father. That's why psychiatrists usually want concrete illustrations whenever patients make especially broad and important statements.

What psychiatrists look for

Except for the telephone call which sets up the appointment, the psychiatrist's first source of information is visual, not verbal. How the patient chooses to look is a statement of how he wishes to be seen, by the psychiatrist for sure, and by others perhaps. Clothes are costumes; they consciously or unconsciously communicate to the psychiatrist information about the patient's self-image, socio-economic class, personality, and tastes.

The psychiatrist has his antennae up for nonverbal clues. For example, when a patient crosses his legs, the psychiatrist mentally notes what the patient is talking about at the moment, since many, though certainly not all, changes of position occur when patients are discussing highly charged topics.

In trying to reach a diagnosis, the psychiatrist has the patient describe his symptoms and everything about them—what they are like, when and how they began, what increases or decreases them, and so on. Precision is crucial.

To illustrate, take one symptom and one small detail: If a patient says, "I'm hearing voices," the psychiatrist might think the patient has schizophrenia, unless he asks for more details. When he does, he finds the patient *only* has hallucinations just before falling asleep. These are called "hypnogogic hallucinations"; they are a variant of normal and not a symptom of mental illness. When people have hypnogogic hallucinations, they are simply dreaming just before they doze off. People with these hallucinations are usually terrified they're going crazy, and so imagine their relief when they discover they're not.* But unless the psychiatrist gets the patient to describe his symptoms precisely, psychiatrist and patient alike might think the patient is schizophrenic.

More than ever, psychiatrists are impressed by how many drugs used in general medicine produce psychiatric symptoms. Steroids, such as prednisone, can trigger a manic or depressive episode, and sometimes a schizophrenic-like psychosis. Inderal, a drug widely used for cardiac conditions, induces depression; so do reserpine and Aldomet, two popular antihypertensive medications. Besides

---

*If hypnogogic hallucinations occur along with the sudden onset of either sleep attacks or collapsing muscles, the patient may have narcolepsy. Yet by themselves, hypnogogic hallucinations are nothing to worry about.

being concerned about addiction, psychiatrists want to know about a patient's use of illegal drugs for diagnostic purposes. For example, the long-term use of cocaine often produces a severe depression, which becomes far worse when the patient stops using cocaine. Sometimes, patients self-medicate: It's not that they take cocaine and become depressed, but that they are depressed and take cocaine. No matter which comes first, once any addiction starts, patients develop all kinds of psychiatric symptoms, making it all the harder to treat the addiction.

Psychiatrists are alert to recurring themes, especially when they pop up out of context. After talking about his father at great length, a truck driver switched topics and described his work: "The hours are long, and by day's end, you feel all washed out. Guys take speed like crazy just to keep going. If my dad ever knew I took that crap, he'd have my balls."

Psychiatrists are also interested in themes that are striking in being absent. A woman entered treatment because of an unexpectedly severe degree of loneliness following a recent divorce. In considerable detail she told me about her ex-husband and about everyone in her family except for her nine-year old son, Eric. When it became clear she was not going to mention the son, I did. She shook, physically as well as emotionally. "I was afraid you'd ask. Five years ago my husband and I were entertaining, when all of a sudden there was a blood-curdling scream from Eric's bedroom. As we raced there I remember thinking that burglars must have attacked him. His door was open, and we saw Eric lying in a puddle of blood. I then noticed a rope tied to the doorknob, and at its other end I saw Eric's testicles and penis. Evidently, he had tied a rope attached to the doorknob around his privates, and then flung the door open to castrate himself." At this point, feelings she had never revealed suddenly poured out: Her guilt over failing as a mother; her anger at her ex-husband for being a poor role model for her son; her pity and rage toward Eric. While speaking, she realized how much she was blaming Eric for her divorce.

The patient's stream of *associations* often illuminate the patient's personality and critical concerns. A middle-aged single man was recounting that when he was ten years old, his father greatly disappointed him by not attending, as promised, the championship Little League baseball game in which the patient was the starting pitcher. In the middle of telling this tale, he complained of not being married. I couldn't see the connection, and said so. He explained that one of his life's great disappointments was not having a son, for whom he could be everything his own father was not.

While listening to the content of what the patient says, the psychiatrist likes to "follow the affect," which means to pursue anything the patient says whenever he becomes more emotional. When patients list a dozen problems, it's hard to know which is the most important, since the patient himself frequently doesn't know. Quite often, however, when rattling off such a list, at one, usually unexpected, point the patient starts to cry or to fumble around. To the therapist that's an invaluable clue that *this,* among all the problems, is the one most worth exploring. A woman kept insisting that nobody liked her—her husband, her kids, her boss, her neighbors; yet it was only when indicating that her parents disliked her that her eyes filled with tears. These tears revealed what her words had not.

The patient's affect (i.e., currently visible emotions) may belie his words. While a patient speaks glowingly of his "great old man," his voice becomes tense. The psychiatrist may simply make a mental note of a possible contradiction and say nothing. On the other hand, he might point out his observations to the patient and wonder aloud if the patient's feelings toward his dad could be "a bit more ambivalent." Whatever the case, psychiatrists look for affect as miners look for gold.

Although the psychiatrist mentally logs any slips of the tongue (or "parapraxes"), at the initial interview he usually will not pursue them. At this early point, pressing most patients on a slip merely compounds their discomfort.

"Screen memories" can help to identify significant psychological themes. The psychiatrist asks the patient to describe "the earliest thing in your life you can remember." One man replied, "From the back side I can picture myself sitting on the floor waiting patiently for my grandmother to roll me a ball." As is characteristic of screen memories, there is no way he could have seen what he claimed to have seen, because he couldn't possibly see his own back. That doesn't mean the event didn't happen, for it could be recalled from an old photograph or movie, or the patient may have slightly distorted an actual occurrence. Later on he revealed that as a child neither parent cared for him very much, and that only this grandmother paid attention to him.

One of the psychiatrist's richest sources of data is his own subjective responses to the patient. Using oneself as a barometer of another must be done cautiously, since the psychiatrist should not confuse his own problems with those of the patient. If a therapist finds all his patients depressing, it's not the patients who are depressed. If the psychiatrist is irritated by most of his elderly patients, then he cannot place much stock in such feelings.

But if that's not the case, if his subjective responses to patients vary considerably, which is usually so, then his feelings toward a particular patient are "legitimate," invaluable data about the patient. If the psychiatrist finds himself being annoyed with a patient who at least superficially appears pleasant, then the psychiatrist starts asking himself what there is about the patient that makes him annoying. On referring a patient to me, another psychiatrist said, "I'd be curious to know how this patient strikes you." After the consultation, I told my colleague, "The guy made me feel I was constantly walking on eggshells." My colleague had felt exactly the same.

Never is the psychiatrist absolutely sure that what the patient says about the rest of his life is true, but the psychiatrist *does* know what happens in his office. When a patient claims that people at work are nasty, one can't know for certain if that's so or if the patient is continually provoking that nastiness. On the other hand, the psychiatrist can see for himself if the patient provokes nasty responses in him. So rather than dismiss his subjective responses to patients as idiosyncratic reactions, the psychiatrist views them as valuable data because they are firsthand evidence of how the patient affects people.

Yet of all the possible things a psychiatrist must look for, nothing is more important than finding out if the patient is suicidal. Since in recent years deaths from suicide have escalated dramatically, especially among youth, more than ever psychiatrists are alert to any hint of a potential suicide. These hints may include profound hopelessness and helplessness, severe depression, previous suicidal threats or actions, a family history of suicide, giving away prized possessions for no apparent reason, reckless self-destructive incidents (e.g., automobile accidents), and alcohol abuse.

If for any reason the psychiatrist thinks the patient might be contemplating suicide, the psychiatrist should ask: "Given how upset you are, I wonder if you have considered committing suicide?" Contrary to myth, inquiring about suicide does not induce people to kill themselves; it does not "put ideas into the patient's head," or make anyone who has not already seriously thought about suicide think about committing it. Another common myth is that people who repeatedly attempt suicide don't commit it. Although the ratio of attempted to committed suicides is ten to one, people who attempt suicide most often are those who are most likely to eventually commit suicide.

Among the many ways psychiatrists evaluate a patient's potential for suicide, there is the obvious question "Why do you want to kill yourself?" But often it is far more revealing to ask, "With all your problems, why do you want to live?" Philosophy aside, if the patient is not precariously suicidal, he may mull over the question, but eventually he will point to something or someone as a reason for living—a daughter, a mother, a husband, God. The more suicidal can't come up with any reason for living.

The psychiatrist's predictions of suicide are fairly accurate, but never perfect. To be sure, psychiatrists know a great deal more about predicting (and managing) potentially suicidal patients than homicidal or violent patients. Nonetheless, psychiatrists keep their ears open for potentially assaultive patients, especially for a history of previous violent behavior, since it is *the* single best predictor of future violent behavior.

The mental status examination (MSE)

As part of every patient's evaluation, the psychiatrist makes *objective* descriptions of the patient's *current* "mental status"—that is, the patient's appearance, speech, behavior, emotions, organization and content of thought, perceptions, memory, judgment, concentration, orientation (to time, place, and person), abstract thinking, and awareness of his condition.

Although the psychiatrist gets most of this information while gathering the patient's history, sometimes he conducts a *formal* MSE, which entails asking a series of standardized questions. For instance, to assess the patient's memory, the psychiatrist might say, "In five minutes from now I'm going to ask you to recall five items: pen, automobile, toothpick, elephant, and orange." Five minutes later, most patients can remember four or five items. To evaluate the patient's ability to think abstractly, the psychiatrist might ask, "What is the similarity between a table and chair?" People who can think abstractly usually reply, "They're furniture"; those relatively poor at thinking abstractly will say, "They're both made of wood" or "I don't see any similarity."

The chief purpose of the formal mental status examination is to provide clues for determining whether a patient has an organic mental disorder, such as dementia or delirium. Because so many organic mental disorders mimic psychiatric disorders, knowing how to perform and to interpret the formal MSE is among the most basic of all psychiatric skills.

Every psychiatrist is shocked the first time he meets a patient who seems quite "with it," only to ask the patient, "What year is it?" and get the reply "1709." Assuming the patient is not joking, this "disorientation" suggests there's something wrong with his brain. When asked the same question, patients with insidiously developing dementias are usually evasive; over time, many learn to hide their impairment by bluffing. "It's the year of our Lord," the patient might say. He might wax philosophical: "Time, time! Who cares about time? That's the problem—everybody's a slave to time." Such charm, such grace, such organicity. Half the time the psychiatrist doesn't have the heart to return to such a mundane question as "What year is it?" Nonetheless, he must, for otherwise he's missing an invaluable diagnostic clue.

The MSE is also helpful because, when recorded in the patient's chart, it becomes the only objective written data about the patient. The patient's history, which is secondhand, is of questionable accuracy; the psychiatrist's psychological formulations are highly speculative. Indeed, many psychiatrists claim that the MSE is the most, and sometimes the only, useful information in a patient's past records.

"Psychoanalytic" versus "scientific" assessments

Although in many respects psychoanalytic and scientific psychiatrists conduct similar evaluations, they differ in several key areas. Perhaps the most fundamental distinction is that psychoanalytic psychiatrists are mainly interested in *why* problems occur, whereas scientific psychiatrists are mainly concerned with *what* problems have occurred. Psychoanalytic psychiatrists want to know the meaning of symptoms; they try to unearth the unconscious conflicts, symbolic importance, and childhood antecedents of symptoms. In contrast, scientific psychiatrists view symptoms as problems in their own right; they obtain detailed descriptions of each symptom.

When a patient complains of insomnia, psychoanalytic psychiatrists focus on why the patient thinks he has a sleep problem and what are the characteristics of the patient's dream life. Does he remember his dreams? Does he have certain recurrent dreams? What do his dreams mean to him? What, if any, nightmares did he have as a child? All these questions are still relevant, but scientific psychiatrists are more concerned with identifying patterns of sleep than with interpreting dreams. They're more interested in facts than in speculations. They will ask how long it takes the patient to fall asleep, and whether the patient awakes in the middle of the night or early in the morning. They want to know if the patient consistently oversleeps or routinely drifts off in the middle of the day.

When a patient says, "On going to bed I feel restless," the psychoanalytic psychiatrist assumes this is a symptom of anxiety, which springs from an unconscious conflict, and that he should encourage the patient to reveal his feelings and thoughts associated with the restlessness. However, by automatically attributing the restlessness to anxiety, the psychiatrist might overlook another disorder, such as a neurological condition called the restless leg syndrome, which is treated quite differently from anxiety. That's why in conducting an assessment, the scientific psychiatrist's first concern is to reach a proper diagnosis. To do so, the psychiatrist asks for a more detailed description of the patient's symptom by inquiring, for example, "Do all, or just some, parts of your body feel restless?" and "Do you feel this *only* at bedtime or does it bother you all day long but feel worse at bedtime?" and "Does it occur *every* night or merely on occasion?" The psychoanalytic psychiatrist goes after subjective impressions, while the scientific psychiatrist tries to elicit objective information.

Psychoanalytic psychiatrists generally view a patient's interpersonal problems with friends, family, and bosses as the *cause* of a patient's mental illness, whereas scientific psychiatrists typically see a patient's interpersonal problems as a *consequence* of mental illness. This distinction is relative, not absolute. If a patient consults a psychiatrist for depression after being fired from his job, the psychoanalytic psychiatrist is more likely to assume that the patient's losing his job triggered his depression. Scientific psychiatrists would seriously consider this hypothesis, but they would entertain the alternative hypothesis that the patient became depressed first, and that so interfered with his work that he eventually got fired. Which hypothesis is correct depends on the case.

Psychoanalytic psychiatrists tend to have a visceral dislike of the patient's family. Exceptions exist, but to such a psychiatrist, if a kid is mentally ill, it is the parents' fault. Psychoanalytic psychiatrists don't overtly blame the parents, yet the accusatory inference is usually there. Many use almost any rationalization to avoid seeing relatives: "It would violate confidentiality," "It would undermine the transference," "The patient wouldn't like it." If asked how he knows if a patient is telling the truth about the family, the psychoanalytic psychiatrist would reply, "Whether it's the truth doesn't matter all that much, because I'm concerned with what the patient *perceives* to be the truth, since for the patient that *is* 'the truth.' " Psychoanalytic psychiatrists frequently see relatives as nuisances, meddlers who are jealous of the close relationship between the shrink and his patient. Many psychiatrists account for a failed treatment by saying, "The family sabotaged the therapy" or "The family has a need to keep the patient sick." Psychiatrists conducting an evaluation either discount what relatives have to say or don't speak to them at all.

In contrast, scientific psychiatrists are more likely to consider family members not as perpetrators of illness, but as victims of it. At least for the more serious mental illnesses, such as schizophrenia, major depression, and manic-depression, modern psychiatrists will blame bad genes far more than bad families. Some relatives deal more constructively with a mentally ill family member than do others, but that's quite different from viewing family members as the cause of the illness. What's more, although scientific psychiatrists are less inclined than psychoanalytic psychiatrists to attribute a patient's *symptoms* to a faulty upbringing, they still feel that problematic *issues* and what symptoms mean to the patient develop largely from familial influences.

When the scientific psychiatrist feels that talking to relatives could provide useful information for the assessment, he will first obtain the patient's permission, and after speaking with them, tell the patient what he was told. Or, depending on the situation, the patient may be present while the psychiatrist talks with the family. When I do not meet relatives during the assessment, I find it helpful to see photographs of them; it makes them "more real."

Because the psychoanalytic psychiatrist is primarily evaluating unconscious conflicts, whatever information relatives could provide is of little interest to him. On the other hand, because scientific psychiatrists are more concerned with making a correct diagnosis, they are eager to gather as much objective information as possible about the patient, especially on subjects the patient is less likely to know about, such as a traumatic birth, a mentally ill second cousin, prolonged toilet training, and an early school phobia.

Since the critical role of genetics in transmitting mental illness is becoming clearer, scientific psychiatrists are increasingly using information about a family history of mental illness to help in diagnosis. It's common for psychiatrists to have difficulties trying to accurately diagnose patients with severe depressions, because the serious depressions of major depression and manic-depression look alike. Statistically, the psychiatrist knows the prevalence of major depression is ten times that of manic-depression, and therefore, everything else being equal, major depression is the most likely diagnosis. But let's say that although the patient has never had a manic episode, his father and brother have. With this strong family history, everything is no longer equal: The patient is far more likely to have manic-depression.

Evidence is also accumulating that a patient's response to psychiatric medication is in large measure genetically inherited. If a depressed patient's depressed mother was helped by the antidepressant Elavil but not by the antidepressant Tofranil, then in all likelihood the patient will respond in the same way. (See Chapter 6.)

Scientific psychiatrists are likely to use the patient's response to drugs as a diagnostic clue. With some delusional patients it is difficult for the psychiatrist to decide if the correct diagnosis is schizophrenia or major depression. How a patient reacts to a medication can resolve this puzzle. For example, since antidepressant medications help patients with major depression but not those with schizophrenia, if a patient improves with an antidepressant, he probably has a major depression; if not, he's more likely to have schizophrenia.

Some scientific psychiatrists criticize this logic, saying that it is like suggesting that since pneumonia improves with penicillin, any illness that improves with penicillin must be pneumonia. Moreover, since antidepressants also help panic attacks, phobias, chronic pain, and some sleep disorders, it would be absurd to figure that everybody who improves on antidepressants is depressed. Nonetheless, most scientific psychiatrists feel it's valid to use a patient's response to medication as diagnostic information, as long as corroborative evidence exists. By itself, no one piece of evidence is ever diagnostic; plenty of confirmatory information must exist before a correct diagnosis can be rendered.

THE PITFALLS OF PSYCHIATRIC EVALUATION

Perhaps the trickiest problem psychiatrists face in evaluating patients is to strike the proper balance between being supportive while acquiring the greatest amount of information. I've seen psychiatrists conduct very supportive assessments, which allow patients to ramble on, but elicit virtually no useful data. I've also observed psychiatrists perform mechanical interviews, as if solely reciting a checklist of symptoms; the shrink barely notices the patient and rarely follows his leads. Blending support and assessment during the initial interview is but one of several major challenges psychiatrists face.

Every psychiatrist realizes that he can fall into the trap of premature closure. Most psychiatrists have arrived at one or two probable diagnoses within two minutes of meeting a patient. Snap judgments like these are unavoidable and inherent to human nature. The chief danger of premature closure is that the psychiatrist skews all further information so that it conforms to, and reaffirms, his initial diagnostic impression; information that doesn't fit his first impression is either downplayed or dismissed. To avoid premature closure, the psychiatrist forces himself to keep an open mind and to consider all other diagnostic possibilities before ruling anything out.

One of my least proud moments during my training illustrates how premature closure may occur. After seeing many patients with severe depressions, I had developed an ingrained image of the depressed patient: self-absorbed, blank face, a low, halting, and monotonous voice, and a dreadfully slow gait.* Into the emergency room walked such a man; he looked forlorn and complained of being extremely unhappy, especially since his wife's death a year ago. He was greatly relieved when I recommended hospitalization. An hour after I admitted him with the diagnosis of major depression, the inpatient supervisor called me to say that the reason this man was unhappy, moved slowly, and stared blankly was that he had Parkinson's disease—not major depression. Patients with major depression and Parkinson's disease physically resemble each other,† yet being in a psychiatric setting, I was thinking solely of *mental* disorders, and the possibility of a *neurological* disorder never occurred to me. I erred by not questioning my first impression and by not systematically considering every other diagnostic possibility; my mental laziness led to premature closure.

Language presents another common pitfall. Psychiatry has the misfortune of having many of its technical words in the popular lexicon. Sometimes a psychiatrist will misunderstand or misconstrue what a patient tells him because the professional and the popular meanings are quite different. A patient said her mother "used a lot of projection," which turned out to mean "put words in other people's mouths." Another patient indicated that after stopping his medication he became "anxious." When I asked what he meant by "anxious," he described nonstop tobacco-chewing movements—a serious neurological side effect of drugs like Thorazine. Normally, when I think of "anxiety," movements of the mouth don't rush to mind. A psychiatrist should never assume that patients use terms as he does. To avoid these misunderstandings, I don't use technical terms with patients, and I ask them not to use them either.

Psychiatrists can be led astray by missing a "calling card"— that is, by not realizing that the patient's ostensible complaint is not his real complaint. The patient may begin with a false complaint that he believes is more socially acceptable than his actual

---

*Frame-by-frame analysis of motion pictures shows that depressed patients have a characteristic walk: In moving forward, they lift their thighs and their lower legs lag behind, whereas most people propel their lower legs and feet forward.
†Patients with major depression and Parkinson's disease also have similar neurochemistries.

complaint. Patients use a calling card as an excuse to get in the door; once in, the patient waits to see whether he will feel sufficiently comfortable to reveal the real, or more serious, problem.

At times the patient himself isn't fully aware he's using a calling card. When being evaluated for insomnia, a man casually mentioned, "I'm going through a divorce, and although it took me a year, my feelings about it are finally under control." Yet later on he started yelling when he mentioned his wife. A normally quiet man, he was stunned by his outburst. "I'm embarrassed," he confessed. "Until now I hadn't realized that what really brought me here was the divorce and not my insomnia."

During evaluations, psychiatrists wonder if, either by omission or commission, the patient is shading or distorting the truth. Does this mean the psychiatrist doesn't believe the patient? No. It means the psychiatrist doesn't take everything a new patient says as gospel, any more than anyone would on a first meeting. When a patient tells me his boss is lousy, I suspect the boss feels differently. Who's right? Who knows? Yet like most psychiatrists, I will usually take my patient's word, unless I have ample evidence to the contrary.

Some patients will deliberately lie, and as a psychiatrist, I will be fooled. I'm no mind reader. If a patient lies or doesn't give me critically important information, he is doing so for a reason; it might not be a good reason, but it is still a reason. Therefore, I often tell new patients, "Look, I realize there might be things you're reluctant to reveal. After all, I'm a virtual stranger. So if you don't want to tell me something, you might wish to tell me what stops you. Perhaps you feel I won't be sympathetic, or perhaps you're ashamed of something. But whatever, the more you can't tell me the more of a problem we have."

While there is a problem with the patient who doesn't give information, there is an equally serious problem with the psychiatrist who doesn't get information. A psychiatrist can always find some legitimate excuse not to inquire about significant problems that he'd prefer to avoid. Sometimes he doesn't ask because he's afraid of what he might be obligated to do with the answer. If a shrink doesn't ask about suicide, he can avoid the hassle of hospitalizing someone. The psychiatrist may rationalize not asking about alcoholism because it might "embarrass the patient" or "inhibit the formation of a working therapeutic alliance," or because "it's not the right time; I'll do it later." Intellectually, the psychiatrist knows better. But if you were the psychiatrist, how would you ask a dignified businessman who's come for a marital problem if he's also a boozer? When you suspect a patient of denying cocaine use, how do you suggest he is lying? How do you inquire about a rape that you must find out about even though the patient understandably resents retelling the story?

For the psychiatrist, performing an evaluation is like being a juggler, keeping many issues in the air at once, without dropping any of them. Given all the technical information he must acquire, all the supportive functions he should provide, and all the formulations he must devise, the psychiatrist finds himself constantly setting priorities. When the psychiatrist is puzzled by something, should he ask about it, or should he let the patient continue? At any given moment, should the psychiatrist provide reassurance or obtain information? Since time is limited, one is always being done at the expense of the other.

COMPLETING THE ASSESSMENT

As an extremely rough generalization, about 90 percent of the information psychiatrists need for determining diagnosis and treatment comes from interviewing the patient and his family. How the psychiatrist gathers the remaining 10 percent has changed as scientific psychiatry has evolved.

From psychological tests to rating scales

Traditionally, psychiatrists often used psychological tests to confirm or refute a diagnosis. These tests consisted of both "structured tests," i.e., those with definite answers, such as the Minnesota Multiphasic Personality Inventory (MMPI)* and the vocabulary section of the standard I.Q. test, the Wechsler Adult Intelligence Scale (WAIS), and of "unstructured tests," like the Rorschach

---

*The classic parody of the MMPI, the North Dakota Bull-Hypothesis Brain Damage Inventory, lists ninety-six statements to be answered true or false. These statements include: (1) I salivate at the sight of mittens. (2) Spinach makes me feel alone. (3) My sex life is A-OK. (4) I like mannish children. (5) A wide necktie is a sign of disease. (6) I have taken shoe polish to excess. (7) I believe in an afterbirth. (8) I have never eaten a fly. (9) My parents always faced catastrophes with a song. (10) I am anxious in rooms that have hairy walls.

("inkblot"), in which there isn't a correct answer; instead the patient can give any interpretation he wishes to what's set before him. Then, as now, psychiatrists have only a superficial understanding of psychological tests; only psychologists are trained to administer and interpret them.

Scientific psychiatrists depend much less than their psychoanalytic predecessors on these tests. The structured tests like the MMPI derive from the analytic, and not from the descriptive, diagnostic tradition, and therefore are not geared to modern psychiatric diagnosis. The primary value of unstructured tests like the Rorschach is to reveal information about the patient's unconscious; however, the quality of this information has far more to do with the quality of the psychologist than with the test itself. Psychiatrists became disenchanted with all psychological tests because to cover themselves, many psychologists would submit test reports whose summaries read, "The patient has a depressive neurosis, a passive-aggressive personality, anxious and phobic features, and an underlying psychotic potential." By diagnosing everything, the psychologist diagnosed nothing. Psychiatrists also felt that most of the time psychological tests would not reveal anything that a good, and much less expensive, interview could not uncover.

Instead of relying on psychological tests, a growing number of psychiatrists are using standardized rating scales for measuring just about anything: depression, anxiety, a sense of self-control. Although a few of these scales call for the patient to make self-ratings, most of the better ones for diagnosis are done by professionals.

In standardized rating scales, whatever is being rated is broken down into its constituent components, with each component being carefully defined or described, and then rated on a scale (e.g., 1–10). For example, a frequently used scale for evaluating depression, "the Hamilton," consists of seventeen items, such as "depressed mood," "guilt," "suicide," and "hypochondriasis." Each item is rated according to its own scale, with each scale going from better to worse. The "guilt" scale reads:

0 Absent
1 Self-reproach, feels he has let people down
2 Ideas of guilt or rumination over past errors or sinful deeds

3 (Patient thinks) present illness is a punishment; delusions of guilt
4 Hears accusatory or denunciatory voices and/or experiences threatening visual hallucinations

The ratings on each of these seventeen items are added to yield an overall score for depression. Although used primarily for psychiatric research, the Hamilton can also be applied clinically, especially as a relatively objective method for monitoring the course of a patient's depressive illness.

At present, most psychiatrists do not employ these standardized rating scales for assessing patients. Yet unlike a decade ago, when psychoanalytic psychiatrists ignored these scales, today psychiatrists in training are learning about them and are more inclined to incorporate them into their clinical evaluation.*

A blood test: psychiatry's golden fleece

Psychiatrists have always yearned for a laboratory test that could diagnose a mental illness. It's almost as if by having such a test, psychiatrists could prove they are "real" doctors.

Not unexpectedly, psychiatrists became quite excited when in 1981 a blood test that seemed to diagnose severe depression entered the marketplace. The Dexamethasone Suppression Test (DST) is simple to administer and relatively inexpensive. Dexamethasone is a synthetic steroid, which the patient ingests as a tablet at eleven-thirty at night. At four the following afternoon, the patient's blood is taken to measure one of the adrenal gland's own steroid hormones—cortisol. In most people, dexamethasone decreases or suppresses the release by the adrenal gland of cortisol. In severe depression, however, dexamethasone does not lower the release of cortisol. In other words, a "positive" DST shows the "nonsuppression" of cortisol and is allegedly diagnostic of severe depression.

---

*In the near future it may be common practice to supplement assessment interviews by having patients sit down in front of a computer that would administer and score a series of standardized rating scales. Such programs are already available. It's also possible that another currently used research tool, the "structured diagnostic interview," will be automated and administered routinely to patients so as to provide another independent and objectified diagnostic assessment.

Unfortunately, the DST isn't what it's cracked up to be. The test is often positive in conditions other than depression, and not all severe depressions yield a positive test. Therefore, the presence or absence of severe depression cannot be diagnosed by the DST; at most it can be viewed as one, among many, pieces of diagnostic evidence. The DST must be interpreted cautiously, preferably by a psychiatrist who really understands it.*

The DST is one of several blood tests, collectively known as a "neuroendocrine battery," which measure the body's hormones affecting the brain. (See Chapter 6.) Although presently limited to research purposes, within several years it may become a standard part of clinical practice.

Latent medical illness and psychological issues

According to one survey, physical examinations (including urinalyses) detected previously undiagnosed medical abnormalities in 20 percent of psychiatric outpatients. That's why psychiatrists are increasingly ordering blood tests to see if a physical disorder, such as hypothyroidism, is masquerading as a mental disorder.

For the same reason, modern psychiatrists want patients with a possible mental illness (as opposed to those with merely problems in living) to receive a physical exam. Although psychiatrists debate whether they or another physician should conduct this exam, in reality this debate is academic, since 98 percent of psychiatrists don't perform physicals on their own patients. Most psychiatrists (like most surgeons, anesthesiologists, neurologists, etc.) prefer that the patient's family practitioner or internist conduct this exam because he is better at performing physicals than they are.

To uncover repressed information, some psychiatrists use so-

---

*That by itself the DST isn't diagnostic of a specific mental illness shouldn't be too surprising, since few diagnostic tests in medicine are ever positive for a single illness. However, the DST might be useful in another way. When severely depressed patients with a positive DST recover, their DST returns to normal. If these patients' DSTs revert to positive, studies suggest they are probably headed for another depressive episode, which could be prevented by promptly restarting antidepressant medications. The evidence for this remains sketchy, but the DST must be measuring some psychophysiologic abnormality, even though nobody knows what. One speculation is that a positive DST reflects a generalized arousal in the brain as occurs with major depression and many other mental disorders.

called "truth serum." The patient slowly receives an intravenous injection of a barbiturate, usually amytal. The drug induces the patient to ramble with fewer inhibitions. During this "amytal interview," patients frequently reveal new, perhaps unconscious, information, such as the young woman who confessed under amytal that she had been raped by her stepfather and that she blamed herself for enticing him. Sometimes amytal interviews can bring out a previously hidden neurological problem.

"Truth serum" does *not* make people tell the truth; subjects can distort facts, embellish events, invent information, and deliberately lie. The same could be said for interviews conducted using hypnosis. It's never clear whether the amytal or the hypnosis makes the patient speak more freely or simply gives the patient an excuse to speak more freely.

FIVE

How Psychiatrists Determine Treatment

The future may teach us to exercise a direct influence, by means of particular chemical substances, on the amounts of energy and their distribution in the mental apparatus. It may be that there are other still undreamt-of possibilities of therapy. But for the moment we have nothing better at our disposal than the technique of psychoanalysis, and for that reason, in spite of its limitations, it should not be despised.
—Sigmund Freud, 1938

That Freud's "undreamt-of possibilities" have become realities are clear, but this does not mean that biology has become more important than psychology; it does mean that modern psychiatrists believe that both play critical, yet *different,* roles in the genesis and treatment of mental illness.

In claiming this consensus exists among today's psychiatrists, I'm not suggesting that all psychiatrists have identical orientations. Some modern psychiatrists are more interested in psychobiology and others in psychoanalysis, but despite these differing interests or orientations, virtually all agree that biology and psychology are important, albeit in different ways. For instance, whereas historically psychiatrists claimed that psychodynamic factors caused symptoms, most of today's psychiatrists would agree with Dr. Robert Michels, a psychoanalyst, who states that psychoanalytic formulations do not address the causes of psychiatric symptoms, but rather what these symptoms mean and symbolize to patients.

More specifically, although an oversimplification, psychiatrists now believe that biology is primarily responsible for the *type* of symptoms found in a disorder (e.g., delusions, insomnia), while psychology primarily determines the *content* and *meaning* of these symptoms. An American and a Russian both have delusions, but the former insists the communists are out to get him, while the latter insists it's the capitalists. Both have a biologically created delusion, but the content of each delusion differs because of psychosocial influences. What a symptom means to an individual also varies from person to person depending on psychosocial influences. One hypochondriac fears his pains mean that he is falling apart, whereas another hypochondriac views his pains as God's retribution.

Similarly, for modern psychiatrists the question of whether the best treatment is drugs or talk has become passé; in determining treatment, psychiatrists believe that psychotherapy and pharmacotherapy are both important, although each accomplishes *different* objectives. Medications reduce or eliminate *symptoms,* such as a schizophrenic's delusions or a manic's spending sprees. In general, psychotherapies do not eliminate symptoms, but address *issues.*

Psychotherapies can accomplish what drugs cannot. They can help patients learn about their mental disorders—their symptoms, dangers, causes, and precipitants. Talk therapies can alert patients to situations which are likely to make an illness recur. By providing an intellectual framework, psychotherapies can enable patients to understand what their disorder means to them. Psychotherapies can improve a patient's willingness to adhere to the psychiatrist's treatment plan (e.g., taking medication); they can foster a therapeutic alliance between patient and psychiatrist. Talk therapies may facilitate social adjustment, interpersonal relationships, leisure-time pleasures, and occupational skills. They may heighten self-esteem, guide ambition, and enhance well-being. Talk therapies may provide insight, especially into how a patient's previous life experiences affect his current difficulties. As frequently occurs, when a patient cannot figure out why terrible things keep happening to him—why people treat him rudely, why his spouse leaves him, why he gets fired from a job—only psychotherapy can help him understand why these events happen and what he can do about them. Psychotherapy enables patients to exert more control over their lives.

TREATMENT STAGING

When today's psychiatrists treat patients, they employ a three-stage process. First, if needed, psychiatrists will prescribe medications or administer electroconvulsive therapy to correct any *biological* abnormalities that give rise to symptoms. Moreover, since patients can best utilize psychosocial therapies if their brains function correctly, psychiatrists make it their first priority to normalize and to stabilize the patient's "biological platform." Their next task is to provide talking therapies that address *psychosocial* issues and problems. Third, the psychiatrist intervenes at the *moral-existential* level by using the doctor-patient relationship to show the patient that he values him as a person.

Treatment's moral-existential aspects begin when the patient first meets the psychiatrist and end when therapy stops. In Chapter 9, when I discuss how doctors feel about patients, I'll examine these moral-existential interventions. In this chapter, I'll briefly describe the commonly used biological and psychosocial treatments, and in Chapters 6 and 7 respectively, I'll detail how psychiatrists practice them.

TYPES OF TREATMENT

With the advent of scientific psychiatry, the main questions confronting psychiatrists in determining treatment have changed. During the psychoanalytic era, psychiatrists thought the only first-rate treatment was psychotherapy, and so their major question in selecting treatment was how much psychotherapy should emphasize insight. Scientific psychiatrists must also make this decision, but since they believe that biotherapies and psychotherapies are both first-rate, their chief question in selecting treatment is which biological and psychosocial treatments to use. Although it is hard to keep track of the ever-increasing number of biotherapies and psychotherapies, the ones used most often by psychiatrists are listed in Table 5-1.

TABLE 5-1
MODERN PSYCHIATRIC TREATMENTS

I. BIOLOGICAL THERAPIES

  A. Medication

    1. Antipsychotics (e.g., Thorazine, Mellaril, Haldol)

    2. Antidepressants

      a. Tricyclics (TCAs) (e.g., Elavil, Tofranil)

      b. Monoamine oxidase inhibitors (MAOIs) (e.g., Nardil)

    3. Lithium

    4. Hypnosedatives (e.g., barbiturates)

      a. Antianxiety agents (e.g., Valium, Librium)

      b. Hypnotics (e.g., Dalmane, Restoril)

  B. Electroconvulsive therapy (ECT)

II. PSYCHOSOCIAL THERAPIES

  A. Individual psychotherapies

    1. Psychoanalysis

    2. Insight-oriented psychotherapy

    3. Supportive psychotherapy

  B. Group

    1. Psychotherapy

    2. Self-help (e.g., Alcoholics Anonymous, Recovery)

  C. Couples/family counseling and therapy

III. BEHAVIOR THERAPIES

    1. Biofeedback

    2. Relaxation techniques (e.g., progressive relaxation)

3. Systematic desensitization
4. Operant conditioning (e.g., "pain clinics")

IV. HYPNOTHERAPY

BIOLOGICAL TREATMENTS

In essence, psychiatrists use five basic kinds of medication: antipsychotics, tricyclic antidepressants, monoamine oxidase inhibitors, lithium, and hypnosedatives.* Because internists prescribe many more types of drugs, mastering these five appears relatively simple. Perhaps so, but the rapidly mounting details and complexities of using each type are staggering. I'll touch on some of these in the next chapter, but for now will merely introduce these psychotropic agents.

Before the modern era of psychopharmacology was launched in 1954, hypnosedatives—mainly barbiturates—were the only available drugs. Since hypnosedatives do not affect the cardinal symptoms of the major mental disorders (e.g., hallucinations, paranoia, grandiosity), psychiatrists prescribe them much less than other physicians. In general, hypnosedatives exert the same effect on everyone: Regardless of a patient's diagnosis or whether he even has a mental illness, hypnosedatives quell anxiety (e.g., Valium) and induce sleep (e.g., Dalmane).

In contrast, the other four types of psychoactive drugs are special because they affect *specific* symptoms of mental illness. When introduced in 1954 as the first antipsychotic medication, Thorazine created quite a splash because, unlike hypnosedatives, it acted directly to eliminate the schizophrenic's hallucinations and delusions. Similarly, tricyclic antidepressants (e.g., Tofranil) help patients with severe depressive disorders, but they don't make normal people feel happier or alleviate everyday human sadness. When "normals" take lithium, they become irritable, yet when

---

*Some of the groups have other names. Antipsychotics are also known as "neuroleptics" and "major tranquilizers." Tricyclic antidepressants are also labeled "psychostimulants"; that's unfortunate, since most psychiatrists consider stimulants to be ritalin, cocaine, or amphetamines like dexedrine. Hypnosedatives are also called "minor tranquilizers," a misleading term because it falsely implies they are less powerful versions of "major tranquilizers."

manics take lithium, their racing thoughts slow down, they're less frenetic, they stop being grandiose, and so on. Just as penicillin helps only patients with infections and does nothing but (possibly) cause side effects in the noninfected, the value of psychotropic agents is restricted to those patients with specific mental disorders.

Generally speaking, antipsychotics treat schizophrenia, and sometimes severe mania. Tricyclic antidepressants treat the severe depressions of major depression and manic-depression; they also prevent panic attacks. Monoamine oxidase inhibitors help patients with major depression and some with a borderline personality disorder. Lithium prevents and attenuates the highs *and* lows of manic-depression. Electroconvulsive therapy (ECT) is used almost exclusively for severe depression.

On the other hand, two highly controversial biological treatments, psychosurgery and megavitamin therapy, are almost never used by psychiatrists. Nonetheless, it's ironic that Dr. Egaz Moniz became the first psychiatrist to win a Nobel Prize (in 1949) for his introduction of psychosurgery. Originally, sections were removed from the front part of the brain; these lobotomies were soon superseded by finer methods that severed nerve connections. Psychosurgery was resorted to in order to reduce violent, severely agitated, or incapacitating compulsive behaviors. Although widely used during the 1950s, by the decade's end the emergence of antipsychotic and antidepressant drugs largely obviated any need for psychosurgery. In 1973, the last year surveyed, fifty-seven American neurosurgeons performed 167 psychosurgeries: one-third for intractable pain and two-thirds for unresponsive obsessive-compulsive disorders and localized brain disease inducing behavioral unrest.

One still hears that psychiatrists are performing thousands of lobotomies for nefarious racist, political, or social purposes, even though for over a decade not a single case of this has ever been documented. Psychiatrists don't even perform lobotomies; neurosurgeons do. In my fifteen-year career, I've never heard psychosurgery suggested as a possible treatment. Nonetheless, the idea of psychosurgery is so ominous and frightening that whenever it's raised, people listen. What most annoys psychiatrists is the portrayal of psychosurgery as just another way psychiatrists routinely "manipulate the brain" by using ECT and psychoactive medications.

Despite numerous anecdotal claims that megadoses of ascorbic acid, niacin, pyridoxine, and vitamin B-12 do wonders for mental illness, there are no controlled scientific studies to confirm such claims and plenty to refute them. Conversely, taking high doses of vitamin A over a long period has occasionally produced symptoms resembling schizophrenia and depression.

PSYCHOSOCIAL TREATMENTS

Clear definitions of psychotherapy have eluded psychiatrists for years. That's partly because there are so many psychotherapies —at least 150—and the number keeps rising. Beside the more conventional psychotherapies, there are gestalt, cognitive, client-centered (Rogerian), Jungian, Adlerian, and transactional therapies, not to mention some of the zanier species like est, primal scream, and rolfing. The sheer diversity of these therapies complicates defining psychotherapy and showing what they all have in common. I'd define psychotherapy as "the informed and systematic application of techniques based on established psychological principles, by professionals who are trained and experienced to understand these principles and to apply these techniques to modify feelings, thoughts, and behaviors which the therapist deems maladaptive."

This definition implies that all psychotherapies have considerably more in common than most advocates of particular approaches usually claim. Overtly or implicitly, all therapies employ a contract between a supposed expert and a person with emotional or behavioral problems called a "patient" or a "client." Ostensibly, therapy derives from a particular theory or set of principles in which both parties have some faith. Regardless of the specific techniques, their use depends on a certain degree of rapport and trust.

Individual psychotherapies

Psychiatrists tend to divide the many psychotherapies that involve a single patient into three basic types: psychoanalysis, insight-oriented psychotherapy, and supportive psychotherapy.

Psychoanalysis applies Freud's technique of "free association" (i.e., saying everything that pops to mind without any self-censorship) to dreams, fantasies, early memories, current experiences, or feelings about the analyst (i.e., transference). Free association is the cardinal rule of psychoanalysis and its most characteristic feature.

The patient lies on a couch; the analyst sits behind the patient to avoid easy eye contact. When asked his reason for this arrangement, Freud explained, "Who could tolerate staring at people eight hours a day?" Another explanation is that if the therapist is beyond the patient's normal visual range, the therapist's non-verbal signals won't influence the patient. The analyst deliberately acts as a "blank screen" and not as a "real person," so that, at least in theory, whatever the patient attributes to the analyst is solely a projection of the patient and not an actual characteristic of the analyst.

Psychoanalysis requires a minimum of three, and usually four or five, sessions a week. Although people often call their psychotherapy which occurs once or twice a week an "analysis," a psychiatrist would not.

Today psychoanalysis is generally recommended for patients with "problems in living" and milder forms of depression, anxiety, and obsessiveness. The patient must be bright, introspective, usually under the age of fifty, a good abstract thinker, and non-psychotic. He should be reasonably adept in at least two of the three main areas of functioning—social, occupational, and recreational. He should also have the time and roughly $18,000 to spend per year. All in all, the ideal psychoanalytic patient has some problems, but in comparison to most psychiatric patients, is a paragon of mental health.

Since most patients don't need, aren't suited to, or can't afford psychoanalysis, *insight-oriented psychotherapy,* also called *psychoanalytic psychotherapy* is the talking therapy preferred by psychiatrists. In this treatment the patient visits the psychiatrist once or twice a week and sits face to face with him. The insight-oriented psychotherapist talks more than the psychoanalyst; the patient does not free-associate. In comparison to psychoanalysis, more attention is paid to the realities of a patient's current life than to his dreams and childhood.

Psychoanalytic psychotherapy is most often used for "problems in living" and "neurotic difficulties." The patient should be relatively sane, introspective, intelligent, psychologically curious, and capable of abstract thought. Patients who are between acutely disturbed periods of major mental disorders may also receive insight-oriented psychotherapy. When psychiatrists mention "psychotherapy," they usually mean insight-oriented psychotherapy, and that is what I'll mean unless I specify otherwise.

Whereas insight-oriented psychotherapy attempts to change the patient by insight into unconscious motivation, *supportive psychotherapy* uses advice, education, persuasion, reason, and other appeals to conscious processes to solve practical problems and immediate life difficulties. To benefit, patients need not be particularly introspective, psychologically minded, curious about motivations, or adept at abstract thinking. When supportive psychotherapy is used for counseling patients with "problems in living" and "neurotic difficulties," there's often a great stress on "learning while doing."

Sessions usually occur from one to four times a month. Patient and doctor sit opposite each other. The therapist, who's fairly active, supports the patient's more adaptive capacities, while minimizing and discouraging his more maladaptive behaviors.

Supportive psychotherapy also is the individual psychotherapy of choice when patients are recovering from, or in the throes of, a major mental illness. On these occasions, therapy provides the patient with emotional reassurance and helps him distinguish reality from fantasy—what is called "reality testing." For example, with a schizophrenic who is convinced Walter Cronkite has implanted a bug in his brain, the psychiatrist would sympathize with how scared he must feel while pointing out that there is nothing implanted in his brain.

When a patient with a major depression insists that his body is rotting of cancer and that his case is utterly hopeless, the psychiatrist does not employ insight-oriented psychotherapy. Instead, the psychiatrist uses supportive psychotherapy—he empathizes with the patient's hopelessness, and then, as a doctor, clearly states that the patient is free of cancer and bound to recover.

Supportive psychotherapy can teach patients to avoid situations which are likely to precipitate symptoms, as well as show them how to cope once they arise. For example, after several bouts of illness, many patients with repeated major depressions become experts at identifying the circumstances that trigger their depressions so that they can quickly get back on tricyclics, and thereby avert a relapse.

Group treatments

When group therapy is recommended, patients often ask, "Do I have to undress in front of everyone?" or "Do I have to say everything that's on my mind?" Although it's nothing like that, given how television, movies, and popular novels depict "group experiences" as confessionals, nude marathons, and orgies, no wonder patients harbor such fears. What many patients don't realize is that there are many types of groups, and some of them—"encounter groups" and "T-groups"—are not even intended for therapy.

Encounter groups do not treat patients, but help "normals" expand their self-awareness and realize their full potential. The chief aim of T-groups—the T stands for "training"—is to train participants in how groups function.* Members observe, for example, how it's natural for people in groups to challenge authority and to compete for leadership. Like encounter groups, T-groups are not for patients but for "normals." Unlike encounter groups, T-groups do not necessarily make members feel better, but they do instruct.

On the other hand, group therapy is a treatment; it helps patients deal with either mental disorders or problems in living. A typical session lasts sixty to ninety minutes, occurs once a week, has six to ten members, and is led by one or two mental health professionals.

Group therapy differs from all other therapies in that it's ideally suited to address *interpersonal* difficulties. The group is a laboratory for showing patients how they affect others, for offering advice on better ways of relating to people, and for experimenting with these behaviors. Once patients become reasonably comfortable using these new behaviors in the group, they can try them out in the real world. Patients claim that groups also help by giving them a sense of belonging to the group and making them aware they are not the only ones in the world facing difficulties.

Beside suggesting regular group therapy, a psychiatrist might

---

*T-groups are also called "process groups."

recommend a "self-help" group, such as those run by Alcoholics Anonymous, Recovery, and various drug programs. Some psychiatrists criticize these groups for their dubious efficacy, their evangelistic nature, and their leadership's lack of formal training. However, many of these self-help groups assist patients, such as alcoholics and drug addicts, whom many psychiatrists don't like or can't help.

The treatment of couples and families

In deciding a treatment plan, the psychiatrist must consider whether family members should be involved in the treatment, and if so, how. When there is a clearly identified patient, the psychiatrist may wish to see the entire family, including the patient, so as to help them weather the crisis of having a mentally ill family member, to reduce tensions that aggravate the patient's illness, and to assist them in being more helpful to each other.

When it's debatable whether there is a single clearly identified patient, the psychiatrist must decide if the patient's major problems reside in the patient, in the marriage, or in the family. If the patient's problems lie mainly within himself, the psychiatrist will recommend individual psychotherapy; if they lie within the marriage or family, the psychiatrist might recommend couples or family treatment. If there are multiple problems, the psychiatrist might recommend individual therapy as well as couples or family therapy.

If the psychiatrist believes the chief difficulties rest within the couple, he then must decide whether to emphasize "couples counseling" or "couples therapy." In trying to improve a relationship, couples *counseling* assumes the couple will stay together, and the psychiatrist stresses practical problem-solving. Couples *therapy* doesn't assume the pair will remain together, but begins instead by identifying each member's wants and needs. After carefully determining his or her own self-interest, if either member wants to part, couples therapy eases the breakup. Most couples, however, find they want to stay together, but now since each party is clearer on the other's needs, they're better equipped to resolve conflicts and to satisfy one another.

When the psychiatrist believes it would be worthwhile to involve a patient's family, he then must decide on whether to emphasize "family counseling" or "family therapy." *Counseling* usually involves helping the family to solve problems, to deal effectively with a member's mental illness, and to minimize psychological trauma to others in the family. Family *therapy* generally assumes that the "problem" lies with the entire family and that the "patient" is a scapegoat of a family's conflicts or simply the most vulnerable member of a "disturbed family."

Behavior therapies

American psychiatrists have had an aversion to behavior therapy, with less than 1 percent ranking it among their top three interests. Scientific psychiatrists, whom one might expect to be drawn to behavior therapy's scientific basis, still tend to view behavior therapy as foreign or suspect. Receiving little, if any, training in it, psychiatrists are inclined to leave behavior therapy to psychologists.

Yet just as many core psychoanalytic concepts, such as the unconscious, have been incorporated into mainstream psychiatric thought, so have many basic behavioral principles, such as positive reinforcement. On top of this, in devising treatment plans, more psychiatrists than ever are considering whether specific behavioral techniques might be useful for specific problems. Ironically, although a major reason psychiatrists have avoided behavior therapy was that it originated in psychology and not in psychiatry or in medicine, modern psychiatry's "remedicalization" has stimulated psychiatrists to use behavior therapy.

Biofeedback techniques can affect the emotional components of medical illness by using electronic instruments which give the patient information about his internal physiologic processes. A patient with tension headaches, for example, tries to identify the tension in his facial muscles while hearing beeps from a biofeedback machine which reflect the degree of this tension. He then experiments with different mental patterns (e.g., he imagines floating in space, humming "Ooooommmm") to see which ones decrease the frequency of beeps, and thereby diminish facial tension and headaches. Biofeedback has also been used for high blood pressure, migraine, and irregular heartbeats.

Psychiatrists teach patients *relaxation techniques,* whereby the patient systematically contracts every muscle in his body and then fully relaxes them. These relaxation exercises can reduce anxiety and induce sleep. They are also used as part of another behavioral technique, *systematic desensitization,* a common treatment of phobias, including those which arise secondarily from panic attacks. After the patient relaxes, the therapist gradually exposes him to the feared object or situation, first in imagination and then in reality. If a patient is phobic about cats, the therapist might say, "Picture in your mind a cat being a hundred yards away, that is, the full length of a football field." Once the patient can do this without becoming anxious, the psychiatrist might say, "Now imagine this cat being seventy-five yards away." This desensitization process is repeated, so that after the patient imagines touching the cat, he may be gradually exposed to pictures of cats, and subsequently to living cats.

In programs designed to treat specific symptoms, such as pain, psychiatrists may employ *operant conditioning,* an ominous term which simply means the patient's positive behaviors are rewarded or reinforced; in these programs, negative behaviors are not punished, but ignored. Operant conditioning, for example, is used widely in "pain clinics," a major, and largely unpublicized, medical breakthrough for helping patients whose organically or psychologically induced chronic pain hasn't responded to conventional medical care. Patients are hospitalized for four to twelve weeks on a pain unit, and then treated as outpatients for about three weeks. Most patients who enter pain clinics have been in such great discomfort for years that their pain has come to dominate their existence: Because they're in too much pain, they can't go to movies, they can't show up for work, they can't talk of anything but pain. Consequently, these programs discourage "pain-related behaviors" and encourage "constructive behaviors." When patients complain of pain to a nurse, the nurse ignores them. When patients go for a walk without mentioning pain, the nurse congratulates them. Because patients receive pain medications only at prescheduled times, they are no longer rewarded with a narcotic-induced euphoria whenever they complain of pain. Gradually, they stop associating this euphoria with pain, so that by the end of the program, patients not only stop talking about pain, they stop experiencing it, or at least most of it. Numerous studies confirm that three to five years after completing these programs, 50 to 80 percent of patients have much less pain, take far fewer medications, make many fewer medical visits, and exhibit considerably more occupational and recreational activity.*

Hypnotherapy

Hypnosis induces a state of hypersuggestability. The patient is relatively oblivious to everything else except the hypnotist's voice. Most people have been hypnotized without realizing it. In driving a long distance at night on a superhighway, many of us "glaze over" and will then suddenly "jerk awake" to attention. When being "glazed over" the driver has been in a light hypnotic trance, focused on the road and oblivious to everything else.

When a patient says, "You can't hypnotize me," I'll agree. To be hypnotized, the subject must be willing to go along with the hypnotist. Although most hypnotized subjects still feel they're in control, they're more inclined to comply with the hypnotist's instructions.

Psychiatrists use hypnosis as an aid for treating bad habits, such as overeating and smoking. When psychotherapy gets "stuck," psychiatrists sometimes employ hypnosis to accelerate information-giving. Patients vary in their ability to be hypnotized: Some find it hard to "relinquish control" to the hypnotist; others may be unsuited for unknown reasons, perhaps neurological.

DEVISING A TREATMENT PLAN

When psychiatrists evaluate patients, the main question usually on their minds is: "Given the many available treatments, which one, or ones, would best meet the patient's needs?" Collectively, these treatments are called a "treatment plan," and in devising it, psychiatrists follow several guidelines.

They first consider whether biological therapies will remedy

---

*Another example of operant conditioning is a "token economy," which is used for treating severely impaired chronic schizophrenics who have great difficulty acting "normally" in the community. As preparation for discharge, whenever these inpatients exhibit socially acceptable behaviors, they receive tokens, which they can exchange for desired goods (e.g., cigarettes) and privileges (e.g., watching TV). This positive reinforcement supposedly "conditions" patients so that eventually they will perform adaptive behaviors in response to the natural rewards from society (e.g., praise) but without needing tokens.

symptoms, and only after that will they turn to psychosocial therapies to help people deal with illness or to live and work better. That scientific psychiatrists take this sequence for granted reflects their beliefs that biological and psychosocial treatments accomplish different goals, and that rather than being mutually antagonistic, biological and psychosocial treatments facilitate one another.

This position differs from the widely held "macho-psyche" view stated as follows in one professional article: "It is much easier to give pills and send a difficult patient away than it is to face up to dealing with the emotions of difficult patients." Scientific evidence has no place in the "macho-psyche" mentality. This "psychological chicken" implies that because something is painful it should be done,* and that if drug treatment alleviates psychic pain easily it must be bad.

Evidence conclusively shows that medications do not increase a patient's passivity, decrease his motivation, or diminish his involvement in psychotherapy. Studies do reveal, however, that properly medicated patients attend psychotherapy more frequently, participate more actively, engage more intensely, and become more distressed when their therapists go on vacation.

A layman who spent a day or two with acutely disturbed psychiatric inpatients would quickly see how medications facilitate rather than inhibit psychotherapy. For instance, wildly delusional and hallucinating schizophrenics are already bombarded by stimuli, and when they are exposed to insight-oriented psychotherapy, they feel even more overwhelmed by this further onslaught of ideas; they're so confused, they are unable to incorporate, process, and use psychotherapeutic insights. However, in usually less than a week of being on antipsychotic drugs, these patients are less distractible, better able to speak and concentrate clearly, and more capable of accepting, organizing, and processing ideas. In short, it's only after being medicated that they start benefiting from psychotherapy.

Severely depressed patients are so absorbed in misery, ridden with guilt, unable to concentrate, and self-preoccupied that even simple questioning can be not only unproductive but harmful. When

---

*"Psychological chicken" is played when "therapy converts" tell their friends, "I bet you won't enter therapy because you're too afraid of what you'll discover about yourself." Most psychiatrists find this tiresome.

I initially evaluated an attorney with major depression, he couldn't answer probing questions like "Are you married?" and "Do you have trouble sleeping?" Four weeks later, when antidepressants had alleviated his depression, he recalled that first session: "All I could think about was feeling worthless, and so when I couldn't answer your very simple questions, I felt even more worthless." Without medication, the patient couldn't even respond to straightforward questions; with it, he could.

If unmedicated severely depressed patients can't deal with simple questions, imagine their difficulties with the enormous complexities of insight-oriented psychotherapy. Unmedicated depressed patients are often confused and almost speechless in psychotherapy. Because part of the illness is to make everything conform to their depressed view of the world, they use psychotherapy for self-flagellation. In trying to conduct insight-oriented psychotherapy with severely depressed patients, well-intended medical students will invariably uncover a sin which the depressed patient supposedly committed twenty years ago. But to the student's surprise, this discovery makes the patient feel worse; to the patient, this recalled sin merely confirms that he's a dreadful person. On the other hand, medical students find that it is only when the patient has recovered with antidepressants that he is able to use insight-oriented psychotherapy constructively.

If the patient did not have a severe (e.g., major) depression, but rather had a moderate depression or merely felt chronically unhappy, obtaining insight and getting things off his chest might be quite helpful. That's one reason making this diagnostic distinction is crucial. Yet as a broad generality, a patient's diagnosis is a more specific and useful guide for selecting biological treatments than for selecting all other therapies. Since biotherapies mainly treat symptoms and psychotherapies mainly address issues, the choice of psychotherapies is less dependent on a patient's diagnosis and more on his specific experiences, traits, and problems.

The patient's previous experiences with therapy greatly affect what treatment plan a psychiatrist will recommend. Tilden's law prevails: "Never change a winning game"—if something works, keep doing it; if something doesn't work, change it. If a patient with a major depression improved before on an antidepressant, the psychiatrist will use it again; on the other hand, if the patient did not improve on antidepressants, after reconfirming the diagnosis, the psychiatrist would most likely recommend something else, such as lithium or ECT.

The same principle applies to psychotherapy. For instance, if a patient has not benefited from insight-oriented psychotherapy on at least three occasions and from three different therapists, then despite the psychiatrist's wish that his own psychotherapy would succeed where others' has not, it's unlikely this patient will benefit from a fourth insight-oriented psychotherapy; the patient needs something else.

Scientific psychiatrists select treatments based more on pragmatic reasons than ideologic or etiologic ones. They are not as inclined as psychoanalytic psychiatrists to recommend a treatment because they feel identified with a specific school of thought, or because they think a particular treatment addresses the original cause of a patient's problem. Although many strokes, for example, are caused by blood clots in an artery feeding the brain, rehabilitation therapy is still crucial, even though it doesn't address the cause of the stroke. Modern psychiatric treatment adheres to the same principle by not insisting that treatment be linked to etiology and by acknowledging that why a problem *starts* is not necessarily why it *continues*. As a teenager I started smoking to feel like an adult; by the time I was thirty-five, my continued smoking was due to habit and hardly to a need to feel like an adult. Knowing why I started smoking was of no help in quitting; another approach was needed. In a similar vein, group therapy may be the best treatment for a lonely patient even though his loneliness stems from a traumatic childhood.

In choosing treatments pragmatically, psychiatrists rely principally on scientific evidence to predict what therapy is likely to work best for a particular patient with particular problems. They also consider what therapies the patient is most likely to accept, to comply with, and to use most effectively. Insight-oriented psychotherapy might be advisable, but it might be worthless if the patient has little psychological curiosity. There's also no point in prescribing a medication unless the patient is going to take it.

Little correlation exists between a patient's expectations of treatment and its outcome. Most psychiatrists know that for biological treatments there is almost no relationship between a patient's improvement and his feelings about drugs or ECT; instead, outcome depends on the patient's particular illness and the overall

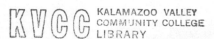

efficacy of its treatments. When actually tested, there's virtually no evidence that the patient's initial (positive or negative) expectations of psychotherapy influence the success or failure of psychotherapy a year later—a finding few psychiatrists know about. Therefore, that a patient likes a treatment doesn't mean the psychiatrist should automatically recommend it; conversely, a patient's dislike of a treatment should not preclude the psychiatrist from recommending it.

FOUR PATIENTS, FOUR TREATMENT PLANS

Given all these guidelines and all these therapies, how does the psychiatrist use all the information gleaned from an evaluation to tailor a treatment plan? How he does so is far more complex than indicated here, and for that matter, all psychiatrists would not reach exactly the same treatment plans I've suggested. Nevertheless, these sketches demonstrate many of the common considerations, questions, and problems psychiatrists face in deciding how to treat a patient.

Stuart Potts

For the seventh time, Stuart Potts, a thirty-four-year-old single Catholic ex-divinity student, was hospitalized. As before, Stuart was having "seizures," which consisted of two to twenty hours of nonstop masturbatory movements accompanied by groans, prayers, flailing limbs, and head-banging. Because his "seizures" were typically in public—this time on the steps of St. Patrick's Cathedral—the police were so familiar with his "act" they would pick him up and simply drop him off at a state mental hospital without first going to a medical emergency room.

All previous neurological exams showed no evidence of Stuart's having any organic problem. He did have a well-documented history of schizophrenia. Although he had been a brilliant high school student, at age seventeen his grades began to slip and he became increasingly reclusive. Weeks before his sister's wedding, he spent day and night making his sister a gift: a stained-glass penis. Two days before the wedding, his father accidentally knocked the gift off a table, and as it smashed into a million pieces, so did Stuart. For the next month he railed against his family, accusing them of trying to destroy him, of turning him into a robot, and of sapping his vital fluids.

God started accusing him of being too preoccupied with sex and telling him that his salvation could come only in becoming a priest. This instruction comforted him: It renewed his life with purpose and direction while allowing for a rapprochement with his family. He enrolled in divinity school, but within two months, he could no longer concentrate. Two other new and unfamiliar voices began discussing his plight, with one saying that Stuart's "prick doesn't work," and the other saying, "If you [Stuart] were a *real* man, you'd go out and use your prick." He did. Stuart picked up a co-ed, took her to dinner, and went to her apartment. They hopped into bed, and when Stuart was about to enter her, he started to "seize" on top of her naked body. Horrified, she ran from the room and called the cops. This episode led to his first hospitalization. Once admitted, he spoke of it with great embarrassment, emphasizing that he felt in a "no-win" situation: If he did have intercourse, he'd be committing a sin; if he didn't, his voices were right, and he wasn't a man.

The next six admissions followed a similar pattern: Dressed like a ragpicker, he would keep to himself, listening to voices comment on his scrawny figure, mock his sexual inadequacies, and insist that he go out with prostitutes. Eventually, he would succumb, but not without considerable guilt. So when he finally did arrive in the prostitute's room, he'd extricate himself from the situation by having a "scizure."

The "seizures" got him admitted, and after they'd stop, Stuart would paint a little, read philosophy and theology, pray, and speak to no one except God and me, his psychiatrist, claiming I was the only staff member with "culture and breeding." To me he'd reveal a litany of self-referential delusions, such as his conviction that the patron saint of travel, St. Christopher, was removed from the universal church calendar, because Stuart had sexual thoughts while traveling. When his parents visited, he'd either have a "mini-seizure," accuse them of "warping" his penis, or give them the "silent treatment." He was diagnosed "schizophrenic."

What should Stuart's inpatient treatment try to accomplish? Modern psychiatrists would say that its chief goal should *not* be to "get to the root of his problem"; doing so would be impossible and the attempt might well be harmful. Although Stuart has long been conflicted over sexuality, it's unclear if this preoccupation is more a cause or a result of his schizophrenia. Most psychiatrists would claim that whereas sexual conflicts did not cause his hallucinations, they had great personal meaning for Stuart and thus determined the content of his hallucinations. But regardless of how crucial sexual conflicts were to his illness, if resolving these conflicts became the goal of hospitalization, he would be institutionalized for years.* Stuart's sexual conflicts had to be addressed, but they could best be treated when he became an outpatient and was in a relatively stable mental state for a longer period.

The overall, yet less ambitious, objective of hospitalization was to help Stuart resume living in the community. To make this happen, his initial treatment plan was:

1. *Haldol, an antipsychotic medication.* To live in the community, his delusions, paranoia, and hallucinations would have to be minimized. His "seizures" would have to stop. Antipsychotics could best treat these symptoms.

2. *Supportive psychotherapy.* While Stuart remained psychotic, I and the staff psychologist would provide reassurance by repeatedly telling him the voices would disappear and that nobody was trying to harm him. He would be taught to distinguish thoughts that were running *inside* his head from imaginary voices coming from *outside* his head. Once his delusions and hallucinations ceased, supportive psychotherapy would help him anticipate and avert stressful situations that triggered his "seizures."

3. *Group psychotherapy.* After his psychotic symptoms were minimized, he should join a supportive group that minimized confrontation. The group's purpose would be to reduce his great discomfort with others, especially women.

---

*Even if offering intensive, insight-oriented psychotherapy were desirable, state hospitals are usually so understaffed they could not do it. But even at the Chestnut Lodge, an extremely well-staffed private psychiatric hospital which specializes in treating chronic schizophrenics with years of intensive, psychoanalytic psychotherapy, fifteen years after discharge, only 14 percent were functioning "good" or better. Those conducting this very extensive investigation concluded that even under the best conditions, intensive, insight-oriented psychotherapy is ineffective in treating most schizophrenics.

4. *Family counseling*. Because Stuart was unable to live on his own, he had to be discharged to live with his elderly parents. Alternating between guilt and rage, his parents were easily provoked by their son into screaming matches; these would usually end by Stuart's having a "seizure." Research shows that exposure to highly emotional situations and "getting things off one's chest" are a major trigger for exacerbating a schizophrenic's symptoms. When families of schizophrenics are taught to minimize emotional eruptions, patients are less apt to become symptomatic and rehospitalized.

Lisa McCann

Life had been kind to Lisa. Born to wealthy Bostonians, blessed with health, wit, and intelligence, she graduated from Vassar with honors, a degree in political science, and a husband—Phil. She entered Yale Law School. He couldn't get into medical school and became a research assistant. Six happy months sped by, until Lisa walked into Beinecke Library to meet her husband. Suddenly, out of nowhere, she was paralyzed by dread. Without realizing it, Lisa was having a widely unknown symptom—a panic attack.

Like most people who first have a panic attack, Lisa was convinced she was going mad. Fearing Phil's ridicule, she concocted a wild tale to explain why she didn't meet him at the library. The next day she was frightened to go outside. When by noon she finally did, she was in constant fear of having another attack.

Over the next month, the mere thought of leaving home made Lisa anxious. She'd invent more and more excuses to avoid class. Whenever she did muster the courage to leave home, she wouldn't venture beyond four blocks; anything farther terrified her. She became increasingly housebound.

Phil was becoming angry that she wouldn't tell him what was troubling her. Fights ensued. Phil would harp away that they were only in New Haven for *her* sake, and now she wasn't even attending school. He'd accuse her of having an affair. As Phil yelled, she sobbed and said nothing.

Phil was fed up and frightened, and dragged Lisa to see me at the student health service, where I subsequently diagnosed her condition as a panic disorder, with its typical three stages: panic attack, anticipatory anxiety, and agoraphobia. The treatment plan was:

1. *Tofranil, a tricyclic antidepressant.* Tofranil prevents panic attacks.

2. *Valium, a hypnosedative.* Even though patients are assured that Tofranil prevents panic attacks, at first they remain anxious about leaving home in fear that another attack will occur. As a stopgap measure for reducing this anxiety, she was given a two-week supply of Valium.

3. *Progressive relaxation.* It takes about two weeks to become proficient at using this technique, which she could then use instead of Valium to quell anxiety.

4. *Systematic desensitization.* If Lisa was still phobic after being on Tofranil for several months, systematic desensitization could be used to eliminate her phobias. Because progressive relaxation is a component of systematic desensitization and Lisa would have already learned this relaxation technique, she would be well prepared to use systematic desensitization.

5. *Supportive psychotherapy.* For the first six weeks I would repeatedly reassure her that the Tofranil does work, that she wouldn't have another panic attack, and that she wasn't going crazy. She would learn that many people suffer from panic disorder, but like her, are afraid to admit it. Supportive psychotherapy would encourage her to leave home and to extend her travels beyond her four-block limit.

6. *Couples counseling; couples therapy?** Initially, couples counseling taught Phil and Lisa about panic disorders and how they could best deal with them as a couple. Meanwhile, I would assess if the marital problems which erupted during Lisa's illness were simply a "side effect" and would go away when she improved, or if they reflected a deeper and more enduring marital conflict. If counseling revealed their problems to be more serious, then ongoing couples therapy would be recommended once matters returned to relative stability.

Robert Aaron

After twenty-five years of marriage, Robert was devastated when his wife, Josie, announced, "Tomorrow morning I'm leaving you

*A "?" placed after a treatment means the treatment will be considered for future use; when no "?" appears, it means the treatment was implemented immediately.

for good. There is no one else. You are a perfect husband, maybe too perfect, but for once in my life, I have to be on my own." Robert was speechless.

By mutual consent, and with considerable pride, they had long agreed on an open marriage. Once a week, Robert would spend the night with his male lover. According to Robert, Josie always approved of his "liberated sexuality." Josie was also becoming liberated—with Howard, their accountant. On a typical day, Robert claimed, he would return home from his engineering firm, play with the kids, and make dinner. According to Robert, most evenings were spent with Josie castigating Robert for not encouraging her budding career as a composer and for being insensitive to her feelings. Robert would apologize and promise to be more sympathetic. (When I questioned Robert about these cardboard characterizations, he insisted they were true and "clear proof that my wife is correct in saying I've ruined the marriage.")

Robert had never taken Josie's criticisms that seriously, and so on the morning of her departure, he was stunned. After pleading to find out what he'd done wrong—"nothing"—and begging her not to leave—"stop always telling me what to do"—Robert helped her move.

Robert became listless. His days were a chore, his nights a bore. He had trouble falling asleep, always thinking that Josie wasn't next to him. Josie would call to acknowledge his unhappiness and to ask a favor—to give her money, to do her income tax, to shop for her. Fearing her wrath, Robert would agree to whatever she requested, believing it was his only way to keep her.

Robert consulted me, saying, "I hope you can help me get Josie back." Although depressed, he did not feel completely helpless or hopeless. Except for insomnia, he did not have biological signs of depression. To me, Robert did not have a mental disorder, but did have two major problems in living: the immediate distress of the separation, and his more enduring masochistic personality. My treatment plan was:

1. *No medication.* His unhappiness and insomnia were not characteristic of a major depression, nor were they serious enough to suggest a moderate depression, or what *DSM-III* calls a "dysthymic disorder"; as a result, no medication was indicated. Sleep-

ing pills could have been prescribed, but neither the patient nor I felt he needed them.

2. *Couples therapy.* An obvious choice, which Josie refused.

3. *Supportive psychotherapy.* This was to help Robert get over the acute crisis and to see if he might eventually profit from more probing psychotherapy.

4. *Insight-oriented psychotherapy?* Given that Robert was a very psychologically minded person with obvious long-standing difficulties, he might seem like an excellent candidate for insight-oriented therapy. There is, however, considerable anecdotal evidence that many strongly masochistic patients become worse with such therapy; they use it to overburden themselves with guilt and to cling all the more fiercely to an ambivalent, punishing relationship. During the once-a-week sessions of supportive psychotherapy, I would occasionally suggest an interpretation, less to be therapeutic and more to see if he used insight constructively or masochistically. For instance:

Maxmen: How do you feel that every time Josie calls she wants you to do something for her?

Robert (seeming annoyed at me for asking): I like it. It shows she still needs me.

Maxmen: Really? What do your friends say?

Robert: They say she's using me. They say I'm a schmuck, but they don't know her as I do; she's truly wonderful, the only person I've ever really loved. (pause) Maybe I am a schmuck. I haven't met all her needs. She has every right to leave me.

This quite typical exchange was dissuading me from suggesting insight-oriented psychotherapy when after our fifth meeting, Robert telephoned me to say he wasn't returning because "I think I'm managing okay and don't need any more therapy. I mean, therapy can't help me get my wife back. . . . Also, I don't think you like her.")

Amy Manning

After a decade of keeping financial records for the National Urban League, Amy was promoted to administer the league's entire national fund-raising activities. Amy had always had weeks of incredible activity, but with this job, she outdid herself. In what was probably a hypomanic period, she was computerizing the office, calling each congressman personally, doubling the number of benefits, writing personal checks for hundreds of dollars, and reorganizing the staff. To her family's growing irritation, she wouldn't return home until eleven at night. She was hardly sleeping, and she didn't mind. There was too much to do.

A month later, her enthusiasm quickly soured. She felt overwhelmed by work. She disliked bossing her former co-workers. ("I've become a slave owner.") Socially, she felt out of step with the organization's higher-ups. Her exhausted body would come home at night while her turbulent mind remained at work. She'd ruminate over her supposed inadequacies and mistakes. Trying to comfort her, Amy's husband would try to put matters into perspective, but nothing seemed to help.

At school, her ten-year-old son broke his leg sliding into second base. Amy blamed herself: "If I were at home more, this would never have happened." She began awakening in the middle of the night, dwelling on how she was failing everyone—Urban League and family alike. A fatigued Amy stopped going to work. More striking for her, she stopped caring about work, and everything else. Her appetite disappeared; she lost ten pounds in seven weeks. Amy lay in bed castigating herself. "I've devoted my life to the civil-rights movement, and now my big chance has come and I've blown it."

Worse yet was the specter of reliving her mother's tortured life. Born in South Carolina, her mother ran away to Harlem at the age of sixteen to become a jazz vocalist. Waiting to be discovered, she waited on tables. After several years as a waitress, she met and married a white man who billed himself as a "record promoter." The day Amy was born, her father disappeared and then her mother went "bonkers." She ran away from the hospital and hitchhiked to South Carolina. When she arrived, she was "hopelessly depressed . . . and after three hospitalizations she committed suicide."

Feeling so hopeless and knowing how her mother had suffered with depression, Amy decided to kill herself. She wrote a note indicating how deeply she loved her family, and saying that she didn't want them to suffer, but couldn't tolerate another day. She swallowed about a hundred antihistamines and waited to die. Amy was rushed to the hospital in a coma, where her stomach was pumped. Hours later, she awoke to see me peering over her. ("My God! I'm in white man's heaven.")

Because I worried she would attempt suicide again, my first decision was whether to hospitalize her. But given Amy's supportive family, her apparently sincere wish to pursue psychiatric treatment, and her promise not to attempt another suicide, I discharged her from the emergency room.

A more thorough evaluation the following day with everyone in the family also revealed that about once a year she'd become very self-critical, bored, and lethargic. This fact, plus her mother's possible manic-depression and Amy's history of periodic hyperactivity, led me to diagnose manic-depression instead of major depression. As a result, my treatment plan was:

1. *Lithium.* If the diagnosis of manic-depression was right, then lithium would be expected to help. Because lithium also prevents future attacks of mania or depression and attenuates excessively high or low moods, it might be prescribed as a "maintenance" drug.

2. *Elavil?, a tricyclic antidepressant.* If Amy's correct diagnosis was major depression, this drug might be used, since on average, of patients with major depression, 72 percent improve with tricyclic antidepressants, 80 percent with ECT, and 22 percent with placebo. In this case, however, because she seemed to have manic-depression, I used lithium alone at first. If her depression didn't improve with lithium, I would add Elavil.

3. *Family counseling.* I wanted them to know the symptoms of manic-depression, to recognize them when they first appear, and to realize that early treatment can attenuate and prevent manic and depressive episodes. I also wanted to teach the family to recognize any clues of suicide, and to understand that the illness was nobody's fault.

4. *Supportive psychotherapy.* Until she pulled out of her acute depression, weekly supportive psychotherapy would comfort her

and ensure she didn't make any major irreversible professional or personal decisions while depression was distorting her objectivity.

5. *Cognitive therapy.* In addition to using regular supportive psychotherapy, I decided to employ "cognitive therapy," a highly specialized and systematic type of individual psychotherapy. Cognitive therapy is an excellent example of how the scientific method can be rigorously applied in the design and study of a psychotherapy. It is used primarily for treating moderate to severe major depressions, especially those which lead patients to adopt, and then to act upon, negative self-images. The cognitive therapist's main task is to challenge every one of the patient's negative thoughts, such as in this example:

Amy: By screwing up this job, I'm nothing.

Maxmen: Were you nothing before the job?

Amy: Of course not, but everything's changed.

Maxmen: Do you really mean that you were *something* before the job, but afterward you became *nothing?* Where did all that something disappear?

For patients with major depression who are still able to concentrate, research strongly suggests that cognitive therapy is as effective as tricyclic antidepressants. Not many psychiatrists know how to perform cognitive therapy, but as evidence mounts, its use is catching on.

6. *Insight-oriented psychotherapy?* Once she had recovered from her depression and had returned to work, she would be sufficiently stabilized to use this therapy best. Insight, especially into her conflict over self-esteem, might prevent her from overextending herself, and perhaps, from exacerbating her manic-depression.

Although many psychiatrists would have devised somewhat different treatment plans for each of these patients, unlike traditional psychoanalytic psychiatrists, today's psychiatrists are inclined to employ more than one therapy. They will use both biological and psychosocial treatments, and involve the patient's relatives. This does not mean that psychiatrists mindlessly force-feed patients with every available treatment; it does mean they are likely to assign more than one therapy per patient, and that each therapy aims to accomplish different and specific objectives.

These illustrations also suggest how psychiatrists might answer one of the questions they're most frequently asked: "What works better—drugs or psychotherapy?" The answer is not simple, and the question is naive. It's like asking, "What works better—medicine or surgery?" As explored further in the next two chapters, whether drug therapy or psychotherapy is superior depends on the patient, his diagnosis, the severity of his illness, his personality, and his social circumstances.

SIX

The Biotherapies

Psychological treatments are good and biological interventions are bad—this seems to be the public's general perception. In social situations, if a psychiatrist just mentions he uses medications or shock treatment, he receives fish-eyed glances. To most laymen, although psychology is "understandable," biology is not; biology seems too complex to comprehend, and too boring to care about. Psychology intrigues; science turns people off. Thus, psychotherapies seem humane, whereas biotherapies do not.

In every movie involving psychiatry that I can recall, the psychiatrist is "good" if he uses psychotherapy and "bad" if he uses biotherapy. In Hitchcock's *Spellbound,* we are supposed to believe that by means of psychoanalysis, a dewy-eyed Ingrid Bergman cures an amnesiac Gregory Peck. In *Ordinary People,* by being available to provide psychotherapy at a moment's notice twenty-four hours a day, a very down-to-earth Judd Hirsch manages to bring hope and meaning to a chronically suicidal teenager. Conversely, whether it's the sadistic psychosurgeons in *One Flew Over the Cuckoo's Nest* or the callous shrink who addicts women to Valium in *I'm Dancing as Fast as I Can,* the biological therapies are portrayed as dangerous relics of "bad" psychiatry.

Paradoxically, biological treatments have thrived in this culturally hostile atmosphere. For during the past decade, psychiatry's greatest advances have been in the biochemistry, genetics, physiology, and pharmacology of mental illness. To understand how the psychiatrist of the 1980s is practicing, one has to understand the biotherapies and their biological bases.

NEURONS AND NEUROTRANSMITTERS

The fundamental unit of behavior is the nerve cell or "neuron." The brain has about one trillion neurons. Neurons consist of a microscopic cell body (or "head") which trails off into an axon (or "tail"), which is smaller in cross section but may be several inches or feet long.* Electrical impulses originating in the cell bodies run through these axons, which in turn transmit them to hundreds, or even thousands, of other nerve cells.

Neurons are the only cells in the body which are anatomically separate from one another. Therefore, to reach a nearby neuron, these electrical impulses don't travel over continuous tissue, but leap over a space between neurons. This leap is accomplished by chemicals called "neurotransmitters," which transmit messages over these tiny spaces which are known as "synaptic clefts."

Neurotransmitters are synthesized inside the neuron and wind up at the axon's end or "presynaptic terminal"; from here neurotransmitters swim across the synaptic cleft, latching onto "receptors" on the edges of adjacent cell bodies. By doing so, these neurotransmitters can affect a nearby nerve cell in many ways: They can trigger its firing, inhibit it from firing, or increase or decrease its ability to respond to neurotransmitters from other nearby axons. The nerve cell acts like a wet sponge: When it fires, it contracts to release its fluids of neurotransmitters; when not firing, it expands and reabsorbs them.

Nerve cells either fire or don't fire, and which they do depends on the quantity and configuration of neurotransmitters reaching its receptors at any instant. Many factors determine whether a neuron fires. The rate of synthesis and release of a neurotransmitter from the first cell could vary. Increases and decreases in the sensitivity of the receptors on the second cell will influence whether it discharges. Something could diminish the first cell's ability to

---

*By definition, axons take electrical impulses *away* from the cell body, whereas "dendrites" bring them *toward* it.

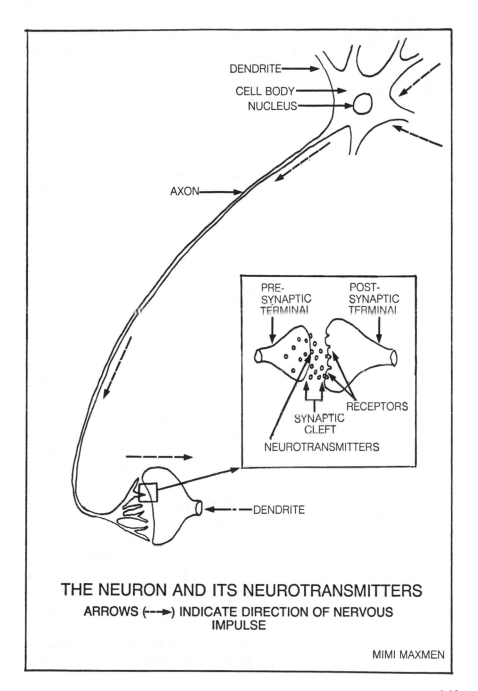

THE NEURON AND ITS NEUROTRANSMITTERS

ARROWS (--→) INDICATE DIRECTION OF NERVOUS
IMPULSE

MIMI MAXMEN

reabsorb neurotransmitters, thereby increasing their concentration at the second cell's receptors. Psychiatric medications reduce symptoms by affecting these mechanisms.

During the past decade, many types of receptors have been discovered, including some that are specific for benzodiazepines, the group name for Valium and Librium. The natural purpose of these receptors is unknown: Evolution did not anticipate the pharmaceutical houses, and the body does not seem to produce its own Valium-like substances. Receptors for enkephalins, the body's own opiatelike narcotics for mediating the perception of pain, have also been identified. Certain types of enkephalins increase during long-distance running, which may account for why so many joggers speak of a "high" while running and a "withdrawal lethargy" after periods of not running. Could it be that health-obsessed marathon zealots have become addicts? Since enkephalin receptors handle morphine and heroin, and since the body contains "Valium receptors," the boundary between what is "natural" and what is "artificial" may be less distinct than many a natural-food fan thinks.

Receptors are commonly affected by only one type of neurotransmitter, and so whether a specific receptor activates depends on its sensitivity as well as the availability of its particular neurotransmitter. Many symptoms of mental illness apparently result from changes in these receptor-neurotransmitter systems, of which four seem especially influential: dopamine (DA), norepinephrine (NE), serotonin (SE), and gamma-aminobutyric acid (GABA).

Although a great deal more evidence is needed before it's clear what these changes are and how they produce symptoms, many psychiatrists believe that schizophrenia involves excessive activity in the dopamine-receptor system. It's known, for example, that when a psychosis closely resembling schizophrenia is produced by large doses of amphetamines, high quantities of DA are released into the synaptic cleft and stimulate DA receptors. Psychiatrists also believe that in severe depression there is a decrease, and in mania an increase, in the activity of the norepinephrine-receptor system. Sleep, and perhaps mood, are affected by changes in the serotonin-receptor system. When stimulated, GABA receptors inhibit neurons and induce calm, and thus anxiety increases when this system becomes less active.

How psychotropic drugs work is not clear, but they appear to "correct" these abnormal receptor-neurotransmitter systems. For instance, antipsychotic medications may block DA receptors from being overstimulated; tricyclic antidepressants may increase, and thereby return to normal, the activity at NE receptors. Valium-like drugs may enhance the normal "calming" activity of GABA receptors. Tryptophan, a natural dietary constituent, especially in warm milk, is converted by the brain into serotonin, which in turn induces sleep. Although other unknown mechanisms must be involved, one way that monoamine oxidase inhibitors (MAOIs) alleviate depression is by preventing the breakdown of DA, NA, or SE.

The body's hormones and neurotransmitters affect each other; these interactions can sometimes influence, or even produce, mental disorders. An underactive thyroid can produce a state similar to depression; too many steroids can induce depression or trigger psychosis. Conversely, during major depression, the adrenal gland releases excessive amounts of cortisol, the body's chief "stress" hormone. Although common sense might suggest that during a major depression the body would be physiologically underactive, in truth, it's in high gear: It's not only overproducing cortisol, but altering a whole series of hormones; some of these go on to influence neurotransmitters and to modify mood and behavior.

Since the major biological signs of depression, such as disturbances in sleep, appetite, and sex, are mediated in the hypothalamus, it's hardly surprising that it is the chief connecting station where neurotransmitters affect, and are affected by, hormones. That's why biological signs of depression are often called "hypothalamic signs."

MIND AND BRAIN

Whether physiological changes play a role in mental illness is no longer debatable: They do. However the details eventually turn out, it's clear that alterations in the body's receptors and its neurotransmitters, hormones, and other chemicals occur in mental illness and produce symptoms. After all, for symptoms of mood and behavior even to exist, at some point there would have to be biological changes. This fact does not dismiss, nor even address, the role of psychological changes.

That's because the brain is not the mind; both exist, but at different levels. The brain is a concrete, physical entity that functions by alterations in receptors and neurotransmitters. The mind is an abstract, mental entity that functions by alterations of psychological "structures," such as the unconscious, the id, and the ego. Changes in the mind and its psychological structures alter the content, meaning, and symbolism of symptoms; changes in the brain and its neurotransmitters alter mood and behavior to produce symptoms.*

Therefore, when people ask what causes mental illness, they must be clear about which "causes" they're talking about. Are they referring to those "caused" by the brain or by the mind? The mind "causes," or more accurately mediates, the meanings and symbols a patient ascribes to a mental illness. That's quite different from the mental illness itself—that is, its symptoms—which are "caused" or mediated by the brain.

WHAT CAUSES MENTAL ILLNESS?

Since mental illness clearly involves abnormal receptors and neurotransmitters, what then causes these pathophysiologic changes to occur in the first place? That abnormal physiologies produce mental illness does not automatically mean abnormal biologies "cause" mental illness.

The abnormal physiologies occurring in mental illness can stem from any one of, or an interplay between, three factors: (1) psychosocial trauma, (2) biological trauma, and (3) genes. When contrasting heredity and environment, it's important to realize that the environment consists of biological, as well as psychosocial, forces.

Biological trauma

By many different means, a person's biological environment could induce the abnormal physiologies of mental illness. During pregnancy, if not afterward, viruses, drugs, malnourishment, physical abuse, or premature birth could help to produce mental illness in the child. For example, in comparison to "normals," schizophrenic patients without a genetic history of schizophrenia tend to

---

*Although changes in the mind and the brain are of a different order, for people to think symbolically, something in the brain must happen. However tenuous, the links between the brain and the mind must exist, even though psychiatrists know almost nothing about them.

have ventricles in the brain which are twice the usual size as well as a high rate of birth complications. Remember that "schizophrenia" is not one illness, but many illnesses that share certain cardinal features. Although genetic factors play a major role in transmitting most of these schizophrenias, in all likelihood, such factors don't produce all of them, and in some cases, nongenetic factors, such as specific types of viruses (namely, "slow viruses") might well be at fault.

Light, natural and artificial, appears to be another biological (or physical) force that contributes to mental illness. Some patients with affective disorders, especially manic-depression, become depressed every fall and winter and recover every spring and summer. These patients' depressions improve with a prolonged exposure to bright artificial light. The antidepressant effect of light is given further credence by the finding that people are more likely to have depressions the farther they live from the equator.

Psychosocial trauma

Psychosocial factors obviously influence the mind, but they also affect the brain. Most scientific psychiatrists believe that in some patients, it is psychosocial and not biological changes that have instigated the physiologic abnormalities of mental illness. How this occurs is largely unknown, but some clues exist.

Dr. Eric Kandel has cleverly devised a way of directly observing how environmental stress alters synapses and neurotransmitters to produce anxiety. He uses the marine snail *Aplysia,* because it often weighs as much as four pounds, consists of only twenty thousand cells, and has neurons up to 1 mm in diameter, the largest in the animal kingdom. Whereas a simple human behavior typically involves hundreds of thousands of neurons, simple behaviors of an *Aplysia* may involve less than fifty. Not only are the *Aplysia*'s nerve cells and synapses virtually identical with those of man, but its behavioral manifestations of anxiety resemble those found in humans. For all these reasons, Kandel conditions these snails in various ways, and because the *Aplysia* is so remarkably easy to study, he can photograph and then see the actual changes in a neuron that are produced by an altered environment.

In more clinical research, evidence suggests that continually being unable to cope—a condition called "learned helplessness"—may induce the abnormal physiologies of depression. For some people, it's quite likely that the death of a loved one or the loss of a job may trigger depression's biological changes.

Genotype and phenotype

Having a gene and having it produce visible effects are two different things. The gene itself is called a "genotype"; whether the gene is expressed—that is, if it actually occurs—is the "phenotype." If there is a gene (or genotype) for an ulcer, whether it develops into an ulcer (the phenotype) depends on diet, stress, smoking, etc. In other words, whether a genotype becomes a phenotype depends on how the person's psychosocial and biological environments affect his genes.

Therefore, to say that mental illness is caused by either genes *or* environment is naive. Even when a person has the gene for a mental illness, that illness won't necessarily occur unless it is the kind of environment that will interact with the gene to produce the illness.

When I began my formal psychiatric training in 1968, psychiatrists debated the cause of mental illness as a choice between "nature" and "nurture." In general, psychiatrists wanted to believe that mental illness was due to a bad psychosocial environment, because then, they assumed, something—namely, psychosocial interventions—could be employed to prevent mental illness. On the other hand, psychiatrists felt that if mental illness was due to bad genes, then short of eugenics, nothing could be done to prevent it.

During the 1970s the simplistic view of "genes versus environment" gave rise to a more complex model whereby mental illness is produced by an *interplay* of genes with the person's psychosocial and biological environments. Consequently, psychiatrists are less apt to believe that if a person inherits the gene for a mental illness, all efforts to prevent this illness are useless. Since, as discussed below, genes do play a critical role in producing the more serious mental disorders, instead of being fatalistic, today's psychiatrists hope that by altering psychosocial and biological environments they can prevent these disorders from occurring, or at least from being too serious.

Contrary to popular belief, scientific psychiatry's emphasis on the genetics of mental illness does not minimize the importance of environmental factors, such as malnutrition, poverty, unhealthy births, and faulty upbringing. Instead, the significance of the environment has changed. For in the new scientific psychiatry, to influence how genes produce illness, it's more vital than ever to alter the environment.

THE GENETICS OF MENTAL ILLNESS

Psychiatrists generally believe that for most, but not all, patients, genetic factors are a necessary prerequisite for developing schizophrenia, manic-depression, and, to a lesser extent, major depression. It now appears that although heredity strongly influences the transmission of panic disorders, as well as many phobic and obsessive-compulsive disorders, it does not seem to produce "generalized anxiety disorders."

The scientific psychiatrist's conviction that genes are a necessary prerequisite for developing most cases of mental illness derives from two types of investigations—those of twins and of adoptees.

Twin studies

By comparing identical or monozygotic (MZ) twins with fraternal or dizygotic (DZ) twins, researchers can identify the relative contributions of nature and nurture in producing a mental illness. Identical (MZ) twins have identical genes, whereas the genes of fraternal (DZ) twins are like those of any pair of siblings. A "concordance rate" is the percent of twins in which both members exhibit the same trait. Because MZ and DZ twins usually share the same environment, the difference in concordance rates between MZ and DZ twins has to reflect the influence of genetics.

For example, the concordance rate for schizophrenia among MZ twins is 31 percent; this means that when one twin of an MZ pair has schizophrenia, 31 percent of the time both members do. In contrast, DZ twin pairs have a concordance rate of 6.5 percent for schizophrenia. (If one sibling is schizophrenic, all other siblings each have a 6.5 percent chance of becoming schizophrenic.) Since there is a statistically significant difference between 31 percent and 6.5 percent, psychiatrists conclude that genes must play a crucial role in transmitting most cases of schizophrenia. Similar methods and findings have also given psychiatrists relatively convincing evidence that heredity plays an equally important role in most other major mental disorders.

While these twin studies show that the major mental illnesses possess genetic etiologies, they also demonstrate that nongenetic factors play a substantial role. Using schizophrenia as an example, if only genes are involved, one would expect that if one member of an MZ pair is schizophrenic, then his twin *must* also be schizophrenic. In other words, the MZ concordance rate would have to be 100 percent. But it isn't; it's only 31 percent.

Geneticists attribute this 69 percent difference to "penetrance," a term used to account for why the genotype does not become the phenotype 100 percent of the time. Penetrance may occur because the abnormal genes were "too weak," or they were interfered with by other genes, or their expression was modified by psychosocial or biological environments. The reasons for penetrance vary depending on the illness, but usually they are unclear or unknown. This prompts some skeptics to claim that "penetrance" is a euphemism for "ignorance," or a loophole for scientists who wish to posit a strictly genetic interpretation to twin studies.

Adoption studies

Because twin studies can't provide definitive answers to the nature/nurture question, in 1963, psychiatrists Seymour Kety, David Rosenthal, Paul Wender, and others launched the first major adoption studies of mental illness. These investigations were conducted in Denmark, because the government had a register of every adoption, including those adults who were separated when they were less than three months old from their biological parents and then legally adopted. These records can be used in many different ways to disentangle genetic from environmental factors.

Applying one method, they found adoptees who were schizophrenic, and then compared the number of their biological and adoptive parents who were schizophrenic. Because biological parents gave the child away so early in life, their psychosocial influence on the schizophrenic adoptee had to be almost nil; only their genetic influence could persist. Therefore, if schizophrenia is genetically transmitted, the biological parents should have a much higher incidence of schizophrenia than the adoptive parents. On the other hand, if schizophrenia is environmental, just the opposite should occur.

The results were striking. Over and over again, the schizophrenic adoptee's biological parents were schizophrenic and his adoptive parents were "normal." These findings provided overwhelming evidence that genes were the principal source of schizophrenia.

Although I've oversimplified their methods and results, I should mention that in addition to comparing the incidence of "schizophrenia," Kety's research group examined the transmission of "schizophrenic-spectrum disorders" (SSD). The schizophrenic spectrum includes schizophrenia, but also includes several disorders which are like, but not identical to, schizophrenia.* Their studies demonstrated that even if a schizophrenic's offspring does not become schizophrenic, the offspring is also at greater risk for developing another SSD.

Adoption studies show that heredity contributes to major depression and especially to manic-depression. Most modern psychiatrists feel there also is a genetically transmitted "depressive-spectrum disorder" (DSD). Psychiatrists differ over precisely which disorders belong to the spectrum, but depression does seem to cluster with alcoholism, drug abuse, panic disorder, and phobia. In other studies, Dr. George Winokur found a genetic link between depression, alcoholism, and antisocial personality—the so-called "hard-core criminal." He showed that about 50 percent of first-degree relatives (e.g., a child, a parent) of depressed females develop some type of depressive-spectrum disorder. Of those who do, virtually all the women become depressed, whereas only half the men become depressed while 25 percent become alcoholics and the other 25 percent have antisocial personalities. These results could mean that culture influences the same DSD gene to produce

---

*An example of these schizophrenic-like disorders is what *DSM-III* labels a "schizotypal personality disorder." These patients, although very weird in how they think, perceive, speak, and behave, are not sufficiently peculiar to meet *DSM-III*'s criteria for schizophrenia. They are not blatantly delusional, but almost: "I'm pretty sure it's my dead mother who visits me every night." Their speech makes sense, but it is so vague, overelaborate, or discursive that it's virtually impossible to follow. Although recent twin studies confirm that schizotypal personality disorder is part of the schizophrenic spectrum, they do not show, as had once been thought, that borderline personality disorder belongs to the spectrum.

more depression in women and more alcoholism and antisocial personality disorders in men.

Genetic counseling

However research eventually clarifies the exact degree and mechanism of genetic transmission, twin and adoption studies have proved that biological relatives of the mentally ill are at greater risk of developing that illness or one similar to it. As genetic evidence mounts, psychiatrists can now provide meaningful genetic counseling—an important advance in the new scientific psychiatry.

In genetic counseling, psychiatrists do not tell the patient whether to mate or to bear children; these decisions are left to the patient. Instead, the psychiatrist helps the patient make better-informed decisions. The psychiatrist gives the patient the best available data and explains what they mean. For example, the patient should understand that any one case can easily defy overall trends, that the environment influences how genes are expressed, that some people develop mental illness without the involvement of genes, and that many unanswered questions remain.

Patients, or relatives of patients, can obtain a formal consultation from an expert in psychiatric genetics by contacting a nearby academic department of psychiatry. The need for genetic counseling can also arise during the course of treatment.

I had been conducting psychotherapy with a thirty-year-old stage director for "inferiority feelings." In the session after he became engaged, he said reluctantly, "She has a schizophrenic brother. If that means our children would have a greater risk of becoming schizophrenic, maybe I should reconsider my proposal." When I told him that speaking statistically, his children had twice the normal risk of becoming schizophrenic, he turned green. "However, another way to look at it," I added, "is that your child's risk of becoming schizophrenic is about two percent, whereas if there were no schizophrenia in her family, your child's risk would be one percent. This hardly strikes me as a big difference, yet what you do is up to you. But in making your decision, don't forget that whether this slightly increased genetic risk translates into a schizophrenic child may be influenced by the child's upbringing."

Genetic counseling also involves informing people about the illness they fear and correcting their misconceptions. In this case, my patient, who assumed that all schizophrenics are hopelessly incarcerated, needed to receive a balanced, yet accurate, picture of schizophrenia, and to know that moderately effective treatments do exist.

Finally, I had to ask if his overt concern about genetics masked a deeper ambivalence about getting married. Historically, psychiatrists have emphasized these types of psychological issues, almost to the exclusion of factual considerations; a patient's request for objective genetic information was treated as a subjective psychological conflict. Today, largely because scientific psychiatrists have greater genetic sophistication, they will address psychological concerns, but only after providing the patient with objective information.

THE BIOTHERAPIES

In essence, of the six basic biological treatments psychiatrists use, one is electroconvulsive therapy (ECT) and the others are medications antipsychotics, tricyclic antidepressants (TCAs), monoamine oxidase inhibitors (MAOIs), lithium, and hypnosedatives. Although there are dozens of drugs within each class, because their chemical structures, clinical indications, and side effects are very similar, most psychiatrists become fully acquainted with, and prescribe, four or five drugs of each type as opposed to "experimenting" with every new medication that hits the market. It's in the same spirit that I'll discuss these medications.

The antipsychotics

Thorazine, Mellaril, Haldol, and Prolixin are prototypic antipsychotic drugs. When Thorazine, the granddaddy of them all, became available in 1954, it radically altered psychiatric treatment in general and therapy for schizophrenics in particular. Two years earlier, a popular psychiatric textbook outlined the most up-to-date inpatient treatment of schizophrenia:

> The patient, on admission should be put to bed, so that his behaviour, his general bodily health and his sleep can be carefully supervised. The peace and quiet of a mental hospital, the orderliness and discipline, the tolerant and understanding attitude of those in charge, and the simplifica-

tion of life, may at once produce a most gratifying change. Habits of a slovenly, untidy and unhygenic nature should be corrected at once, and episodes of violence should be treated with explanation, suggestion, analysis, or where necessary, by hydrotherapy* and [sedative] drugs. . . . When necessary, tube-feeding should be resorted to without undue delay.

The bowels and bladder should be carefully regulated, and the skin made to act freely. Sleep must be promoted by open-air treatment, baths, warm drinks at night; or when necessary, by hypnotics [i.e., sleeping pills], such as hyoscine, paraldehyde, sulphonal, veronal, etc. . . .

Almost nothing from this excerpt would be found in a contemporary textbook, and that's mainly because of antipsychotic drugs. I, like many psychiatrists who never practiced in the pre-Thorazine era, wonder how our predecessors managed without them. Previously, all the drugs psychiatrists had were hypnosedatives, and all they did was to slow patients down and put them to sleep; they couldn't touch delusions, hallucinations, or any other psychotic symptoms. With Thorazine, however, delusions and hallucinations lost their intensity and often disappeared. Back-ward patients who'd been hiding from devils for decades suddenly left their corners and began to speak. At long last, what they said was being understood by relatives and friends; they could also effectively participate in psychotherapy. These drugs have enabled hundreds of thousands of schizophrenics to live in the community instead of being incarcerated for life.

Antipsychotic drugs have been called "major tranquilizers." That's misleading and inaccurate. Not only is antipsychotic action their main and distinguishing feature, but many of the newer ones don't even tranquilize. When first prescribed, some antipsychotics like Thorazine will sedate. But this soporific effect wears off

---

*Hydrotherapy is usually performed in "wet packs," so named because after lying down, the patient is tightly wrapped in bed sheets and then drenched with ice-cold water. Dressed as a mummy, the patient soaks for twenty to forty minutes. Although wet packs sound (and look) dreadful, many patients enjoy them. Like many others, one teenager found them to be so soothing she would deliberately misbehave just to get herself into wet packs, where she'd relax and study algebra. Today, wet packs, like other types of hydrotherapy, are rarely used.

within two weeks. Schizophrenics on a whopping 3,000-mg-a-day dose of Thorazine for several weeks are usually quite alert and active. (A typical total daily dose of Thorazine for a hospitalized schizophrenic is 400 to 800 mg.) Assuming you're not schizophrenic, if you ingested just 100 mg of Thorazine, you'd be very groggy and probably fall asleep; if you took 3,000 mg of Thorazine, you'd wake up, but a day later. On the other hand, if you took Prolixin, you would remain alert. If you were a schizophrenic on Prolixin, your psychotic symptoms would be reduced, but you would not be drowsy. Thus, to call these drugs "major tranquilizers" is to misunderstand what they do.

In general, psychiatrists select an antipsychotic agent which sedates as little as possible, but enough to guarantee the patient's safety. If a patient is calm, psychiatrists prescribe a relatively nonsedating antipsychotic, such as Prolixin. On the other hand, a patient who is convinced he's a bird and wants to fly out a window or one who feels compelled to beat up a fellow patient for being a sinner is likely to receive a sedating antipsychotic drug like Thorazine. Although sedation is not its chief reason for being used, until Thorazine's antipsychotic effects take hold, the drug's sedative properties can prevent people from getting hurt.

Many other factors go into the psychiatrist's decision to prescribe one antipsychotic drug over another: the patient's previous history with a drug, how the patient's genetic relatives have responded to a drug, and a drug's side effects. With a few exceptions, all antipsychotics induce the same side effects, but there is considerable variability in how frequently each antipsychotic gives rise to each side effect. For instance, Mellaril produces a more uncomfortable dry mouth than other antipsychotics, but Mellaril also causes fewer neurological side effects; just the opposite is true for Haldol and Prolixin. No drug is devoid of side effects, and they all have their pros and cons. Patients should always ask their psychiatrist about the type and frequency of side effects for each drug under consideration.

Contrary to myth, antipsychotic drugs do not mask schizophrenic symptoms, but rectify at least one of their major pathophysiologic causes. Since the schizophrenic's symptoms result partially from receptors' being overwhelmed by dopamine, by blocking these receptors, antipsychotic medication normalizes a patient's abnormal biochemistry. Therefore, antipsychotic-drug use is not a "crutch." People who take such drugs are not "running away from their problems," but facing them. They are confronting their schizophrenia and correcting its abnormal pathophysiology. Telling a schizophrenic that using Prolixin is a crutch is like telling a diabetic that using insulin is a crutch.

The single most frequent cause for the rehospitalization of chronic schizophrenics is that they stop their antipsychotic medication. Within a year of discharge, 70 percent of chronic schizophrenics who don't take their medication are readmitted, whereas 40 percent of those who remain on medication are rehospitalized.

If you observed an acutely disturbed schizophrenic who was starting to take antipsychotic medications, you would usually see his delusions and auditory hallucinations gradually recede. If a floridly psychotic patient is totally convinced a hospital is zapping his brain with x-rays, after a day or two on an antipsychotic drug, he might say, "I wish the hospital would stop it, although today there seem to be fewer rays." After four days on the drug, the patient might say, "I think I'm becoming immune to those x-rays. In fact, sometimes I'm not altogether sure they're even sending them." By day seven, the patient might confess, "That whole business about the hospital sounds a bit crazy. It still occurs to me, but I no longer believe it." After two to three weeks, if the delusion is of recent origin, it usually vanishes. (Long-standing delusions are more refractory.)

Although antipsychotic medications are clearly beneficial, they do *not* cure schizophrenia. These drugs work best against the disorder's acutely appearing and "wilder" symptoms, such as delusions, auditory hallucinations, and incoherent speech. They are less effective against schizophrenia's chronic and less flamboyant symptoms, such as social withdrawal, flat emotionality, impaired family and job performance.

A minority of schizophrenics will do as well without antipsychotics, but what distinguishes these patients is largely unknown. Therefore, when selecting therapies for previously untreated schizophrenics, psychiatrists have no way of predicting these exceptions, and so they usually prescribe antipsychotics.

These drugs can also alleviate many conditions other than schizophrenia, such as certain types of delirium, drug-induced psychosis, and mania. Thus, a patient who is prescribed an antipsychotic medication should not leap to the conclusion that he has schizophrenia. On the other hand, only schizophrenics should take these drugs for more than a month or two. For the story of antipsychotic drugs also has a dark side—*tardive dyskinesia.*

About 15 percent* of patients who take antipsychotic drugs continuously for over two years (though it can be as little as six months) develop involuntary, bizarre movements of the mouth, limbs, and hips. Most often tardive dyskinesia appears as "tobacco-chewing," lip-smacking, and "fly-catching" movements of the mouth and tongue. Less often, there are hip jerks or slow, undulating motions of the hands or feet. These movements typically erupt within a few days of decreasing or stopping antipsychotic drugs and subside only when the patient sleeps or is put back on antipsychotic medication.†

Unless detected early, half the time tardive dyskinesia is irreversible. Although other drugs may occasionally counteract it, once this draconian side effect occurs, there is usually *no* good way to eliminate it. The best way to avoid tardive dyskinesia is to avoid antipsychotic drugs altogether. Except for treating schizophrenia, they should never be used for more than two or three consecutive months. What's criminal is that all too many patients receive antipsychotics who shouldn't, usually from nonpsychiatric physicians who mistakenly believe they are merely "tranquilizers" for "nervousness."

When the drug is given for chronic schizophrenia, doctor and patient must decide, as with any medication, if the treatment is worse than the disease. At some point, most schizophrenics must

---

*Depending on the patients investigated and the methods used, studies report that tardive dyskinesia occurs in anywhere from 5 to 56 percent of patients taking antipsychotic drugs. Nonetheless, the most accurate figure for inpatients, the so-called "mean prevalence," is probably closer to 15 percent.

†Whereas side effects usually occur while somebody is *on* a drug, in tardive dyskinesia it occurs when somebody is going *off* a drug. This peculiarity may partly account for why it took over a decade for a full awareness of tardive dyskinesia to filter down to most psychiatrists. Although the cause of tardive dyskinesia is unknown, a popular theory holds that because antipsychotic drugs block DA receptors, these receptors eventually become "supersensitive" to DA so that when antipsychotics are decreased or withdrawn, they can't handle the onslaught of DA; as a result, these receptors degenerate, resulting in tardive dyskinesia.

choose between the risk of tardive dyskinesia and the risk of recurrent madness and institutionalization. Most choose the risk of tardive dyskinesia.

In reality, this choice isn't quite so dreadful. If tardive dyskinesia becomes too troublesome, the patient can take slightly higher doses of an antipsychotic drug to suppress his abnormal movements. In the long run, however, more severe symptoms of tardive dyskinesia will erupt, which only higher doses of medication can control.

That only antipsychotic drugs cause tardive dyskinesia has further increased the importance of psychiatric diagnosis. If the patient who might be diagnosed as schizophrenic has any significant signs of mania or depression, the psychiatrist may prefer to use lithium or an antidepressant, since these drugs don't produce tardive dyskinesia.

Tricyclic antidepressants

Depressive disorders are the most common mental illnesses treated by psychiatrists in their offices. Therefore, it is fortunate there are so many different types of effective biological treatments. These include monoamine oxidase inhibitors, lithium, and electroconvulsive therapy, as well as some newer drugs, the tetracyclics (e.g., Ludiomil), triazolopyridines (e.g., Desyrel), and one benzodiazepine, Xanax. Which of these a psychiatrist recommends depends on the circumstances, but most often he will prescribe a tricyclic antidepressant (TCA), such as Elavil and Tofranil.

As with all of these antidepressants, TCAs treat the *disorder* of depression; they do not alleviate the isolated *symptom* of depression. Tricyclics work best for depressive disorders which have "biological signs," such as appetite and weight loss, middle-of-the-night and early-morning insomnia, inability to experience pleasure and interest, decreased libido, and a diurnal mood variation in which patients feel worse in the morning and better as the day goes on.

Whether or not the patient *feels* depressed, if he has these biological signs, TCAs will be effective. That's because no matter if psychological or biological events induce the abnormal physiology of depression, once this abnormal physiology occurs, it gives rise to the biological signs of depression, and once these biological signs occur, TCAs are effective because they correct the abnormal physiology of depression.

Whether TCAs help depends on the existence of these biological signs and *not* on whether the depressive disorder was precipitated by an environmental event. Too many patients deny themselves proper treatment with TCAs under the mistaken assumption that biotherapies won't work if the "cause" of their depression is "understandable." Quite often patients with a major depression will say things like "Of course I'm depressed; my wife left me. Antidepressant drugs won't help my depression because they won't bring her back." TCAs won't bring the wife back, but they will stop his pervasive inability to experience pleasure, his insomnia, his agitation, his total lack of energy, and all the other symptoms of a depressive disorder. With TCAs he will still miss his wife, but as a "normal" person, not as a depressed one. Without TCAs the person usually suffers for six to nine months—the usual duration of a biologically untreated depression—but with TCAs he will be fully recovered in four to six weeks.

Because major depressions often manifest atypically, physicians and mental health professionals sometimes miss the diagnosis and fail to prescribe potentially helpful TCAs. This usually occurs when sadness or unhappiness (i.e., the symptom of depression) is not the most prominent feature; the patient may not even feel depressed. The most striking symptom may be hypochondriasis, delusions, hallucinations, physical pain, or an inability to experience pleasure. The depressed patient can also appear totally demented: He can't concentrate or remember what happened five minutes ago. Many elderly people get written off as hopelessly "senile," when in fact their "pseudodementia" is a severe depression which can be fully reversed with TCAs.

Although TCAs are completely successful in treating over 70 percent of all major depressions, the most common reason they don't work is that the patient is taking an inadequate dose and for an inadequate duration. Doses vary depending on the drug, but for Elavil and Tofranil, the patient must receive at least 150 to 300 mg a day. Even then, determining a therapeutic dose is tricky because patients can vary up to a hundredfold in how much of the drug they swallow gets into the blood by absorption through the gut. Consequently, a psychiatrist could not determine if his patient was getting the right dose—that is, until recently. Psychiatrists can now obtain fairly accurate blood levels for some, but not all, TCAs. By finding out if the patient's blood level is too low or too high, the psychiatrist can readjust the TCA's dose into a therapeutic range.

Whatever the proper dose, the patient must be on it for at least ten to fourteen days before his depressed mood begins to lift; for many patients it may take four to six weeks. Prematurely giving up on a TCA is a common error: Some patients who are still depressed after four weeks on TCAs will improve by six weeks. Patients are frequently demoralized because they assume that antidepressants work as fast as sedatives. Since within thirty minutes of popping a Valium one feels calmer, it's hardly unreasonable for a patient to assume he will feel happier within thirty minutes of taking an antidepressant. But that is not what happens.

When patients start on a TCA, their improvement follows a typical pattern. After three or four days, insomnia usually improves. By five to seven days, appetite returns. The patient's diurnal mood variation fades around eight days, and by ten days his libido and ability to experience pleasure reemerge. About then, hopelessness and helplessness recede. Finally, after ten to fourteen days, depressed mood, excessive guilt, and suicidal ruminations begin disappearing. Thus, TCAs are effective, but slow.

This ten-day-to-six-week waiting period is usually excruciating for the patient and his relatives. The patient's mind is imprisoned by depressive preoccupations. For months he may think of nothing else and constantly repeat these thoughts to loved ones. One patient kept telling her husband, "I'll never get better. At least you shoot a sick dog. You should do the same to me." After hearing this a thousand times, he started to believe her.

During this waiting period, beside feeling bad for the patient, psychiatrists feel helpless; they know the drug will work, but until it does, they're frustrated because they can't do much to hasten the patient's recovery. Feeling scared and desperate, the patient and his family are relieved by the psychiatrist's repeatedly telling them that there is light at the end of the tunnel.

Moreover, the psychiatrist must be alert to any clues of suicide, because 15 percent of patients with severe depression kill themselves. Ironically, the very medications that help this potentially fatal disorder, TCAs, are among the most lethal of all psychoactive drugs. If swallowed at once, a ten-day supply of a therapeutic dose can be fatal.* Thus, if a psychiatrist is worried that a new patient might commit suicide, he may prescribe only a few days' supply of medication at a time and ensure that someone other than the patient administers the drug.

Monoamine oxidase inhibitors

Q: What do aged cheese, chianti wine, chicken livers, broad beans, pickled herring, yogurt, yeast extracts, beer, "cold tablets," "pep" pills, hay-fever medications, and cocaine have in common?

A: Patients on monoamine oxidase inhibitors (MAOIs) who take any of these substances may develop a "hypertensive crisis," in which their blood pressure soars, causing a splitting headache, chest pain, fever, vomiting, and, rarely, a stroke.

Q: If these MAOIs are so dangerous, why aren't they taken off the market?

A: They were. When first introduced, MAOIs triggered these hypertensive crises, and since nobody knew why, they were banned. Eventually, researchers discovered that foods with tyramine, a naturally occurring amino acid, as well as these drugs, were the culprits. Once these causes of hypertensive crisis became known, MAOIs were commercially reintroduced.

Q: Are these drugs relatively safe to use?

A: Yes—as long as one avoids these foods and drugs. Most patients know what to avoid, and so today it is uncommon to hear about an MAOI-caused hypertensive crisis.

Because initially psychiatrists were so frightened by these hypertensive crises, even now, many clinicians have never used MAOIs. Such concerns also stymied research into whether these

---

*In comparison, overdosing on a two-month supply of Valium (or Valium-like drugs) can induce a coma, but it won't be fatal. When combined with other psychoactive substances, such as alcohol, the danger of a lethal overdose with all types of psychiatric medication increases substantially.

drugs have any special value, and only since the mid-1970s has any substantial evidence emerged.

MAOIs are a class of antidepressants which psychiatrists often use when TCAs don't work. If one lumps together all patients with major depression, TCAs are slightly more effective than MAOIs. Nevertheless, some patients with major depression will improve on MAOIs but not on TCAs.

Moreover, patients with so-called "atypical depression" are helped equally by MAOIs and TCAs. Some, but not all, of these patients have borderline personality disorders (see Chapter 3). Patients with atypical depressions are usually females whose lives are emotional roller coasters and who respond flamboyantly to environmental changes; they tend to be "rejection-sensitive," chronically unhappy, dependent, demanding, and histrionic. Their biological signs of depression are just the reverse of those in major depression: They sleep and eat too much rather than too little; they feel best in the morning and dreadful by nightfall. Unlike patients with major depression, these people function—sometimes quite productively. They are frequently overwhelmed by anxiety, phobias, and panic attacks. Many psychiatrists claim that these patients, especially if they have panic attacks, do better on MAOIs than on TCAs.

Like TCAs, but by different means, MAOIs correct the abnormal physiology of depression, at least in part by increasing the brain's norepinephrine. Like TCAs, MAOIs usually take at least ten to fourteen days before they lift a patient's depression. And as with TCAs, an overdose of only a two-week supply of MAOIs can be fatal.

At times, just a small dose (15 mg) of an MAOI such as Nardil is sufficient to bring about a dramatic improvement. More frequently, the patient needs between 60 and 90 mg a day. But when MAOIs are effective, they are strikingly effective: The patient feels "energized" and "alive"—quite often for the first time in his life. Right now, however, we still need to figure out which groups of patients will benefit most from these drugs.

Electroconvulsive treatment

Probably no single psychiatric treatment in common use has created as much turmoil as electroconvulsive treatment (ECT). In the article "Electroshock Therapy: Let's Stop Blasting the Brain," a neurology resident writes in *Psychology Today* that ECT "is remarkably widespread, demonstrably ineffective, and clearly dangerous. It causes brain damage . . . and often permanent loss of memory. . . . " In the newsletter of the American Psychological Association, an internationally known psychologist says, "I'd rather have a small lobotomy than a series of electroconvulsive shock."

Despite such outcries, ECT is highly valued by psychiatrists. By restricting the use of ECT to those patients most likely to benefit—those with severe depressive disorders—the actual use of ECT has slightly declined since 1974. Nonetheless, more than 100,000 patients a year currently receive ECT.

Research strongly suggests that in general, ECT is *the* most effective treatment for severe depression. (Dare I say, "Living better electrically"?) Studies reveal that in patients with major depression, between 72 and 80 percent improve with ECT, 65 to 72 percent improve with tricyclics, and 23 percent improve on placebo. Of the seven well-controlled investigations comparing ECT with tricyclics, four showed no difference and three favored ECT. ECT is even more advantageous if the severely depressed patient is delusional. Despite all this evidence, TCAs are routinely tried first because ECT usually requires hospitalization; drugs are also used first because people fear ECT, and, at least historically, for good reason.

For many years ECT was gruesome. The patient was plugged into a wall socket for a few seconds; he would violently convulse for thirty seconds and awake five minutes later. Although the patient did not feel the seizure *per se,* he was unanesthetized and aware of everything else, including the fractures of his spine, limbs, and jaw that often resulted from the seizure. Patients normally received one treatment for twenty to thirty consecutive days.

Today, ECT is considerably safer. Usually six to ten treatments, one every other day, are given. (In emergencies, when drugs don't work, typically three ECTs will be administered to patients who are dangerously manic, catatonic, or suicidal.) In addition, the methods for administering ECT have greatly increased its safety.

If you were to observe ECT, this is what you would see:

The patient is pretreated with atropine, which dries oral secretions and prevents irregular heart rhythms. Once on the table, the patient receives an intravenous, short-acting anesthesia (e.g., pentathol) so as to avoid any discomfort during the procedure itself.

(In most settings, the psychiatrist performs ECT along with an anesthesiologist.) After going under, the patient is intravenously given a temporary muscle paralyzer (e.g., succinylcholine), thereby eliminating the possibility of fractures during the seizure. Until the muscle paralyzer wears off four minutes later, the anesthesiologist mechanically respirates the patient. Once fully oxygenated, the patient is ready for the treatment itself.

The psychiatrist places two electrodes on the patient's head, either one on the right and left forehead (called "bilateral ECT"), or one on the front and back right (i.e., nondominant) side of the head (called "unilateral ECT"). He then applies between 0.1 and 0.5 second of the lowest possible voltage (70 to 130 volts) that can produce a seizure. Two to three seconds later, the patient abruptly contracts every muscle for ten to twelve seconds. This "tonic phase" is immediately followed by a "clonic phase," when the patient seizes for thirty to fifty seconds. Yet because of the muscle paralyzer, all you would see during this clonic phase is a slight tremor of the eyelids. Five minutes later the patient awakes from the anesthesia, alert and without pain. The patient doesn't remember the shock, nor does he complain of any discomfort. The entire procedure—from when the patient gets the anesthetic until he wakes up—takes roughly fifteen minutes.

Invariably, those who witness ECT for the first time find it underwhelming; they are surprised these treatments are so undramatic. Patients are also surprised they don't feel anything, and, of course, they shouldn't—brain tissue is free of pain fibers. A recent survey of patients who received ECT revealed that half of them found going to the dentist more upsetting and frightening than ECT. Most of them felt ECT was helpful, and almost none felt worse.

The most dangerous aspect of ECT is not ECT itself, but the anesthesia. Yet regardless of cause, the mortality rate from ECT is one in 60,000 treatments, whereas from tonsillectomy, it's one in 18,000. In a report of 259,000 treatments, Barker and Baker found a mortality rate of 0.0036 percent.

Ever since fractured bones and cardiac arrhythmias have been virtually eliminated, the chief concern about ECT is if it causes permanent memory loss. Many patients, especially if treated with modern techniques, have no confusion or memory loss at all. On the other hand, some clearly do: Within two, and sometimes up to four, weeks after the last treatment, a patient may exhibit such severe confusion and memory loss that he can't recognize his wife or children, can't name the hospital or the day of the week, can't find his room, and sometimes is urinating into wastepaper baskets. However, this gross confusion *always* clears up. Moreover, during the past decade psychiatrists have virtually eliminated this immediate post-ECT confusion by using unilateral, instead of bilateral, ECT.

Nevertheless, over the six months following treatment, about 10 to 30 percent of patients will complain of slight memory loss. They'll claim, "Ever since that shock treatment I can't remember phone numbers quite as I should," or "I keep forgetting so-and-so's name." The apparent memory loss is relatively minor, but annoying. Nonetheless, there's every scientific reason to believe that ECT has nothing to do with this long-term memory loss. Research comparing patient's memory before, and then six to nine months after, ECT shows absolutely *no* change. How come? It may be that the instruments for assessing memory aren't sensitive enough to detect the change. Since, as seen in "pseudodementia," severe depression by itself can produce memory loss, maybe their memory was impaired *before* they received ECT. (Indeed, when patients with pseudodementia receive ECT, their memory dramatically improves.) Being preoccupied with other concerns, perhaps they were unaware of a failing memory, and later on blame ECT. After all, we're always forgetting a face or a phone number. Normally we blame it on "getting old," but if a person has had shock treatment, ECT becomes the obvious culprit. Despite the very dubious possibility of long-term memory impairment, there has been no good evidence that ECT, as presently administered, causes brain damage.

In emergencies, ECT can be life-saving. Not infrequently a psychiatrist is faced with an inpatient who is so depressed he is on the brink of starving to death. It is almost impossible to force-feed such people; they refuse all medications, and even if they took them, they would die before the drugs took effect. Unless prompt measures are taken, these patients will die. Only ECT can work quickly enough to save them.

Except in these life-and-death situations, patients must consent in writing to receive ECT. Although an understandable precaution, giving consent can pose serious problems. ECT works best for depressed patients who have delusions. But if the patient is delusional, how can he give informed consent that's meaningful? The law assumes people are rational; psychiatry does not. When, as often happens, a delusionally depressed patient consents to ECT "because I deserve to be punished," legally that patient may receive ECT. That may be consent, but it's hardly informed. Even without delusions, patients who are seriously enough depressed to require ECT are usually overwhelmed by indecisiveness. Consequently, they can barely make any decision, much less a rational one. Since a major symptom of serious depression is profound hopelessness, some patients will not consent to ECT, being convinced that *nothing* will help them.

Because seriously depressed patients are prime candidates to commit suicide, Dr. Darold Treffert claims the law's "protection" of patients from ECT illustrates how "patients can die with their civil liberties intact." Cynicism aside, inherently, severe depression makes it impossible to fully respect a patient's legal right to refuse treatment, as well as his legal right to obtain *proper* treatment.

Although the legal, ethical, and clinical aspects of consenting to ECT are extremely difficult to resolve, in reality, pragmatism resolves the issue. When a patient has not responded to antidepressant medications and his family will not grant consent to administer ECT, eventually, consent is given. They will agree to ECT because the only other choice is to watch their loved one suffer in a severe depression and possibly commit suicide.

Realizing that a small minority of psychiatrists "shock everybody," laymen have every reason to ask whether, given the circumstances, ECT is the best, or the only decent, treatment. When laymen question a recommendation of ECT, some shrinks feel their professional integrity is under attack. But sometimes the psychiatrist's apparent defensiveness is actually his irritation at patients or relatives for taking so long—a week, perhaps—to reach a decision. In frustration, I've heard many a psychiatrist, including myself, mutter in private, "I wish they'd shit or get off the pot. The patient's suffering and clogging up a bed that another patient desperately needs." Most psychiatrists understand a family's reluctance to rush into ECT, but they would recommend that if a family wants a "second opinion," they should get one promptly to avoid prolonging the patient's agony.

Another charge against ECT is that since nobody knows how it works, it shouldn't be used. Psychiatrists argue that that's irrelevant. Physicians have used all types of drugs, including aspirin, morphine, and barbiturates, without knowing how they work.

Even though psychiatrists, like other physicians, choose treatments because they work, the question of how ECT works still remains. Most psychiatrists believe the seizure itself is therapeutic, since sub-seizure bolts of current do not affect depression. That patients get better just to avoid future shock treatments is not borne out by research, since patients receiving "sham ECT"—that is, the entire ECT process but without the electrical shock—believe they've received ECT yet remain depressed. Although consistent biochemical responses to ECT have not been identified, ECT might trigger all the brain's neurons to fire their particular neurotransmitters, thereby correcting the deficiencies of neurotransmitter activity normally found in depression.

Lithium

Lithium was used by the ancients and by Henry VIII for treating gout. Yet it wasn't until 1949 that its antimanic properties were discovered by an Australian, Dr. John F. Cade. Despite being used safely and extensively throughout Europe during the 1950s and 1960s, it wasn't until 1971 that lithium made its commercial debut in America.*

Because lithium resides in rocks and water supplies, Cade thought it might account for the therapeutic properties of medicinal springs. Two Cleveland psychiatrists speculated that a relatively high concentration of lithium in a city's water supply might correlate with a low incidence of manic-depression. It doesn't.

Lithium is a salt, like regular table salt. Once lithium was used as a salt substitute, but was quickly taken off the market because it readily caused toxicity—upset stomachs, vomiting, diarrhea, finger tremors, and sometimes kidney damage and coma. This may occur because there is a very narrow range between lithium's therapeutic and toxic effects. Thus, until a patient stabilizes, psychiatrists will order serum lithium levels up to three times a week

---

*A major reason for this delay was that because lithium is a naturally occurring substance, American drug firms could not patent exclusive rights to sell lithium. At most they could only patent the commerical names of lithium products.

to ensure the dose is high enough to be effective, yet low enough to avoid toxicity.

Lithium is definitely indicated for the prevention and acute treatment of both the highs and the lows of manic-depression. It might also be helpful for the prevention and acute treatment of major depression, as well as for the mini-highs and mini-lows of "cyclothymic disorders." Evidence further suggests that lithium alleviates mood-related symptoms (e.g., grandiosity, euphoria, sadness) in schizophrenia, minimizes premenstrual tension, reduces alcoholism, and controls violence and aggression in some emotionally unstable and explosive personalities.

When "normals"—that is, college students—take lithium, they get irritable and twitchy. That's not the case with manic-depressives. In fact, the only reason manic-depressives stop taking their lithium is that they miss the ecstasy of mania. On the other hand, when patients are low, lithium is a godsend.

Lithium has also been a fiscal godsend. During the past decade it has saved $1.28 billion in productivity alone, and has saved an additional $2.88 billion in direct mental health costs. Not bad for an eight-cent tablet!

Hypnosedatives

These medications include daytime sedatives like Valium, Librium, Ativan, Xanax, and Tranxene as well as prescription sleeping pills (hypnotics) like Dalmane, Restoril, Quaalude, and chloral hydrate. Alcohol and barbiturates (e.g., Seconal, Amytal, Tuinal) also act as hypnosedatives. These chemicals are grouped because they all depress the brain to produce overall calming and soporific effects. In many respects, whether a drug is officially a "sedative" or a "hypnotic" depends more on marketing strategy than on pharmacologic activity.

Although psychiatrists are most often associated with prescribing hypnosedatives, in reality internists and general practitioners use these drugs most often, since about half their patients suffer from mild anxiety and depression. In contrast, "nervous" patients consulting psychiatrists typically receive psychotherapy and not medication, and if they do have a drug-responsive mental disorder, they'll get psychoactive agents other than hypnosedatives.

Hypnosedatives are the only psychiatric medications that cause psychological or physical addiction. Patients don't get "high" on them. When abruptly stopped, only hypnosedatives have the potential to produce withdrawal symptoms. Tolerance—that is, the need to take more of a drug to get the same effect—does not develop to the therapeutic actions of antipsychotics, TCAs, MAOIs, or lithium—only to hypnosedatives.

Roughly four times the normal therapeutic dose of hypnosedatives is physically addicting. A daily antianxiety dose of Valium is 15 mg, but if 60 mg or more is taken daily for several weeks, addiction has probably set in. Addiction to hypnosedatives is considerably more dangerous than addiction to opiates in one major respect: Unlike the case with opiates, abrupt withdrawal of hypnosedatives leads to seizures, and in 10 percent of cases, to death.

Tolerance to their sedative and hypnotic effects occurs within days. Except for benzodiazepines like Dalmane and Restoril, sleeping pills lose their effectiveness in five to seven days. If taken nightly for roughly six weeks, virtually all hypnotics, including Dalmane and Restoril, will disrupt normal physiologic sleep, and thereby aggravate rather than alleviate insomnia.

While aware of the addictive potential of hypnosedatives, psychiatrists generally feel that when used episodically and briefly, they can mitigate anxiety safely and effectively in selected circumstances. Sedatives quell the anxiety of patients with severe depressions and help patients with chronic and abnormally high levels of anxiety. Hypnosedatives also palliate "anticipatory" anxiety, especially as a consequence of panic attacks. In all these situations, however, hypnosedatives should be used sparingly and monitored carefully.

In recent years, doctors and patients are using hypnosedatives with far greater caution. Hypnosedatives are still overprescribed, but not as much as generally assumed. From 1971 to 1977, the number of prescriptions for sleeping pills declined from 41.7 million to 25.6 million. From 1973 to 1981, the number of prescriptions for both hypnotics and sedatives declined by 30 to 65 percent. As this marked decline in the use of hypnosedatives has occurred, another major problem with psychiatric medications has arisen.

THE MISMEDICATED SOCIETY

Many scientific psychiatrists believe we are not so much an overmedicated society as a mismedicated society. By "mismedicated society" I mean that all too often people who are not taking medication would benefit greatly from doing so, and that people who are taking medication should be on either no medication or a different medication.

For example, a recent survey showed that 34 percent of 217 patients with major depression received antidepressant medication, and only 12 percent of the total took antidepressants in large enough doses for a long enough time. Although the proper dose for most TCAs is usually 150 mg or more per day, in another survey, 77 percent of patients on TCAs were taking less than 100 mg per day. Inadequate doses of TCAs do nothing to help a patient's depression, but can still cause every one of the drug's side effects.

We constantly hear about one type of mismedication: Movies like *I'm Dancing as Fast as I Can* show temporarily nervous people becoming permanently hooked on sedatives and sleeping pills. But another type of mismedication that we do not hear about regards those patients with genuine anxiety syndromes who would be helped by sedatives, but don't receive them; according to one survey, only 40 percent of these people use one sedative, and even then, just occasionally. (Indeed, only 40 to 70 percent of persons with clearly designated anxiety disorders receive any psychotherapy or biotherapy.) Only 59 percent of patients with panic disorder receive any drug, and if they do, only 8 percent get the correct one—TCAs. This finding strongly suggests that these patients are receiving hypnosedatives when they should be on TCAs.

Like other psychiatrists, I keep seeing mismedicated patients. Some are being treated with antipsychotics which may cause tardive dyskinesia, when they should be either on no drug, or on lithium or TCAs, which don't cause tardive dyskinesia. I've seen hypochondriacal patients become addicted to hypnosedatives, when they would probably improve with TCAs or MAOIs. I've seen many people try to alleviate a depression by medicating themselves with cocaine, amphetamines, alcohol, or marijuana. Once again, they're on the wrong drug.

In the midst of so much antidrug hysteria, it is hard to convey the message that in so many respects we are a mismedicated, more than an overmedicated, society. Those antidrug crusaders who issue blanket and misinformed condemnations of all psychoactive drugs scare many people away from getting the help that psychoactive drugs can provide.

SEVEN

Psychotherapy

Discussing what happens in psychotherapy and how it works—the main topics of this chapter—is easier than one might expect. Although each psychotherapist has his own way of conducting the various psychotherapies, I think most psychiatrists would agree on certain generalities about psychotherapy. Before presenting these, however, I must dispense with the "root" myth of psychotherapy, because it constantly distorts what people expect from psychotherapy.

THE "ROOT" MYTH

Many patients come to treatment saying, "I want to get to the root of my problem." This notion should be buried. There is no such thing as *the* root of a problem. At best, there are *roots,* but never *a* root. This myth gives patients the false expectation that psychotherapy will cure them when it uncovers a single, all-important childhood trauma.

When patients indicate they want therapy to "unearth the root of their problem"—I suddenly picture myself with hoe and spade—what they actually want is to feel better. They are confusing means with ends. Whether it's unearthing roots or acquiring greater self-understanding, these are means, not ends. No patient enters therapy saying, "My life is fine and I don't wish to change, but I'm coming here *solely* to learn more about myself." Understanding the origins of a problem does not automatically solve it. An alcoholic may understand that he started drinking as a teenager because it was the thing to do, but having this insight hardly deters his drinking.

If psychotherapy does not work as in the movies—that is, by inducing a grand catharsis when the shrink delivers a single, devastating insight into the patient's root problem—then how does it work?

HOW PSYCHOTHERAPY WORKS

For psychotherapy to be effective, there must be a "therapeutic alliance." Psychiatrists believe that for a therapeutic alliance to exist, there should be mutual trust and respect between therapist and patient. Neither need approve of everything the other says and does. Such automatic acceptance would discourage the critical examination of psychological issues. In a therapeutic alliance, doctor and patient are partners in pursuit of the patient's well-being. The therapist is not expected to run the patient's life or to be his "friend," but to offer insights and perspectives that may help the patient exert greater control over his own life. Therapeutic alliances are rarely perfect, but when they are reasonably good, psychotherapy can work; when they are not, psychotherapy cannot work.

Research comparing individual, group, and couples therapies demonstrates that successful treatment depends far more on the fit between patient and therapist than on the specific form of therapy. Some patients prefer psychiatrists who talk a lot; others prefer psychiatrists who talk very little. A good therapist for one patient may be a lousy therapist for another.

With an effective therapeutic alliance as a prerequisite, psychotherapy involves five related steps: gathering data, forming hypotheses, making interpretations, acquiring insights, and working through.

Gathering data

While the patient provides the psychiatrist with information, just having to articulate problems out loud "forces" the patient to clarify them. After all, it's hard to solve a problem without knowing what exactly needs to be solved.

In gathering information, the psychiatrist uses his own feelings toward the patient. Once the psychiatrist is reasonably certain that his reaction is not idiosyncratic but one that most psychiatrists would have, the psychiatrist views it as "legitimate" data about the patient. For example, a normally reserved psychiatrist finds himself wanting to hug a patient. But instead of doing so, the psychiatrist views his urge as a psychological clue. He will ask himself questions like "What is there about this patient that brings out my protective instincts?"

Forming hypotheses

After obtaining some basic information, the psychotherapist constantly formulates and reformulates hypotheses to account for the patient's difficulties. He is in a good position to do so, since he is uninvolved in the patient's personal life and can devise hypotheses that are relatively fresh and objective. The psychiatrist examines every new piece of data to see if it confirms or refutes his hypotheses. Whenever a psychiatrist questions a patient, he is testing the validity of a hypothesis. When a psychiatrist conducts psychotherapy, a large part of what he does is this continual generating and testing of hypotheses.

Psychiatric theories are critically important in formulating these hypotheses. Although I am simplifying a bit, psychiatrists employ these theories in one of two ways: The psychiatrist can fit the patient to a preconceived theory, or he can devise a theory that fits the patient.

Because they believe psychoanalysis is a universal theory of the mind, psychoanalytic psychiatrists are especially prone to use data from a patient to show how the patient fits psychoanalytic theory. For the psychoanalytic psychiatrist, the question is not *if* the patient has an oedipal complex—the theory says he does—but *how* it manifests.

Because to the psychoanalytic psychiatrist the theory is never wrong, the patient has not improved until he genuinely sees how the theory applies to him. Until that happens, the patient is "resisting."

Indeed, when a patient gets better by psychoanalysis, the analyst typically credits the theory, not himself. In the analyst's eyes, since his theory is both ingenious and right, if the patient improves it is because the analyst, a "mere" skilled technician, has properly implemented this all-powerful theory; if the patient does not improve, then it can only be because the analyst has incorrectly applied the theory.

In what I call a "seek-and-ye-shall-find maneuver," the psychiatrist keeps pursuing information that will eventually corroborate the theory. If, as happens often enough, a psychiatrist keeps suggesting to the patient that he is "terribly anxious"* about the psychiatrist's up-coming vacation, the patient will eventually become anxious. Recounting a previous bout of psychotherapy, a patient told me, "My therapist kept insisting that my real problem was my unconscious hatred of my father. I didn't agree, since I always got on well with my dad. But after a while I started to wonder if my therapist could be right. After all, he is an expert. So in therapy we spent weeks talking about my father, and the more we did so, the more I recalled that my father spanked me once, or when he forgot to take me to the movies—minor stuff like this. Eventually, I was convinced my father was a menace, and gullible as I am, for two years I 'worked out my feelings toward my father' by not speaking with him."

Psychiatrists can employ seek-and-ye-shall-find maneuvers in many ways, not just in rendering psychoanalytic formulations, but also in making a diagnosis and in evaluating a medication. For example, when a patient on the antidepressant Tofranil says he feels "so-so," a biologically oriented psychiatrist may falsely interpret the patient's response as a therapeutic triumph. Practicing *any* kind of seek-and-ye-shall-find maneuver is poor psychiatry.

Nevertheless, seek-and-ye-shall-find maneuvers are most likely to happen under particular circumstances. They occur far more often when the psychiatrist has a fervent ideological commitment

---

*Psychoanalysts habitually speak in hyperbole: Patients are never "anxious," but "terribly anxious"; they never have "castration anxiety," but "overwhelming castration anxiety." When analysts talk among themselves, they will not say "the patient suffers from repressed rage," but that "the patient has the worst case of repressed rage I've ever seen." I don't know why analysts invoke so much hyperbole, but my hunch is that by describing a patient's psychopathology as so terrible and unsolvable, the analyst protects himself: If the patient doesn't improve, nobody can blame the analyst; if the patient does improve, then the analyst must be a genius.

to a specific theory, especially a relatively abstract one, since the more abstract the theory, the more the same clinical data can be interpreted to fit that theory. When patients are feeling especially miserable, psychiatrists are more likely to resort to seek-and-ye-shall-find maneuvers. Not infrequently, the psychiatrist may believe he is not "doing enough" for the patient, and so he may push the patient even harder to accept his hypothesis, thinking, "If only I can get information to confirm my hypothesis, then, and only then, I can alleviate the patient's misery."

Many psychiatrists would argue that whether a particular theory is "true" for a particular patient is irrelevant. If the psychiatrist makes the patient fit his theory—no matter which theory —as long as the patient authentically feels the theory applies to him, helps him understand why bad things keep happening, and affords him a way of doing something about them, then the theory is accomplishing its mission.

Some psychiatrists prefer to work within the restraints of an established theory like psychoanalysis, whereas others use theories more eclectically. In formulating hypotheses that primarily derive from the patient and not from a theory, the psychiatrist may draw from many theoretical concepts, use those which fit and reject those which don't. Thus, in contrast to the approach of the psychiatrist who adheres to a universal theory of the mind, under this approach whether a patient has an oedipal complex becomes an open question; the answer depends on the patient. Classical theory maintains that at some point during psychotherapy the patient consciously or unconsciously loves his shrink; under an eclectic approach the psychiatrist will consider this possibility, but does not automatically assume it to be true.

The psychiatrist's hypotheses may include concepts derived from established psychological theories or from no specific psychological theory. In either case, the psychiatrist continually formulates, tests, and reformulates hypotheses, as in this example:

Isaac Grant was an unmarried thirty-year-old successful stockbroker who complained of a generally unhappy life. "I'm single and without prospects. I don't like being a stockbroker; it's boring and without challenge. At parties I'm ashamed to say what I do. If I had any balls, I'd do what I've always wanted to do, and that's to be a full-time novelist."

By our fourth meeting Isaac and I agreed that he had long-standing fears of taking risks, whether in asking women for dates, moving away from home, choosing stocks, or becoming a novelist. For the moment, the issue became: How come Isaac doesn't take risks?

I kept raising hypotheses in my head which might answer this question. Suddenly it dawned on me that I was doing three-quarters of the talking, and so I asked myself, "How come?" What's more, I was doing all the work in therapy that *he* should have been doing. For instance, around the outset of every session I would ask him, "Have you had any thoughts about the previous session?" He would say, "No." I then would ask, "What would you like to talk about today?" and he would say, "Whatever *you* want to talk about." Despite telling him many times to bring up issues he thought important, I was carrying the ball for him; no wonder I was talking so much. Could this shed any light on why he didn't take risks?

Maxmen:	I've noticed that instead of you raising issues, you always have me do it.
Grant:	You're right. I'm lazy that way. But I do that all the time; it's another way of not taking risks. I guess that's bad.
Maxmen:	"Bad"?
Grant:	Because you'll think I'm not trying to get better.*
Maxmen:	But if this really worries you, and you know I want you to bring up issues, then why don't you?
Grant:	Because if therapy doesn't work, it won't be my fault; it'll be yours. That's pretty stupid, isn't it?
Maxmen:	But since you're not stupid, I suspect you are not taking risks for other reasons.

*I could have picked up on his being more concerned with gaining my approval than with getting better, but instead I stored this observation for future use in formulating another hypothesis. Although I chose to follow-up on another theme, other therapists may have chosen the former. Hardly a minute passes during psychotherapy when the psychiatrist doesn't face such a choice. Part of being a good therapist is knowing which themes to pursue at the right time and in the right way.

Grant   (trying to needle me by throwing out hackneyed formulations): Maybe it's my need to fail; maybe it's my fear of success? How in the hell should I know?

Maxmen: Take a risk! Speculate.

Grant: I can't.

Maxmen: Really?

Grant: I can't, because I don't want to look foolish. In everything I do, I always want to *appear* above everything to hide that I don't *know* anything. I'm constantly fooling people into believing that I know more than I do.

Maxmen: And if people get to know you . . . ?

Grant: I don't let them; if I did, they'll see nothing's there. All image, no substance. As long as you raise the issues, I don't have to confront being a fake.

What started with "my doing all the talking" and with Grant "not taking any risks" led to Grant's facing his deeper fear of being a fake. One might say, "Big deal! Now his feelings of being a fake are only worse. Why is this helpful?" It's helpful because now Grant and I knew what we were dealing with; his fear of taking risks was not a fear of failure, success, or castration, but a fear of being a fake. Having formulated this hypothesis, we now knew *what* fear to examine, which led Grant to see that he had far more substance than he realized.

Sometimes the hypotheses are formulated primarily by the psychiatrist, and at other times more by the patient. In this situation, however, Grant and I collaborated in devising a hypothesis for why he avoids taking risks. During this interaction, we also see how the formation of a hypothesis can spill over into an interpretation.

Making interpretations

Technically speaking, an interpretation is a statement or observation the psychiatrist makes to heighten the patient's awareness of psychological material. This material may be conscious or unconscious; an interpretation may clarify what has been vague or provide a new slant.*

Psychiatrists often make interpretations by thinking aloud.† In doing so, they're not trying to be know-it-alls, but to engage the patient in a collaborative examination of something new which they think might benefit the patient.

Examples of interpretations are: "This sounds like the kind of guilt you might try to ignore." "A son can't be oblivious to his parents' divorce." "Could you really have hated your mother that much?" "Is it possible your father had some redeeming features?" "Your mother seemed unable to acknowledge you could accomplish anything on your own." "I noticed that after you mentioned a great many personal tragedies, your eyes only began to tear when you mentioned your son's leaving home." "You look annoyed whenever I praise you."

The timing and delivery of interpretations are crucial. Interpretations are least effective when the psychiatrist guns down the patient with rapid-fire, devastating "insights," which the patient experiences as coming from nowhere. Because this type of "wild analysis" makes for good TV, many laymen enter treatment expecting that "wild analysis" makes for good psychotherapy. As they soon learn, it doesn't. Even when interpretations are correct, unless they make sense to the patient, they are useless. Unless the patient has enough time to consider an interpretation, he can neither assimilate it properly nor use it constructively. An interpretation is most likely to be accepted by a patient when the patient himself is close to realizing it. Ideally, the psychiatrist guides the patient right to a point where the patient can make the interpretation himself. More often the psychiatrist makes the interpre-

---

*What I'm calling an "interpretation" of *conscious* material, some psychiatrists call a "clarification." They restrict the use of the term "interpretation" to making the unconscious, conscious. For simplicity's sake, I've used "interpretation" for both conscious and unconscious material.
†Dr. Roy Schafer points out that "the risk of his (the therapist) being misunderstood by the patient . . . is increased in proportion to his reliance on nonverbal communication." A frown, a blank stare, or a pair of upwardly rolling eyes may convey something to the patient, but usually not as clearly as words do. Moreover, nonverbal interpretations are emotionally evasive, whereas words establish a record.

tation, and when he has sufficient evidence to support his interpretation, if he makes it at the right time and in the right way, the interpretation's validity will usually be obvious to the patient.

The psychiatrist should present the interpretation more as an offering to be considered than a fact to be consumed; it should be phrased so that the patient feels free to reject or modify it. There's a big difference between the comment "You are guilt-ridden about your son's death" and "I wonder if you sometimes feel guilty about your son's death."

I always tell patients that when an interpretation doesn't make sense, they should say so: The patient may have misunderstood me, I may have stated it incorrectly, the patient may be "denying," or I may be wrong. Pseudo-agreement between me and patient wastes my time and the patient's. To do my job effectively, I need to know how and why my interpretation doesn't feel right to the patient.

Yet no matter how a patient responds to an interpretation—whether he agrees, disagrees, changes the subject, becomes discombobulated, or gets angry—the therapist uses this response as information to guide treatment. When the therapist is virtually certain that his interpretation is right, and the patient rejects it, the therapist normally stands his ground and sees what evolves.

For instance, Francine Mathews, thirty-five years old and unmarried, entered treatment with a major depression which arose after her father's death. For two years she had been at the beck and call of her debilitated, insatiably demanding, and never-pleased father. His final words to her were "If you would take better care of me, I would not be dying."

Maxmen: It surprises me that you deny feeling any anger at your father.

Mathews: The man was bitter about dying. Can you blame him?

Maxmen: He can blame you, but you can't blame him?

Mathews: He had every right to blame me: He was dying, not I.

Maxmen: So?

Mathews (angrily): What do you mean "so"? If I'd nursed him better, he'd still be alive.

Maxmen: Really! Does that mean *you* caused his death? No wonder you're not angry at *him*!

At the start of this session I suspected she was angry at her father for his nastiness and ingratitude. Although I was partly correct, the patient's responses showed that she was more angry at herself.

Psychiatrists interpret dreams in the same way they interpret any other information. Dreams do not have *a* correct meaning. What counts is only what the dream means to the dreamer. (After all, it is *his* dream.) Most psychiatrists do not believe there is a universal language for dreams—a tree does not always represent a penis, nor does a house always represent a uterus. To interpret a dream, most psychiatrists have the patient first describe the dream in great detail, then discuss the personal meanings of, and feelings stimulated by, every detail in the dream. Finally, patient and psychiatrist try relating this information to the dominant psychological themes and problems in the patient's life. Although dreams are interpreted as is any other material, they have the advantage of being, as Freud claimed, "the royal road into the unconscious."*

Many of the psychiatrist's comments are interpretations of the "transference"—that is, the feelings and attitudes which patients displace or transfer onto a therapist from significant people in their (early) lives. Many patients are surprised and embarrassed to discover the existence, and power, of these feelings. By identifying them, by finding out how they get to be distorted, and by pinpointing their source, psychiatrists can make interpretations based on the transference to help patients realize how they might hold similar misperceptions about people in the "real" world.

A major advantage of psychiatrists' interpreting information which occurs *in* the session or pertains to the doctor-patient relationship is that the therapist can speak of it firsthand. When the

---

*Psychiatrists will use their own dreams to understand more about the patient and his therapy. In one such dream, a teenager, dressed in the same style as a patient, sits on her psychiatrist's lap and then walks away. In reality, the patient was a high-powered attorney who had been acting like his daughter in therapy, but recently had begun to behave more maturely. The psychiatrist felt his dream pointed out that he was still treating her like a little girl, and that he should acknowledge that she was grown-up and relate to her accordingly.

psychiatrist interprets information that occurs *outside* the office (e.g., during childhood, at home), the psychiatrist never really knows if, or how much, the patient has distorted what happened. That's one reason why so many interpretations are based on transference.

Acquiring insight

Although they are related processes, interpretations are made by therapists, whereas insights are acquired by patients. Acquiring insight is more than a strictly intellectual endeavor. To be meaningful, three things must happen. First, there is the *intellectual* awareness of the insight. Second, this awareness is accompanied by an *emotional* recognition. To work, an insight must not only *sound* right, it must *feel* right. Third, the insight must translate into *action*. Talk is cheap. When a patient realizes he has an "authority problem" but doesn't change his behavior toward authorities, the insight is useless. When a patient implements an insight outside the session he finds out what makes it hard to change and which of his fears are justified.

Barbara, a highly accomplished and socially active middle-aged woman, had "succeeded" at everything in life except one: She tried and failed at a dozen antismoking programs. So with the hope of quitting, she entered psychotherapy. Loaded with insights about why she smoked—to feel sophisticated, to imitate her much-beloved mother—forty-eight hours after going "cold turkey," she gave in and lit up. Barbara's insights were not sufficient; only when executing the changed behavior did she acquire the insights sufficient to quit. At the next session she described everything going on in her mind when she succumbed: "Out of the blue, I started thinking about my life as a teenager. That was thirty years ago. I was miserable. No friends. Never a part of anything. I felt unconnected, just like now when I'm without a cigarette. I never realized where this unconnected feeling came from and have always felt vaguely haunted by something. Now I guess I know what it is: I'd forgotten that lonely teenager, but she's still very much inside me. I think having a cigarette has been my way of keeping her away." This fuller understanding led Barbara to feel far less pressured to smoke, and so when she abstained again, she did so for good.

Working through

Contrary to the popular view that one swift, devasting insight turns a patient's life around, acquiring insight is the beginning of a therapeutic process, not its end. This process, called "working through," is the most crucial, yet least recognized, part of psychotherapy. Just because a patient has once carried out an insight doesn't mean it has become ingrained in his behavioral repertoire. Working through is essential, since it is how a new insight becomes an enduring pattern; it involves (a) examining, and then eventually understanding, the many psychological angles to an insight, and (b) changing behavior *repeatedly* until implementing the insight has become second nature.

For example, Charlie Sharp, a single thirty-five-year-old bank teller, realized during therapy that he habitually avoided touchy situations, which caused feelings to fester and led minor annoyances to mushroom into tumultuous problems. One day he was invited to a dinner party he'd gladly have missed. His previous pattern would have been to put off the host with a "maybe," to waste six days worrying about what to do, and then to attend the deadly dinner "because it's too late to decline and I didn't want to hurt the host's feelings."

But now Charlie had insight. Because he and I, his therapist, were fully aware that typically he would fall into a neurotic trap with such a dinner invitation, we both knew that he now had a clear and conscious choice to handle the invitation constructively. If Charlie repeated his old pattern, he could no longer use the excuse of not understanding his problem. It would not mean that Charlie was "bad" or of weak character, but that Charlie and I would need to figure out why he found it so hard to politely decline the invitation. As it turned out, however, between the pressure he experienced from within and the support (if not pressure) he received from me, he was primed to risk a new and more constructive way of dealing with the situation.

So the first time around, he threw caution to the wind and turned down the invitation. Charlie felt proud, as well he should have. I felt it was a great start, but knew it was just a start. If the insight was to "take hold," if it was to translate into a natural and enduring pattern of behavior, it had to be worked through.

Soon afterward another situation occurred which struck me, but not Charlie, as posing essentially the same psychological problem. Working through began here. A friend of Charlie's had bought some hockey tickets without getting any for Charlie. At the next psychotherapy session, he said that the more he had thought about this, the more it irked him.

Sharp: I'm always doing things for him, but he never reciprocates. I'm sure he likes me, but he takes our friendship for granted.

Maxmen: What did you do about this?

Sharp (meekly): Nothing. It's too late. The tickets are already bought, and what's the point of bringing up my hurt feelings *now*? He'll think I'm nuts for dragging up a week-old issue. I would sound like a crybaby.

Maxmen: Why a "crybaby"?

Sharp: Because people who complain are crybabies.

Maxmen: Oh?

Sharp: Well, in my family they were. With six siblings you didn't complain, and being the youngest, that was especially true for me.

Maxmen: Why? What would happen?

Sharp: You were seen as pushy. I recall that if I asked for anything, all day long they would give me the "silent treatment." I can't blame them, since I always seemed to be asking for things.

Maxmen: And always seemed to be pushy?

Sharp: Yes. (pause) I don't like pushy people; they're insensitive. (pause) Do you think I'm pushy?

Maxmen: No, but I wonder if you do.

Sharp: I guess I do, or I would have already asked my friends about those tickets. It's like that dinner-invitation bit. I keep thinking that I'm that insensitive little brat. So

183

> I keep bending over backward to be polite, and the more I bend the more I become furious, which only confirms that I'm a brat.

Maxmen: Are you a brat?

Sharp: Of course not, but then I should stop acting like I'm afraid I am.

If Charlie Sharp had received "assertiveness training," he would be taught to change his usual behavior mainly by learning concrete techniques and skills, whereas in insight-oriented psychotherapy, he seeks change primarily by acquiring a greater understanding of his feelings and motivations.

In this example of working through, Charlie realizes that the dinner invitation and the hockey-ticket situation are both variations of a common theme, but that dealing successfully with the former does not mean that he will automatically do so with the latter. Over time he will discover that the more he contends with these situations the easier each becomes. That is true in part because, as illustrated here, Charlie is becoming increasingly able to identify his inner fear that he is a pushy brat; and so in the future, whenever he feels he is being pushy, he will be better prepared to view this feeling for what it is: an old neurotic pattern and not a legitimate concern.

In working through, the patient repeatedly practices in the "real" world what he's learned in therapy. This practice helps the patient see for himself what difficulties, practical or emotional, might get in the way of converting insight to change. By frequently doing so, the patient finds that his newly acquired insights lead to feelings of competence and self-mastery, feelings which many claim are essential for psychological well-being.

As working through progresses, patient and therapist gather new information, and as this happens, the five steps in psychotherapy that I've delineated repeat themselves. Once therapy has been launched, during every session, each of these steps occurs as each issue is discussed. As a result, therapy consists of constant reexaminations of issues, and with each cycle of exploration, new understandings and behaviors evolve.

PERSONAL QUESTIONS

Listed in no particular order, here are the personal questions patients most often ask psychiatrists: "Are you married? If so, do you have children?" If not, a few patients will muster the courage to ask, "How come?" If you're not married—or perhaps even if you are—gay patients ask if you're gay. Some patients, especially Jews and Catholics, want to know your religion. "Do you talk about me to your colleagues?" "Do you talk about me to your spouse?" "Do you think about me in between our sessions?" "Do I appear in your dreams?" "Do you like me?" "Am I your favorite patient?" "If I were not your patient, would you want me as a friend?"

How a psychiatrist responds to these questions depends on his training, his personality, the type of psychotherapy he's conducting, the kind of patient he's treating, the exact circumstances at the time, and habit. For example, in conducting psychoanalysis, the psychiatrist wishes to be a "blank screen" for the patient's projections, and so he does not want to reveal private information that would define himself. In supportive psychotherapy, the psychiatrist may reveal a good deal about himself, since by being a "real" person and not a "blank screen," the psychiatrist helps the psychotic patient test reality and the neurotic patient deal with concrete issues.

On social occasions, people who are in insight-oriented psychotherapy will often ask me, "How come my shrink gets offended if I ask a personal question?" or "Is it all right to ask a psychiatrist something personal?" I can't speak for every therapist, but most psychiatrists do not mind personal questions; this does not mean, however, that they will answer them. Laymen understandably get their impression because their shrink refuses to give a direct answer or replies with a "Why are you asking?" What laymen misperceive is the psychiatrist's motive.

When a patient asks a personal question, I will answer it, but I also know that patients ask these questions for a reason, which may or may not be clear to them or to me. Therefore, if I am to answer the patient's question properly, I need to know why he is asking it.

Like many psychiatrists, I have a stock approach to personal questions. Whatever the question—suppose it's "Do you talk about me to your colleagues?''—my standard reply is: "I'll be glad to answer your question, but before I do, I'd like to know why you're asking." If the patient replies, "I want to know if you think my case is interesting," I ask why that worries him. He might say, "Because you seem bored with me." The issue is not whether I discuss the patient with colleagues, but rather the patient's concern that he bores me. Therefore, we need to examine our relationship and not be detoured into talking about what I say to colleagues. Indeed, more often than not, the patient's question is a means to get to another issue. When I'm asked, "Do you have children?" the patient is actually concerned with whether I understand what it's like for him to be a parent.

When conducting psychotherapy, psychiatrists do not feel they must always be completely open and honest with patients. Although rarely, if ever, is there a reason to lie to a patient, psychotherapists must be careful in *how* they are "open and honest." Should the psychiatrist tell his patient he is thoroughly disgusting? If a patient's political beliefs offend the psychiatrist, should he say so? Should the psychiatrist tell a patient that he becomes deeply depressed every time he sees him? Such "truth-dumping"—all in the name of being "completely open and honest"—is frequently done by therapists who believe that the patient will change only if the therapist stirs things up. This belief may or may not have validity, but it runs dangerously close to being the therapist's intellectualization for being sadistic.

Psychiatrists do not believe that just because the patient divulges highly personal information, therapists should reciprocate. After all, therapy is for the patient, not the therapist. This does not mean that the therapist is a better, wiser, or saner human being, but that if therapy is to succeed, it should be respect, and not personal information, that is reciprocated.

How much a psychiatrist reveals about himself has little correlation with how much warmth he communicates or how much distance he creates between himself and the patient. For instance, the famed psychoanalyst Harry Stack Sullivan's favorite way of responding to a psychotic patient's hallucination was "I don't see it" rather than "It isn't there." This nuance illustrates how a psychiatrist can show genuine respect for a patient's experience while he maintains "therapeutic distance."

Although everyone knows of the stereotypic analyst who says

nothing but "Uh-huh" three times an hour, less recognized is that many patients object to therapists' being too talkative and too self-revealing. Patients will tell their psychiatrist, "You talk so much, I can't get a word in." Or "I end up not taking enough responsibility for my therapy." Or "You act too much like a friend and not enough like a doctor." Or "Although I appreciate your compliments, I'm worried that your liking me may color your objectivity."

As therapists go, I'm relatively talkative, as much by temperament as by choice. However, I must admit that despite the many complaints about psychiatrists' behaving as near-mutes, I also have seen many patients object to psychiatrists who don't maintain enough professional distance. Yet no matter how much or how little a psychiatrist talks, the therapist's decision to reveal personal information ultimately rests on whether he believes it will help or harm the patient.

THE THERAPEUTIC ATTITUDE

This section could also be titled "How to Get the Most from Psychotherapy," since patients can gain the most from psychotherapy by adopting the "therapeutic attitude." Although psychiatrists emphasize different aspects of the therapeutic attitude, most agree that those I'm about to mention are important.

To me, the most crucial element in having a therapeutic attitude is *curiosity* about why feelings, thoughts, and events occur. Good therapists, to paraphrase H. L. Mencken, make the unknown worth knowing about* by helping patients become intrigued by their own psychology. Too often psychological curiosity is stymied by reflexive value judgments. The patient becomes more concerned with placing blame than with asking why. To illustrate, the following exchange took place during the fifth session between me and a middle-aged teacher, Dan Berman:

Maxmen: It seems that every time I give you a compliment, you point out one of your supposed faults.

---

*I can't think of a better criterion to judge anything than the ability to "make the unknown worth knowing about"; to me, it is the hallmark not only of good therapy, but of good art, good teaching, good science, good writing, and so on.

Berman: That's bad, isn't it?

Maxmen: But what I'm curious about is why you do this.

Berman: Yes, I'm always blaming myself for everything, and that's a terrible habit that I've got to break.

Maxmen: Now you're blaming yourself for blaming yourself.

Berman: You're right. That's the wrong thing to do.

Mr. Berman's persistent viewing of issues as being either "good" or "bad" kept blocking psychological exploration. Effective insight-oriented psychotherapy requires the patient to suspend, but not dismiss, value judgments and to adopt temporarily an ethically neutral stance for self-questioning and self-evaluation. Later in the same session, the frequent difficulties in adopting a therapeutic attitude were illustrated:

Maxmen: You seem to focus on whether something is good or bad, when it might be more constructive to examine why that something occurs. For example, when I point out that you respond to compliments by criticizing yourself, instead of blaming yourself, you would gain more by asking yourself, "Why do I do this?" or "What could this mean?"

Berman (with tears welling up): So you think I'm not a good patient, that I'm not trying hard enough. Well, you just don't know how much I've struggled, how tough it's been for me even to see a psychiatrist.

Although I was entertaining hypotheses about why he was converting a neutral suggestion into a personal attack, my immediate task was not to interpret the reasons for this distortion, or for his defensive tantrum, or for his self-pity, but to reassure him that I understood how he felt and was on his side.

Maxmen: I realize how very difficult it was for you to see a psychiatrist, and I certainly regret if what I said hurt you. Do you have any suggestions for me about how I could have phrased things differently?

Berman   (pause): No, not really. (pause) I think I'm overly sensitive to criticism.

Maxmen: Why is that?

Berman: I don't know, but it's weird this comes up, since I've been noticing that whenever my boss makes a suggestion . . .

Once the patient felt understood, he was ready to join me in psychological exploration. He less often made automatic value judgments and more often examined why things happen, and thus he was adopting a therapeutic attitude.

Having a therapeutic attitude also involves the patient focusing on how he can change himself instead of on how others should change. We have far greater control over ourselves than we do over others. In the next example, the psychiatrist shifts the focus from a sister to the patient.

Patient: My sister constantly makes me feel guilty for not visiting her more often.

Psychiatrist: Should you feel guilty?

Patient: Heavens, no! I see her more than anyone else in the family. Everybody knows she's a real pain in the ass; she doesn't listen to anyone. I just wish she'd stop making me feel guilty.

Psychiatrist: But if you have nothing to be guilty about, the problem is not that she provokes guilt, but that you believe her. So why do you believe her?

Throughout therapy, the psychiatrist tries to instill the therapeutic attitude as well as offer the patient specific suggestions for getting the most from therapy. The psychiatrist might say, "In thinking about therapy between sessions—something I'd strongly recommend—some patients set aside a definite time for doing so; others jot down a few notes right after a session to refresh their memories. I've generally found that patients benefit most when, after thinking about the previous session, they come to the next one with specific issues in mind for discussion." If the psychiatrist does not provide any guidance, the patient should ask for some.

HOW PSYCHOTHERAPY GOES ASTRAY

Dr. Jay Haley cited studies indicating that 50 to 70 percent of patients on waiting lists get over their emotional problem without psychotherapy. Since that's a higher success rate than psychotherapists get, Haley concluded that shrinks must go out of their way to fail. The big flaw in his reasoning is that people on waiting lists are not a very good control group, since those in dire need of help make it their business to get treatment; those who remain on waiting lists and don't receive help probably have milder problems. Nevertheless, therapies do fail, and knowing how to diminish the chance of this occurring is important for both psychiatrist and patient.

Dr. Hans Strupp, the dean of psychotherapy researchers, surveyed seventy experts on psychotherapy, who suggested the most frequent reasons for psychotherapeutic flops are that the patient lacks motivation, or that the therapist promises more than he can deliver, lacks respect for the patient, improperly assesses the patient, incorrectly assigns the patient to psychotherapy, has excessive psychopathology (especially hostility and seductiveness), or doesn't convey enough hope to the patient.

When supervisors at a program well known for teaching psychotherapy were asked what mistakes residents most often made, they reported, in order of frequency, wanting to be liked by the patient, an inability to "tune in to" the patient's unconscious, premature interpretations, excessive intellectualization, inappropriate transference interpretations, uncalled-for and stereotyped "analytic" stances, insufficient appreciation of countertransference feelings, an inability to tolerate the patient's aggression, difficulties coping with silence, and avoidance of setting a fee. In contrast, the mistakes least often observed were lack of interest, excessive voyeurism, conscious dislike of the patient, excessive personal revelations, dissembling, therapeutic nihilism, being seductive, lacking empathy, competing with the patient, and lacking psychological-mindedness.

I could go on citing such lists, but I'm not sure how instructive they are, except to show how little agreement exists on why therapy fails. Professionals even find it hard to agree on how to rate psychotherapeutic skills. Therefore, if the experts can't approximate a consensus, let me advance some ideas about a few major reasons psychotherapy goes astray.

As I mentioned in Chapter 1, psychotherapists often miss the boat by constantly "explaining" the patient without showing they also "understand" him, or that there even is a difference between understanding and explaining.

Patient:	Ever since I broke up with my boyfriend a week ago, I've been feeling miserable.
Psychiatrist:	Have you felt this way before?
Patient:	Yes, when my father died.
Psychiatrist:	What might that suggest?
Patient	(skeptically): Do you mean that it's my father I *really* miss?
Psychiatrist:	Isn't that what you've just indicated?
Patient:	No. I said the feelings were similar, but that's not why I'm feeling crummy right *now*. I'm feeling awful now because my boyfriend is gone.
Psychiatrist:	Aren't you denying the impact of losing your father?
Patient:	You keep insisting that I'm missing my father, when I keep telling you that I miss my boyfriend. Why can't you understand me?
Psychiatrist:	But I do. Childhood traumas often leave indelible scars.

In this dialogue of the deaf, the psychiatrist's interpretations may be true, but they are only explanations; they do not show that he understands what the patient feels. This causes patients to feel removed from the therapist and to withdraw into themselves. If, right at the start, the psychiatrist had said, "It must feel dreadful to miss your boyfriend," and if he also had spent a couple of moments acknowledging the patient's sadness, the patient, sensing the therapist was on "her side," would be more receptive to the psychiatrist's interpretation.

As this patient objects to the psychiatrist's explanations, the therapist is likely to claim the patient is "resisting" or "denying," thereby aggravating the situation with even more explanations.* By implying that the patient doesn't know his own mind, the psychiatrist is blaming the patient for the lack of therapeutic progress. Whether the patient responds by feeling guilty or angry, therapy goes astray.

Indeed, when therapy goes badly, psychiatrists frequently blame the patient, most often claiming the patient "wasn't motivated." Psychiatrists will say, "The patient fears change," or "The patient needs to be sick," or "The patient wants to suffer." But if a patient "isn't motivated," it's the psychiatrist's job to motivate him. If the psychiatrist can't motivate the patient, I believe, unlike most of my colleagues, that the psychiatrist has failed. Perhaps no psychiatrist could do better, but this hardly diminishes the psychiatrist's responsibility to motivate the patient. If a patient feels his psychiatrist blames him for the failure of therapy, he should definitely discuss this with the psychiatrist.

I cannot stress enough that when patients feel uncomfortable about raising anything touchy—objecting to an interpretation, admitting feelings of love, affection, or distaste for the therapist, expressing dissatisfaction with therapy, or indicating a wish to stop treatment—it is imperative for them to bring these issues to the psychiatrist's attention. If the patient is afraid that raising an issue will anger the therapist, he might introduce his statement with "I'm reluctant to bring this up because I'm worried you'll be angry with me, but . . ." and then go ahead and raise the specific concern: "I don't think this therapy is going anyplace." By first pointing out the feared response, the patient has effectively undercut the therapist's potential anger. Too many psychotherapies fail because doctor and patient are not discussing matters of great concern to the patient.

Therapists often play the "X-Y game," in which if the patient says something is X, the therapist will say it is actually Y. If the patient indicates he has a serious problem with his boss, the ther-

---

*When therapists have a strong ideological commitment to a particular theory, a patient who questions an explanation is challenging not just an explanation, but a psychiatrist's entire belief system.

apist insists his real problem is with his parents. After all, if the psychiatrist agrees with the patient, who needs the psychiatrist? If the patient claims to hate his mother, the shrink says, "Aha! Deep down you really *love* your mother."

Be careful whenever psychiatrists insert the phrase "deep down." Invariably its use "deskills" the patient. The psychiatrist employs "deep down" to "prove" the truth lies directly opposite where every shred of evidence points. The term "underlying" is similar to "deep down," in that an "underlying" problem is something the patient couldn't possibly discover on his own. "Really" is another popular buzzword for demonstrating that the problem is never what the patient thinks it is. Laymen also use these buzzwords for psychological one-upmanship.

When a patient enters therapy saying, "My chief problem is getting along with my wife," the psychiatrist not infrequently suggests that his *real* problem is getting along with his mother. The patient begins to fret over his newly uncovered problem, but draws solace by reasoning, "Thank goodness for therapy; without it I never would have realized my terrible problem with my mother." After several months of therapy, the patient revises his outlook on his mother and credits therapy for the improved relationship. Having discovered and resolved a problem he never had, the patient is back where he started—worried about his relationship with his wife.

Psychiatrists certainly do find patients who enter psychotherapy having focused on the "wrong" problem, such as the man who goes for a sleep problem, which immediately disappears after he has wept inconsolably about his parents' deaths. Where the X-Y game leads therapy astray is not when it reveals other dimensions to a patient's problem, but when the patient's original problem goes unaddressed and the patient abdicates all independent judgment.

For this reason, modern psychiatrists are more inclined to have the patient define and specify his goals for psychotherapy. If he delineates and explicitly indicates these goals, a patient is less likely to find therapy disappointing, since the therapist can say whether these goals are attainable and can guide therapy to accomplish them. Because a major reason therapy flounders is that clear goals no longer exist, I periodically have patients redefine what they still hope to achieve in therapy.

TERMINATING PSYCHOTHERAPY

Strolling through Leyden in 1908, Freud analyzed Gustav Mahler in four hours. Freud acknowledged that Mahler was exceptionally quick to catch on to psychoanalysis, but analysis in those days rarely extended beyond a year. As psychiatrists kept discovering more and more things to analyze (since it was becoming clearer that shorter analyses didn't work), they increasingly felt that more and more work was "required" to "cure" the patient. (For the psychiatrist, longer analyses were also more profitable.) In 1937, when analyses typically took two to three years, Freud wrote *Analysis Terminable and Interminable,* in which he warned against the ever-increasing length of psychoanalysis. Prophetically anticipating the biopsychosocial integration characteristic of the new scientific psychiatry, he reemphasized that fundamental biological factors produce aberrant behavior and can't be altered by psychological interventions. These truths, he claimed, were not sufficiently appreciated by his colleagues, leading them to underestimate the inherent limits of psychoanalysis and to draw it out interminably. Freud's warnings went unheeded. Today not only do most psychoanalyses last five to seven years, but so do many insight-oriented psychotherapies; they can often drag on for a dozen or more years, if not for life.

That people remain in therapy forever used to bug me: The patient had to be spineless, and the therapist, although maybe great at starting therapy, had to be lousy at terminating it. I've mellowed. If some thrill to opera, break dancing, and golf, surely others have every right to spend all their time and money talking about themselves. It is, after all, their time and their money.

Although it's not my style, I could understand how people could view interminable therapy as a way to keep mentally fit, just as we view going to a health club as a way to keep physically fit. Like bodies, psyches wear down; they're continually frayed by new strains and stresses. So why not devote an hour or two a week to a psychological tune-up?

The final stage of psychotherapy, which psychiatrists call "termination," typically begins two to eight weeks before the final visit. (In therapies lasting several years, termination may begin as long as three to six months before.) Under ideal circumstances, the goals of therapy have been accomplished and psychiatrist and patient agree the time is ripe to end therapy. During termination, patients are to work through any remaining problems, consolidate gains made previously in therapy, avert potential difficulties, and become more independent of therapy and the therapist. At the final session, the psychiatrist reminds the patient that his door is always open; the doctor and patient exchange fond memories, offer good wishes, and say goodbye. Although this is how termination is supposed to happen, it is the exception when it does.

Therapy often stops for external reasons: Patients can no longer pay, or they or the psychiatrist may move away or have incompatible schedules. At times, neither patient nor psychiatrist is completely sure if the reasons offered by the patient for ending are truly external or excuses; frequently, they're both.

In either case, the psychiatrist usually does not fully approve of the patient's leaving treatment. I'd guess that 10 to 20 percent of all psychotherapies end with the psychiatrist's full endorsement. Another 10 to 20 percent of the time psychiatrists feel ambivalent about the patient's terminating. The rest of the time psychiatrists think it's a lousy decision. When patients, as psychiatrists say, "terminate prematurely," psychiatrists usually blame the patient.

For example, Manhattan psychiatrists in private practice pooled their reasons for why thirty of their outpatients terminated prematurely. (They could give more than one reason per patient.) The psychiatrists cited 87 percent of the patients leaving as a way of "acting out" a conflict in treatment, usually related to transference, or a fear of aggression, sexuality, or an overdependence on the therapist or on therapy. They believed 57 percent left because of maladaptive character traits, such as "masochism," "a need to fail," or "negativism." The psychiatrists conceded that 40 percent dropped out because of "reality factors," such as the patient's moving away. With only 37 percent of the patients did the psychiatrists feel that the therapist himself was partly responsible, largely because of countertransference difficulties. The psychiatrists usually claimed that three of these four general categories played a significant role in the patient's quitting psychotherapy too early.

When psychiatrists explain to colleagues (and to themselves) why their patient acted out* in leaving treatment, they usually say things like "Ever since he started confronting feelings toward his father, the patient became so terribly overwhelmed by anxiety, he abandoned treatment." Or "The transference was too hot for the patient, so he suddenly claimed poverty and stopped therapy." There is often a "macho" ring to their explanations, as if they're saying, "If only the patient had enough guts, he could have stood up to the pressures of therapy."

The psychiatrist can usually make a patient feel self-conscious about stopping treatment. Since patients and psychiatrists know there are always more problems to resolve and more issues to explore, a psychiatrist can merely say, "Have you wondered if you're leaving therapy to avoid certain conflicts?" and the patient can't help but question if he is right to leave treatment.

In a commonly used "seek-and-ye-shall-find maneuver," psychiatrists induce many patients to feel far more upset about leaving therapy than they would be otherwise. In theory, patients *must* be upset about terminating treatment, and if the patient is not upset, the psychiatrist is often sure the patient is repressing strong feelings. To prove his point, the psychiatrist may comment, "You must have feelings about leaving therapy," or "It's quite normal to find termination very difficult." Hearing this, many patients reason, "Ending treatment doesn't feel like that big a deal, but since the shrink must know what he's talking about, I must be denying a lot of feelings."

Patients are not as easily swayed, nor are psychiatrists so manipulative, as I've implied in the two previous paragraphs. But I mention these interactions because it is my distinct impression that with the best of intentions, psychiatrists prolong therapy far too often and don't give enough support to a patient's need to "fly on his own."

That termination can be highly traumatic for some patients is certainly true. But since termination is usually initiated by patients and not therapists, ending treatment is often more traumatic

---

*Psychiatrists often misuse the term "acting out" to describe any misbehavior, for which "acting up" would be a more accurate term. Technically, "acting out" refers to a person's misbehaving to reduce anxiety that stems from repressed childhood conflicts, which have been aroused by the patient's unconscious feelings toward the therapist.

for therapists. After all, it is the therapist who is being ditched, whose services are no longer useful or needed, and whose income suffers. And no matter how tactfully the patient explains his reasons for leaving therapy "prematurely," to various degrees the psychiatrist will feel he has failed the patient.

Worse yet for the therapist is when the patient suddenly stops treatment without giving a reason. Sometimes the patient cancels an appointment, promises to reschedule, but never calls back. When the patient terminates without warning or explanation, the psychiatrist may become annoyed and angry about the patient's abrupt disappearance and apparent lack of courtesy. He may blame himself: If he had won the patient's trust, the patient would have confided in him. He may feel he failed the patient, but most assuredly, he is frustrated because he doesn't have a clue as to what went wrong.

Sometimes the psychiatrist does not want to stop treatment even though he is fully aware the patient is not getting any better and even though he dreads sitting through unproductive sessions. The psychiatrist continues because he fears ending treatment would do more harm than keeping it going. He is not so much "treating" the patient as "maintaining" him. If the psychiatrist ends therapy, the patient may correctly feel that the therapist is giving up on him or that his case is hopeless. In these situations, the psychiatrist is in a genuine quandary, because there is no sure way of knowing if he is still treating the patient for the sake of his patient or his pocketbook. Concerned they are seeing a patient only to make a buck, psychiatrists sometimes stop seeing a patient when continued contact would be beneficial.

Some therapies don't really end as much as fizzle out. Both parties go through the motions, although since some long-past imperceptible moment, therapy stopped being therapeutic. To the patient, treatment is floundering. The psychiatrist may hammer away at the patient's "resistance," but if the patient continues to find therapy unproductive, then regardless of who's at fault, therapy is no longer worthwhile.

When a therapy fizzles, it's often because the psychiatrist has exhausted his bag of tricks. Even the best psychiatrists have limited psychotherapeutic repertoires. Once the patient has seen the full act and there's nothing more to see, therapy may become routinized, predictable, and boring.

A therapy that's fizzled is not necessarily a therapy that's failed. As a friend told me about terminating his therapy, "Despite things petering out near the end, we had two very good years." Wondering if he felt that overall therapy had been worth it, he replied, "Sure. Look, we'll always have Paris."

There's usually been enough "Paris" for psychiatrists to tell patients that if they ever wish to return for one or more sessions, they should feel free to do so. Leaving the door open eases termination for patients (if not for therapists). For the same reason, instead of stopping all at once, some therapists prefer tapering the frequency of the last sessions; this allows patients to see what it's like to fly on their own before treatment ends, as well as defusing the impact of the final visit.

Leaving aside professional considerations, in many circumstances the therapist deeply regrets losing an intimate. When termination occurs, the psychiatrist often feels a bit like the patient's teacher, parent, priest, and friend all rolled into one. So even when a patient leaves treatment before the psychiatrist thinks he should, the psychiatrist's warm feelings toward the patient usually override any bruises to his professional ego.

DOES PSYCHOTHERAPY WORK?

The answer is: "Yes, but."

Yes, but to answer this question scientifically is almost impossible. The answer depends on the types of patients, diagnoses, psychotherapies, therapists, goals, and circumstances; it would also depend on who's the judge: Is it the patient, his friends or family, the therapist, or an uninvolved rater/clinician? A study of twenty-two cases of insight-oriented psychotherapy and fifteen cases of psychoanalysis revealed that in comparison to patients and independent judges, therapists overrated their success; they also overlooked and misperceived their patients' dissatisfactions with the outcome of treatment. Research judges gave lower ratings to therapy than both patients and therapists. These findings only begin to demonstrate why evaluating psychotherapy is a scientific nightmare.*

---

*Psychotherapy research also poses ethical problems which change from generation to generation. For instance, in 1960 an experiment on the outcome of

Yes, but psychotherapy has side effects and hazards. Most psychiatrists agree with famed psychoanalyst Abraham Kardiner when he wrote, "Freud was always infuriated whenever I would say to him that you could not do harm with psychoanalysis. He said, 'When you say that, you also say that it cannot do any good. Because if you cannot do any harm, how can you do good?'" Barely glued-together patients often become psychotic when receiving insight-oriented psychotherapy. Suicide, morbid ruminations, an overdependence on therapy or the therapist, and paralyzed decision-making are frequent side effects of psychotherapy. As in determining if drugs work, a major consideration with psychotherapy is whether its potential benefits outweigh its potential risks.

Yes, but it depends on what's meant by "work." The goals of pharmacotherapy and psychotherapy differ; the former alleviates symptoms, the latter alleviates intrapsychic and interpersonal problems. In the most extensive and expensive ($1 million) study of its kind, the Boston–New Haven Collaborative Study has been comparing the effects of Elavil (a tricyclic antidepressant) with various psychotherapies in the treatment of moderately depressed outpatients. All the results aren't in, but apparently Elavil is better than psychotherapy for symptom relief, while psychotherapy helps more with social adjustment. No one expects group psychotherapy to cure diabetes, yet it clearly helps patients deal with their diabetes. The same applies for helping patients deal with mental illness. Unfortunately, up to now most research has judged

---

psychotherapy with schizophrenics was deemed unethical if it had a control group that did not receive psychotherapy; by 1968 it was considered unethical to have a group that *only* received psychotherapy.

In evaluating any psychiatric treatment, one should consider the "humanist" fear that drug therapy is tantamount to "mind control," whereas psychotherapy doesn't involve mind control. Yet when patients take a drug, they know it will affect them, but when they receive psychotherapy, they often don't have the vaguest idea how it's affecting them. The influence of drugs is clear and overt, whereas the influence of psychotherapy is insidious and covert. By stimulating specific receptors in the brain, psychoactive medications can only affect particular symptoms; drugs cannot alter an individual's overall personality or force people to adopt a particular philosophy or to perform a specific complex act. Lacing the city's water supply with a drug that makes people kill is not only impossible, but hardly worth the effort. Goebbels did not have to use drugs to turn people into savages. And if you really want to use mind control, don't bother with drugs, or even with psychotherapy—try advertising.

psychotherapy's efficacy by how well it squelched symptoms, and therefore may have missed psychotherapy's greatest benefits.

Yes, but to ask if psychotherapy works is like asking if a restaurant works. A "good" restaurant may satisfy your palate, improve your health, or delight your eye; it all depends on what you expect and on what you pay. You wouldn't compare McDonald's with Lutèce. Each is splendid at what it does. The same for psychotherapy. It does what it does, and when it does it, it does it very well. There are good and bad therapists just as there are good and bad restaurants.

So, yes, psychotherapy does work, *if* the right type is used for the right purpose and with the right expectations in mind. Unless psychotic, every patient can determine if psychotherapy is accomplishing its mission, since every patient can tell if it is helping him deal more effectively with his illness, improve his social relations, or bolster his self-esteem.

EIGHT

Public Psychiatry

Who treats a majority of patients with mental disorders? It's not psychiatrists; it's not even mental health professionals. In truth, a majority (54.1 percent) are treated by primary care physicians, roughly a quarter (21.5 percent) receive no treatment at all, and only 24.4 percent are treated by mental health personnel. Three times as many patients with mental disorders are treated by the general medical sector as outpatients than are treated by the mental health sector as outpatients *and* inpatients. On the other hand, mental health professionals treat a greater proportion of severely ill patients, and not on Park Avenue.

For the typical psychiatrist does not have a full-time private practice. Most psychiatrists have several jobs, and for several reasons: to escape the isolation of private practice, to be around colleagues, to pursue a variety of interests, and to make a living; there simply aren't enough wealthy people to fill most private practices. Therefore, during a normal week a typical psychiatrist spends twenty-five hours in private practice, five hours in teaching students, and twenty hours in something called "public psychiatry."

"Public psychiatry" is a relatively recent, and ill-defined, term which refers to a wide range of *publicly* funded psychiatric services to people who otherwise could not afford them, especially the indigent and chronically ill. These activities include the treatment of psychiatric and substance-abusing patients in public clinics, emergency rooms, state hospitals, Community Mental Health Centers, nursing homes, and inpatient units. Public psychiatry often entails consultation to schools, prisons, or courts, as well as the administration or evaluation of government-funded treatment programs. Because medical schools are frequently intertwined with publicly funded treatment facilities, much of the teaching, research, and clinical service performed in academia involves public psychiatry. Roughly a third of all work done by psychiatrists is in public psychiatry.

Public psychiatry is highly political. Its sole justification is that it serves patients that private psychiatry does not, and cannot. These millions of patients have genuine mental disorders and not everyday angst; for them, treatment is a requirement, not a luxury. The success of public psychiatry largely depends on the allocation of government funds and resources.

Because it is so political and affects so many people, virtually every day newspapers report a scandal or controversy in public psychiatry. As I'm writing this, a headline in today's *New York Times* about a state mental hospital reads: "Abuse Cited in Death of Creedmoor Patient."

Amid the politics and controversies of public psychiatry, it is easy to overlook that contemporary public psychiatry would not have been possible without advances in scientific psychiatry. During the 1950s and 1960s, psychoanalytic psychiatrists created a movement known as "social psychiatry," which was based on the theory that by "treating society," mental illness would diminish and mental health would flourish. This notion fizzled fast when it became clear that (a) nobody, especially psychiatrists, knew how to treat society, and (b) psychiatric expertise was limited to treating patients. As a result, social psychiatrists started examining their own work less ideologically and more scientifically.

In the 1950s, research in social psychiatry was demonstrating that long-term incarceration had devastating effects on patients. However obvious this might seem today, in the 1950s psychiatrists were inclined to attribute almost all of the chronic mental patient's deterioration to the natural course of schizophrenia.* This

---

*In general, chronic mental patients and patients in state hospitals have been schizophrenics.

research showed that the cold, mechanistic routinization of long-term stays in state mental hospitals further induced patients to become socially inept, emotionally restricted, and behaviorally weird. Furthermore, this "institutionalization" could be avoided by using more active treatments on inpatient units, and more important, by discharging patients as soon as possible.

Yet releasing patients earlier and maintaining them in the community longer would have been impossible if it hadn't been for the introduction of antipsychotic medications in 1954, and subsequently of antidepressant medications and lithium. Thus, scientific psychiatry married social and biological psychiatry, giving birth to modern public psychiatry.

THE STATE HOSPITAL

Today's state mental hospitals are not the snake pits of yesteryear. Nor are they the Hilton. When you first walk through the locked doors of a "modern" state hospital, you're likely to be accosted by a scrawny "bag lady" who invades your "body buffer zone" and begs for a cigarette. If you offer her a cigarette, in a second, ten patients will accost you for cigarettes. If you don't offer her a cigarette, she might curse you, growl unintelligibly, wander off dejectedly, or pester you to talk with her, very often to the exclusion of everyone else. Before you realize it, one patient wants to know if you're the "new doctor" on the service, while another propositions you. And yet, no matter how much these patients assault your sensibilities, you're not frightened by them. You feel sorry for them.

Leaning against the drab institutional green walls are isolated patients staring blankly into space, muttering to themselves, boxing with hallucinations, undulating their arms, or shouting obscenities. Within an hour they will so fade into the walls you'll hardly notice them. But initially, you're struck that they are oblivious to your entrance. Engage one in a conversation, and he might not respond. You end up talking to yourself; you feel foolish and frustrated for failing to get through. Of course, you haven't failed any more than anyone else, but you might not know that, and even if you did, it's of little comfort. Sorry, but your good intentions and warm smile can't penetrate this chronic schizophrenic's private world.

A staff member tells you, "Don't take this patient's lack of response personally. He does this to everyone. The most skilled psychiatrists can't get him to talk." You begin to sense the frustration of those who work with these patients all the time. For a moment, you even contemplate the frustration of actually *being* one of these patients.

These frustrations are not nearly so bad if one works or lives at a fancy long-term private mental hospital, such as Chestnut Lodge, where all the patients have their own bedroom, decent cuisine, lovely grounds, plenty of therapy, and enough privacy. Yet, Chestnut Lodges are for the wealthy. Most chronic schizophrenics reside in state hospitals, where the food is slop, ten patients may share a dorm, therapy is scarce, and privacy is nil. Although working with chronic schizophrenics is frustrating enough, doing so in dreary, understaffed, and overcrowded state hospitals makes it terribly depressing.

Consider, therefore, if you would like to work in such a place, day in and day out. I doubt it. More than being around these patients, it is having to be responsible for them, and with so few resources, that makes this work so demoralizing. The patients' anguish is great, their behavior off-putting, their personalities bland, and their futures bleak; many go for months, and often for years, without making the *slightest* improvement. Their futility becomes yours. In short order, if you're a staff member with halfway decent self-esteem, ambition, or talent, you find another job. Many staff members remain because they can't get another job, or because they acquire a perverse satisfaction in being superior to these patients. Leaving aside the patients, would you like to be around this kind of staff?

On your tour you cannot help but observe psychiatric aides. You notice them because they are probably the only people you can see who are doing anything for the patients. Psych aides make things run and prevent anarchy. They feed, clean, and dress the patients. They play Monopoly with patients and talk to them. When a patient defecates in his bed, spits out his meal, bangs his head against a wall, or slugs someone, it is the aides who come to the rescue. If you're an aide, after a while all this gets to you. Eventually, some aides become institutionalized themselves; they start acting like patients. They sit for hours, especially on the night shift, transfixed by a flickering TV set. They don't talk with patients, they yell at them. If, as a guest, you object to their bossy tone, they will, in a surly tone, inform you, "What these patients need is *order*," and by implication, "Don't tell us how to do our jobs." Just as schizophrenics become overwhelmed by stimuli and withdraw into themselves, aides get overwhelmed by the ward's stimuli and retreat for sanity into the nurses' station. The demoralization of many psychiatric aides is compounded because most state hospitals offer them little professional or economic incentive.

A large proportion of state-hospital psychiatrists are foreign-born. Many barely speak English, and few understand the nuances and idioms of American speech; that's a major problem, since psychiatry depends so much on clear communication. Their cultural values and assumptions are often quite different from their patients', as when a thirty-year-old patient who wants to live away from his parents finds that his Indian-born psychiatrist feels he is being disrespectful to his parents. Many foreign-reared psychiatrists feel strongly that Americans place too little value on family ties and too much on independence. Although these psychiatrists vary tremendously, in general their psychotherapy is relatively authoritarian, it doesn't reflect American egalitarian and democratic instincts. They often flounder with more abstract psychological tasks, but they may also offer patients perspectives that American-born psychiatrists may not. Moreover, foreign-born psychiatrists usually master the concrete skills of diagnosis and prescribing medications, which are of most importance for helping patients in state hospitals.

The positive picture

Many psychiatrists would say I've unfairly described the patients, staff, and facilities of state hospitals, and have needlessly and irresponsibly frightened laymen from using state hospitals. Nevertheless, I not only believe that my portrayal of a *typical* state hospital is accurate, but that most psychiatrists, even though they would be reluctant to say so in public, would agree with me. On the other hand, the psychiatrists who object to my description have a point: The picture is far more complex.

Condemning the callousness of state hospital aides is easy. But callousness is an occupational hazard. It develops in everyone, regardless of discipline. Psychiatrists often feel like telling their critics, "Of course I know that most of these places, and the staffs that work in them, are awful. Yet before rushing to judgment, *you* try working there, and I bet you'll become just as callous.''

What's amazing is not that aides become callous, but that so many remain dedicated and sensitive. What's amazing is not that treatment is often substandard, but that so many staff members, from aides to psychiatrists, are so inventive and effective with so few resources.

An important product of this inventiveness is that many state hospitals provide services which many other, and supposedly better, psychiatric hospitals do not. There are many inpatient units in state hospitals that specialize in treating violent patients, running token economies (see Chapter 5), and offering patients experimental biotherapies and psychotherapies.

Over the past three decades, a smaller proportion of psychiatric patients are being admitted to state hospitals, and those who are admitted are discharged much sooner. Of all patients who entered any type of (inpatient or outpatient) psychiatric treatment, in 1955 about half went to a state hospital, whereas in 1975 only 9 percent did. Until 1955, patients admitted to state hospitals usually stayed for several months, several years, or a lifetime; today, half of the patients are discharged within a month, a quarter leave in six months, 15 percent are released after a couple of years, and the rest live, and eventually die, on back wards.

The less frequent and briefer use of state mental hospitals evolved as part of a trend to treat patients in the community. During the past twenty years, general medical hospitals have become major providers of psychiatric services, so that today it is common for acutely ill patients to be admitted to the psychiatric inpatient units of general medical hospitals and chronically ill patients to be admitted to state facilities. General medical hospitals also played a major role in keeping patients out of hospitals by greatly expanding the psychiatric care in their emergency rooms.

EMERGENCY PSYCHIATRY

Psychiatrists don't like emergencies. Granted, nobody does. But for psychiatrists, that's especially so. Emergencies run against their contemplative grain. In comparison to other physicians, psychiatrists like to mull over a problem instead of jumping in and medicating it. In addition, psychiatrists often feel impotent to handle emergencies.

In a typical situation, a psychiatrist is entertaining friends at home on Friday night. The phone rings. It's a patient. "Christ!" the psychiatrist thinks. "I'm a bit drunk; I'm not all that sharp; I hope the patient doesn't notice. What can I do over the phone, anyway? I can't stop someone from killing himself, from going bananas, from breaking up with a girlfriend, or from plunging into utter despair. What clever little insight can I once again pull out of a hat? Will this be a patient who simply wants to talk? If so, I understand his loneliness and I do want him to call if he needs to, but I still resent the intrusion into my personal life. If I were an internist, all I'd be expected to do would be to spend a minute telling the patient to take drug X; but as a psychiatrist, I'm expected to spend a long time talking. Maybe this will be Mrs. Furman suddenly wanting me to solve a problem we haven't solved together after three years of psychotherapy. Maybe it will be Mr. Walters, that angry/scared father telling me his son is back on drugs and demanding that I do something about it—*now!*"

The psychiatrist's concerns may be exaggerated, since many calls are merely to change an appointment or to refill a prescription. But other calls justify the psychiatrist's dread of them.

Indeed, many psychiatrists feel the most emotionally taxing job they can do is work in a big-city hospital emergency room, which is why ERs are usually staffed by psychiatric residents; they generally are far better at handling emergencies than most highly experienced private practitioners.

On average, psychiatric residents work the night shift in the ER once every seven to ten days, and the day shift once a week. The resident performs his normal duties the day before, and after, being on night call. Although the psychiatrist a patient sees at night usually has but two hours of light sleep, emergencies stimulate his adrenaline and he is surprisingly alert. It's not until the following day that the exhaustion catches up with him.

In a very informal survey of psychiatric residents they told me the most rewarding aspects of working in the emergency room are helping patients in serious crises, getting quick results, and saving people's lives. The most demoralizing aspect of nighttime work in the ER is the loneliness of being the only psychiatrist available for emergencies. They become very distressed by having to keep five to ten severely disturbed patients waiting for hours; they can see only one patient at a time, and quite often, they can't see the next patient until they finish the mountains of paperwork on the previous one. Another time-consuming headache is trying to hospitalize patients; few beds are available, and even when they are, doctors on call at night are already so busy they are reluctant to add to their workload by accepting new patients for admission. Beyond these practical concerns, the ER evokes more profound emotions in the psychiatrist, such as those expressed by this resident:

"The ER is a microcosm of everything that's wrong with society. It's filled with the homeless, the hungry, the mad, and the heartbroken. Every discontent that exists finds its way to you, and when it's 4:00 A.M., and you're exhausted, and all you can see is rows and rows of crying and frightened people lined up to see you— at this point it all seems so futile. I can't begin to provide what they need. I feel so goddam helpless. The only thing that gets me through the night is knowing I'll be off duty at 8:00 A.M. . . ."

On the plus side: "In the ER you feel like a *real* doctor. The patient comes in and you solve his problem. Psychotherapy takes so long, but here the results are quick. . . . What's most gratifying is when you *talk* a patient out of doing something very destructive. This happened last night. This nearly psychotic guy wants to kill his best friend after catching him and his wife in bed. The patient has this revolver, and so I tell him, guns make me nervous and would he please, at least for now, give me his. To my surprise, he does. I then dissuade him, in a way that allows him to save face from killing the friend. What I said and how I said it made all the difference. It felt so great to be a psychiatrist. I was drained, but nothing is as thrilling for me as when I can do this sort of thing."

The psychiatrist faces assaultive patients in the ER every night. I've seen a delirious encephalitic stab a psychiatrist with a Bic pen. (Some claimed he "flicked his Bic.") I've seen a seventy-year-old manic woman slash a nurse with a letter opener. I've seen a 300-pound bully, supposedly on PCP ("angel dust"), fight off three cops who dragged him into an ER; after the cops left, he broke the receptionist's arm. Twice I've seen psychotic patients shoot their way out of the ER. Psychiatrists quickly learn in the ER that assaultive patients have little respect for medical degrees.

Although violent patients usually benefit from medications, many will fight, often fanatically, to refuse them. For them, continuing to fight is a matter of honor; to stop in the absence of overwhelming opposition, a disgrace. Psychiatrists detest such confrontations and find it distasteful to use force to give patients medication. Justifiably or not, psychiatrists often view their resorting to force as a professional failure to handle the patient peacefully. Nevertheless, sometimes it is essential to inject patients with a drug to spare everyone—nurses, doctors, other patients in the ER, and the patient himself—from getting hurt. When subduing a dangerous patient, on rare occasions, psychiatrists in the heat of battle may pounce on a patient or slug him. The psychiatrist can often prevent everyone from being harmed by giving the assaultive patient medication relatively early before matters get out of control. The psychiatrist prefers not to be alone with a highly combative patient, but to have five huge guards beside him so that the patient sees he's being given an offer of medication he can't refuse; in this way nobody gets hurt, because the patient can take the medication without a fight and without losing face.

Suicidal patients present other problems for ER psychiatrists, but the issue of a person's "right to suicide" isn't among them. People *absolutely* determined to commit suicide do so; they don't see a psychiatrist. The only people contemplating suicide who do consult a psychiatrist are, almost by definition, *ambivalent* about suicide.* The psychiatrist's overall aim is to tip the balance by helping these patients consider issues and options they have overlooked in their suicidal ruminations.

Most of the suicidal patients psychiatrists see in the ER suffer from various types of serious depression, schizophrenia, alcoholism, early dementia, adjustment reactions of adolescence, bereavement, or other major losses. Consequently, they have not,

---

*About 50 percent of patients who kill themselves have visited their physician within three months of committing suicide, usually with vague complaints of physical symptoms, depression, and hopelessness. At this point they are on the verge of considering suicide or are highly ambivalent about it; in either case, they are reaching out to the physician for help.

as is widely believed, "run out of options." The patient might feel that way and even say so, but his condition so clutters his thinking that he can't see his options. Every psychiatrist has been thanked by countless patients who were glad the shrink cared enough to stop them.

Obsessed with why they should die, suicidal patients lose sight of a reason they should live—something the ER psychiatrist tries to find for the patient. For example, after days of thinking about killing himself, a student decided to see a psychiatrist, who happened to be me, at a nearby hospital's emergency room. During the past four months, his father had died, his apartment had been burglarized, he had lost a scholarship, his girlfriend had dumped him, he had lost $5,000 worth of negotiable bonds in the mail, and two days previously, his mother had died. Eventually, I asked him, "Given all the miserable things happening to you, how come you haven't already killed yourself?" He was stunned; the question had never occurred to him. After thinking awhile, he whimsically, yet seriously, explained, "Look, I would have done myself in long ago, but the only thing that keeps me going is that I can't wait to find out what dreadful thing will happen next. I guess I take pride in being a survivor." More than anything else, recognizing this pride and realizing its full importance are what pulled him through the crisis.

Ironically, although critics continually charge that psychiatrists hospitalize too many people, in reality their biggest problem is getting patients admitted. The average occupancy rate for all American psychiatric hospitals in 1979 was 85 percent; in Manhattan in 1982 it was over 92 percent, and in five major Manhattan hospitals it was over 100 percent. I had a patient who, in the space of a week, set three fires in his mother's home, was rescued twice by the police when he threatened to jump from a seventh-story window, and was caught running naked on Madison Avenue in mid-January. During this week he was dragged to four different emergency rooms, where his mother, who was recovering from a stroke, was told that her son wasn't sick enough to justify hospitalization, "especially since we have to keep our one available bed open for real emergencies."

A family member cannot merely sign a few papers to commit a kooky, or even a truly mentally ill, relative to a psychiatric hospital. In most states, patients can be hospitalized against their will only if they are in immediate danger of harming themselves or others. Although psychiatrists are better at predicting suicide than homicide, in any one case, the psychiatrist has no surefire way of predicting either. As a result, because attorneys who defend patients' rights are on the premises of most psychiatric hospitals, attorneys can spring most patients from the hospital unless the psychiatrist can present a judge with compelling evidence that the patient is dangerous.

The civil-libertarian concern over patients' being "hospitalized against their will" assumes the patient is relatively rational. To see if this assumption was merited, Dr. Howard Owens and I studied the forms that psychiatric patients in New York State must fill out indicating the reasons they wish to hospitalize themselves voluntarily. Half the reasons made sense. The other half did not: "I want to be in the hospital to get my shoes shined," or "I like flowers," or "My teeth need fixing." If this is voluntary—and legally it is—then what is voluntary and involuntary makes little sense.

A major decision a psychiatrist makes in an emergency room is whether to hospitalize someone. Very often the psychiatrist has just met the patient and does not have enough time to do a thorough evaluation. Even when the psychiatrist does know the patient and has had weeks to consider hospitalization, the decision can still be difficult because there are so many psychological, social, familial, ethical, legal, occupational, clinical, administrative, and financial considerations.

PSYCHIATRIC HOSPITALIZATION

In 1979, the average daily census for all American psychiatric hospitals was 233,384. Of these, 59 percent were in state hospitals, 12 percent in Veterans Administration Hospitals, 10 percent in general hospitals, 6 percent in private psychiatric hospitals, and 4 percent in Community Mental Health Centers; the remainder were in residential treatment facilities like those for children and the retarded. Thus, although from 1969 to 1979 the number of patients residing in state hospitals declined by 60 percent and increased in general hospitals by 30 percent, a majority of psychiatric inpatients are still *lodged* in state hospitals.

In contrast, slightly more psychiatric patients are *admitted* to general, and private mental, hospitals than to state hospitals. That's largely because a higher proportion of the chronically ill are admitted to state hospitals and remain there much longer, whereas a patient's first few hospitalizations are more likely to be in facilities other than state hospitals.

Psychiatrists do not like to hospitalize patients, mainly because when this occurs they are seeing someone they know in severe pain. Some psychiatrists also feel they have failed if they must hospitalize one of their outpatients. Hospitalizing a patient is surely no sign of success—at best, it is nobody's fault; at worst, it is the psychiatrist's fault. Therefore, a psychiatrist may feel vulnerable whenever he admits a patient, since the hospital staff might think he has botched the job.*

The desire of psychiatrists and patients to avoid hospitalization is understandable, but not always justified. Inpatient treatment can accomplish many things that outpatient treatment cannot: Better evaluation can be done because the patient is being monitored continually and by a variety of mental health professionals; treatment can be more intensive, frequent, and varied; medications too risky to start on outpatients can be safely started with inpatients.

Although it is widely assumed that being admitted may affect the patient's career, social standing, and self-esteem, very often *not* admitting the patient does more harm. Not uncommonly, a patient's major depression so diminishes his productivity at work that eventually he's fired; but if he had been hospitalized earlier, his job could have been saved.

Patients often worry that hospitalization will hurt their future employment, yet in my experience, that's infrequent. If a patient has a job and is then hospitalized, the psychiatrist will get the patient's permission to speak with his employer. The psychiatrist usually tells the boss, "Mr. Smith has had a depression that caused his work to fall off. Fortunately, there is good treatment for depression and he was smart enough to get it. He will be discharged soon, and I'm sure you'll notice that he and his work are

---

*For psychiatrists in private practice, hospitalizing a patient is often a hassle that is without commensurate financial renumeration; moreover, with many hospitals, especially in academic centers, the patient's private psychiatrist must hand over control of the patient's hospital treatment to the psychiatrists working full-time on the unit.

markedly improved. Treat him normally, and don't worry about saying the wrong thing. Do that, and Mr. Smith will do just fine.'' If given the chance, employers like doing well by the patient as long as it doesn't interfere with work.

When hospitalized patients lose or can't get a job, it's usually because of how they *behave* and not because they were hospitalized or have a psychiatric diagnosis. All too often patients invoke the stigma of mental illness and of psychiatric hospitalization as an excuse for being unemployed. These stigmas surely cause some patients to lose jobs, but not nearly as often as patients claim. If patients act normal, they will be treated normally; if they act like mental patients, they will be treated like mental patients. Meanwhile, since these stigmas do exist, most psychiatrists tell patients to avoid mentioning their illness and hospitalization, and some psychiatrists, myself included, have no qualms about a patient's lying, if—and I stress *if*—he has good reason to do so. (Today it is illegal to ask potential employees if they have a history of mental illness.)

The first time patients are admitted to a psychiatric hospital they invariably ask these questions and receive these answers:

Q: Can I have visitors?

A: Yes, but only during visiting hours. Visitors are restricted only if the patient doesn't want any or in the unusual situation when the staff feels a particular visit would harm the patient.

Q: Are the doors locked?

A: The chances are fifty-fifty. Private hospitals, especially those which accept only voluntary admissions, have fewer locked doors than public hospitals. In reality, whether the doors are locked is not that important, since even on "open-door" units, patients cannot leave unless they have the staff's approval. The patient's potential dangerousness determines if he is permitted to leave the unit, and if so, with whom (e.g., nurses, other patients, relatives, by himself).

Q: Can I get a weekend pass to go home?

A: In most hospitals you can, but usually nearer the end of hospitalization to prepare for discharge.

Q: Can I go to work while hospitalized?

A: This depends on the hospital, the patient, and the job. If the patient is always at a daytime job he will miss most of the hospital's treatment. Patients can usually return to work when the staff feels they are in less need of daytime treatment, and are ready to focus more on readjusting to life in the community.

Q: What do you wear as a patient?

A: Street clothes. Some staff wear street clothes, others wear medical garb.

Q: What is the average length of stay?

A: For patients having their first psychiatric hospitalization, about 30 percent are discharged within a week and 80 percent within a month. While almost half the admissions to state hospitals stay twenty-nine or more days, half the admissions to public general hospitals stay seven days or less. This last statistic is deceptively low, since many admissions are for detoxification of drugs or alcohol, which requires only several days. On the other hand, for treating a major depression, the most common reason for first-time admissions to a psychiatric hospital, the average stay is around twenty-two days.

Q: Would it help to stay longer?

A: Probably not. Research conducted during the 1970s convincingly showed that in the first year or two following a patient's release, his adjustment to community life, the severity of his symptoms, and the chances of his readmission were the same whether he was hospitalized for three weeks or for three months.*

Q: Will I have my own room?

---

*Another distinction between psychoanalytic and scientific psychiatry is that formerly it was axiomatic among psychiatrists that the longer a patient's hospitalization the more beneficial the treatment. In contrast, scientific psychiatrists no longer believe that, when hospitalizing patients, "length equals strength."

A: Probably not, but you might. It depends on the hospital. Most often patients shared a room with another patient, although it's common to have anything from zero to five roommates.

Q: Are the wards co-ed?

A: Yes.

Q: What kind of patients are on this ward?

A: In 1975, the primary *(DSM-II)* diagnosis for all psychiatric inpatients were as follows: 27 percent were schizophrenic, 25 percent were depressed, 19 percent were alcoholic, and the rest were divided equally between "personality disorders," "neuroses," and "organic brain syndromes." Private and general hospitals have relatively more patients with depression, whereas state hospitals have relatively more patients with schizophrenia. Patients often find that how comfortable they feel with other patients relates more to social class than to diagnosis.

Q: But are the patients dangerous?

A: Not really. If a patient does pose a serious threat, he is transferred to a special unit for violent patients or he is monitored continuously by a nurse, or if necessary, a guard.

Q: What type of therapy will I receive?

A: The quality and types of therapy differ enormously depending on the unit, the patient, his diagnosis, and his circumstances. On a reasonably good unit, a patient may receive individual psychotherapy three times a week, group therapy twice a week, family or couples therapy once a week, and occupational or recreational therapy every day. Once or twice a week, all patients and staff meet to discuss problems that affect everyone. Eighty to 90 percent of patients receive psychotropic medication.

Q: Do I have to take medication?

A: Although the law is in flux, in general a psychiatrist can force you to take medications only in an emergency.

Q: Must I attend therapies that involve other patients, such as group or occupational therapy?

A: On most units there is some flexibility, but in general patients are required to attend most therapeutic activities. Initially, many patients are reluctant, and some even refuse, to discuss their problems with other patients. Quite soon, however, they get to know their fellow patients, find them sympathetic and supportive, and feel comfortable talking to most of them. You would be silly not to attend these activities. If you wish, you can just listen; you are under no obligation to reveal anything that you feel is personally sensitive.

Q: Who will be my psychiatrist?

A: Either your outpatient psychiatrist or a psychiatrist who works full-time in the hospital. In academic centers, he is often a resident in the first year of his psychiatric training. Although relatively inexperienced, he is carefully supervised by a senior psychiatrist.

Q: Will my psychiatrist conduct all the treatment?

A: No. After discussions with you and the staff, your psychiatrist determines your overall treatment program, orders laboratory tests, prescribes medication, and performs some of your individual psychotherapy. Psychologists may do psychological tests, psychiatric social workers will keep in touch with your relatives and conduct family/couples therapy, and any of these professionals, as well as nurses, occupational therapists, and recreational therapists, will provide some of the individual and group psychotherapy.

Q: Will I be cured by the time I leave the hospital?

A: No. In general, the chief criterion for discharging a patient is his ability to reenter the community. After hospitalization, you will still need treatment, but it should start before you're released. Outpatient treatment will consolidate the many gains you have made in the hospital and resolve the problems that remain.

COMMUNITY MENTAL HEALTH

During the past three decades, public psychiatry has emphasized treating patients in the community, and whenever possible, on an ambulatory basis. Yet this would never have become a widespread reality if it weren't for the Community Mental Health Centers Act of 1963. Pushed through Congress by President Kennedy, the act helped to refurbish state hospitals, to train ancillary personnel, and to aid the mentally retarded. However, the centerpiece of this legislation was the nationwide establishment of Community Mental Health Centers (CMHCs), each center servicing 70,000 to 200,000 people.*

CMHCs do not offer new types of treatment, but new ways of delivering and paying for them. This is no mean feat. The establishment of CMHCs has made it possible for millions of low- and middle-income people to receive high-quality psychiatric care. Indeed, there is probably a CMHC serving you right now, whether you know it or want it. For the first time, CMHCs provided this country's over two million chronic schizophrenics an excellent treatment alternative to warehousing in state mental hospitals.

Psychiatrists provide the same treatments inside CMHCs as they do outside them. By law, CMHCs offer five services: (1) inpatient, (2) outpatient, (3) partial, or day, hospitalization, (4) emergency care, and (5) consultation and education. Some CMHCs also provide child, drug and alcohol, and geriatric services. These services, while usually under the direction of a psychiatrist, are frequently offered by other mental health professionals.

CMHCs try to prevent and to reduce the damaging effects of mental disorders by being convenient geographically and economically, by affording consultation and education to community groups, by detecting and averting potential psychiatric problems (e.g., spotting and treating child abuse), and by integrating the services of general hospitals, state hospitals, CMHCs, ERs, day or night hospitals, and outpatient clinics.

---

*CMHCs provide treatment for mental disorders. They do not, however, provide mental health, since nobody knows what mental health is. Certainly a more accurate term for CMHCs would be "Community Mental Disorders Centers," but that might not induce people to seek their services. Semantics aside, the first-line providers of community mental health are hairdressers and bartenders; only their "failures" go to CMHCs.

This integration function is critical, because psychiatry's private sector can never be more than a hodgepodge of services. Anytime a patient enters any inpatient or outpatient facility in the geographical jurisdiction of a CMHC, the CMHC can offer the patient a full range of follow-up services. On the other hand, a private psychiatrist does not always have access to hospital beds, occupational training centers, emergency services, or day hospitals.

THE STATUS OF PUBLIC PSYCHIATRY

The emergence of CMHCs and the scientific psychiatry which made them possible have greatly improved the status of public psychiatry within the profession. During the era of psychoanalytic psychiatry, a shrink's status was directly related to how much insight-oriented psychotherapy he conducted. Since many patients seen in public psychiatry are too ill for this type of therapy, public psychiatry held little appeal for the self-respecting psychiatrist.

The launching of CMHCs soon after 1963 started to change the profession's attitudes toward public psychiatry. CMHCs were a new source of money, which medical schools could now use to expand their departments of psychiatry. Consequently, those working in public psychiatry often had academic affiliations, which they had not had before.

Yet the big change in attitude evolved as scientific psychiatry evolved. Today, psychiatrists are interested by more than insight-oriented psychotherapy; they value many professional activities and therapeutic interventions. Those working in public psychiatry, especially in CMHCs, find it exciting to manage crises and to handle emergencies. Public psychiatrists have many more opportunities to practice the medical side of psychiatry, something the profession values more than ever. Psychiatrists intrigued by the careful use of *DSM-III* diagnosis and of psychotropic medications find these tasks more germane to public than to private psychiatry. Although the patients in public psychiatry may be sicker than those in private practice, the psychiatrist still gets to work with the relatively healthy families of such patients.*

---

*Dr. Marge Smith has observed that CMHCs have changed how psychiatrists view family members. In the 1920s and 1930s, the days when a Jimmy Stewart

Beyond strictly clinical considerations, psychiatrists interested in politics and government are right in the thick of it when they work in public psychiatry. That is especially true for psychiatrists in top administrative positions; they tend to have relatively lower status in academia, but any day they can pick up a newspaper and read about themselves or their programs. And if they pick up today's newspaper, they are bound to read about the biggest social controversy in modern psychiatry:

DE-INSTITUTIONALIZATION AND THE HOMELESS

The purpose of de-institutionalization was to avoid the adverse effects of chronic state hospitalization by keeping and treating patients, whenever possible, in the community. By decreasing the number of patients in state hospitals, money spent on state hospitalization could be reallocated to outpatient clinics. In principle, de-institutionalization was a fine idea; in practice, the public and even many psychiatrists feel it was a noble enterprise that flopped.

More specifically, popular gospel holds that state hospitals suddenly dumped patients onto the community, and then, because of a lack of government money and poor planning by psychiatrists, community-based treatment facilities could not handle the onslaught of discharged mental patients. As a result, hordes of prematurely released mental patients have been roaming the streets, picking at garbage cans, accosting children, and sleeping in alleys. There emerged a new social malady—the homeless. If the mental health system would do its job correctly, the homeless would disappear. But since the mental health system has merely substituted alleys for hospitals, de-institutionalization is a failed policy.

The problem with this gospel is that it rests on three false assumptions.

The first is that most of the homeless are psychiatric patients. In 1981 a study of the homeless at New York City's men's shel-

---

would talk to a rabbit named Harvey, psychiatrists saw family members as *victims*. During the psychoanalytic era, especially from 1940 to 1975 or so, psychiatrists viewed family members as *perpetrators* of the patient's illness. Today, as psychiatrists struggle to maintain patients in the community, they desperately need families to take care of the patient, and so they tend to view family members as *saviors*.

ters revealed that only a third were ever admitted to a psychiatric hospital, and only 22 percent of the total group had ever been admitted to a state mental hospital. Of this 22 percent, about half were released more than five years before the survey. Only 15 percent of the total were felt to be homeless because of mental problems, whereas nearly a third had severe chronic medical problems. Two thirds seriously abused drugs or alcohol; over half had been in jail, and about a quarter had been imprisoned for major offenses. Studies throughout the country show similar findings. Thus, contrary to myth, most of the homeless are *not* former mental patients.

The second myth is that state hospitals suddenly flooded the community with large numbers of mental patients. In truth, state hospital populations were gradually dwindling ever since Thorazine was introduced in 1954, and then there was a somewhat steeper decline from about 1968 to 1975, at which point the census in state hospitals leveled off. While state hospital populations were diminishing, admissions to all kinds of psychiatric facilities were rapidly increasing. Thus, although exceptions exist, state hospitals did not suddenly dump masses of patients into the community.

Myth number three is that the homeless emerged primarily because of de-institutionalization. The facts, however, are that the problem of the homeless arose long after de-institutionalization had run its course. For example, in New York State, de-institutionalization had been completed by 1973–74, the very same years that the population of New York's homeless was at its lowest! It wasn't until 1979 that the number of homeless began to climb, and in 1982, the number shot up. Thus, although the problem of the homeless is genuine, it was not caused by de-institutionalization.

The Director of Quality Assurance for the New York State Department of Mental Hygiene, Dr. Stanley Hoffman, suggests that the number of homeless began to rise in 1979 mainly because of the oil crisis: People started to abandon the automobile and to leave suburbia for the cities (i.e., "regentrification"); in turn, up went the cost of urban housing and down went the number of single-room occupancies in which the poor and marginally adjusted had lived. Hence, the homeless. In 1982, reductions in federal social programs made matters worse.

Since most of the homeless are not mental patients and de-institutionalization has had little to do with the problem, it seems that mental patients and mental health systems are being blamed for problems which are principally due to social and economic dislocations.

In no way does this mitigate the serious lack of funding for treating the severely ill. State hospitals, which house over half of all chronic schizophrenics, cannot provide decent care when, as typically happens, there is one psychiatrist for over 200 patients. Properly taking care of these patients, therefore, is as much a problem of politics and economics as it is of psychiatry.

At the same time, even with enough money, it is not true that all state mental hospitals could be closed and everybody could be treated in the community. It can't be done, at least not yet. We don't possess enough basic knowledge of how to treat schizophrenics, who are the vast majority of state hospital residents.

Unfortunately, much of the debate over de-institutionalization has focused on *where* these patients are treated—in state hospitals or in community clinics—which is more a political than a psychiatric issue. Instead, the key therapeutic question is *how* to treat these patients, and the key answers will come not from the politics of public psychiatry, but from the investigations of psychiatric research.

Finally, it would be a mistake to assume that de-institutionalization has failed. Problems with it surely exist, but still, most patients discharged from state mental hospitals are not begging on street corners. Yes, many have repeated and brief hospitalizations, which have given rise to the "revolving-door" phenomenon. And yes, many of these patients do not obtain proper treatment in the community. Yet, for all its many deficiencies, the policy of de-institutionalization has spared millions from becoming the emotionally blunted, socially inept, and behaviorally unappealing creatures that once crammed our state hospitals.

NINE

How Psychiatrists Feel About Patients

"Doc, you gotta fix me," Jack Jonas demanded. "I've been waking up and hitting my wife with a pillow for absolutely no reason; once I even used a lamp. This oughta stop, don't you think?" As his new psychiatrist, I agreed.

"You better be straight with me," he continued. "We American Nazis ain't stupid. Two weeks ago we made forty dollars selling swastikas to Yale kids. With the money we bought and painted lampshades with the words 'official Jew skin' on them." He smiled.

Fumbling for words, I pointed out, "Excuse me, Mr. Jonas, but in all fairness, you should know that I'm Jewish. I wonder if you'd feel more comfortable with a non-Jewish therapist."

"Hell no, that doesn't matter. You're a doctor." With that reassurance, the Nazi and the Jew began therapy.

Jack was all contradiction. Since when do Nazis seek psychotherapy—and with a Jew, no less? He looked like a contradiction. Like a truck with twinkling headlights, his soft, babylike features did not belong on his dumpy frame. Although twenty-seven years old, he spoke with the enthusiasm and naïveté of an adolescent. "I love my job. You might say I'm a specialist mechanic: I fix engines, especially the big motherfuckers. I'm damn good at it, too! Haven't missed a day since I dropped out of [high] school. Engines keep the trucks rolling, and that keeps America rolling.

The future lies in transportation." Jack meant everything he said.

With the same youthful zeal, he was a thoroughly egalitarian racist. Trying to win my approval by showing an interest in medicine, he said with pride, "Doc, I've invented a transplant toy. You can put together the arm of a nigger, the leg of a spic, the balls of a kike—any combination you like. The thing I like best is pulling it apart."

My stomach growled. I could not believe Jack was for real, but he was and very much in earnest. He spoke of his transplant toy as a child shows off his very first bike. Meanwhile, I was wondering how I could help this baboon without becoming a lampshade. My goose pimples were on the march, spurred less by his lurid descriptions than by his total obliviousness to his effect on me. Finally he noticed I didn't share his enthusiasm, and that disappointed him.

As if nothing had happened, he went on to explain why he had created the transplant toy. "My dad invented things and wanted me to do the same. He was quite a guy. Taught me fishing, how to shoot. Taught me how to fuck till a bitch's eyes bleed. Sorry, doc. The point is, we did everything together. Mom died when I was born, so Dad raised me all by himself. He did absolutely everything for me—everything. He hated Jews, but he'd work for them because I needed clothes. Five years ago I needed a kidney transplant and he gave me his."

His voice softened. "Then he got an infection and died."

Jack looked very alone, and he cried.

PERSONAL AND PROFESSIONAL VIEWS OF PATIENTS

Personally I felt Jack was a slime; *professionally* I not only felt comfortable treating him, I enjoyed doing so. I'm sure many psychiatrists would feel the same. For psychiatrists, such conflicting personal and professional views may coexist, each at a different level; to understand how this occurs is to appreciate some of the complexities of how psychiatrists feel about patients.

As doctors, psychiatrists are trained to heal and not to judge. They are accustomed to putting aside their personal feelings about patients, and do so more from reflexive habit than from conscious effort. Therefore, automatically bracketing off my contempt toward Jack came naturally. At the time, I was fully aware I detested him, but as best I can tell, it never interfered with his treatment.

Personal feelings, especially negative ones, can always contaminate a psychiatrist's therapeutic endeavors. When the psychiatrist's feelings toward a patient are hazy, the psychiatrist may find it difficult to see how they are affecting therapy. But in Jack's case, my personal feelings toward him were so blatantly clear, I had no trouble knowing what they were and making sure they did not interfere with treatment.

More traditional psychiatrists would insist that my even calling Jack a "slime" was, as a colleague of mine said, "unprofessional and a problem of countertransference, since Jack is not a slime; he is sick." Yet other psychiatrists, myself included, would say that Jack is a slime *and* sick. We do not consider *everything* distasteful about patients to be psychopathology; we still make personal judgments about patients, and still have personal feelings about them as people. Like all psychiatrists, we strive not to let these personal feelings and judgments harm treatment. (On those rare occasions when a psychiatrist believes that his personal feelings toward a patient will significantly interfere with treatment, the psychiatrist is ethically bound to send the patient to another therapist.) What concerns psychiatrists is not that they have personal feelings about a patient—it's hard not to—but that they are unaware of these feelings; when this occurs, not only can these feelings interfere with treatment, but the psychiatrist cannot use them as data about the patient's psychology in order to facilitate therapy.

A psychiatrist's personal feelings about a patient do not automatically determine the outcome of therapy. The psychiatrist can so like a patient that he overlooks the patient's difficulties and deficiencies. Conversely, a therapist may detest a patient, but help him. For instance, Jack Jonas's treatment, whose sole aim was to stop his violent sleepwalking but *not* his bigotry, was a complete success.*

---

*Rightly or not, I did not treat his racism for three reasons. First, racism is not a mental disorder, nor, by itself, a symptom of one. It is a belief system, from which (I feel) none of us is totally immune. Like many psychiatrists, I'm not eager to alter people's belief systems, no matter how offensive. Second, had I even wanted to "treat" his racism, I wouldn't know how. There's no good evi-

I've heard many people say, "I really wish I knew how my psychiatrist feels about me. Yet because he is a psychiatrist, he won't give me a straight answer." There is, however, a straight answer: *In most situations, how the psychiatrist feels about a patient is the same as how the patient feels about his psychiatrist.* By the end of treatment, Jack felt about me as I felt about him: We liked each other, but only in a professional context.

WHAT PSYCHIATRISTS LIKE IN PATIENTS

Psychiatrists do not either like or dislike patients. Instead, they like patients in a variety of personal and professional ways, each for different reasons. In general, a psychiatrist's personal views about a patient are based on standards similar to those he uses in choosing friends, whereas his professional outlook on a patient hinges on whether the patient gets better.

In these respects, Jack's case is dramatic. Although personally I felt him despicable, to my great surprise, I ended up liking him. Why? Because he made me feel I was an effective therapist. Was my professional ego that desperate? I'm afraid so. However, I'm not alone.

Psychologist Dr. William Schofield surveyed 377 psychotherapists from various disciplines—psychiatry, psychology, and psychiatric social work—and he consistently found that therapists best liked patients for whom they felt their therapy was highly effective. In other words, for the psychiatrist, *the Good Patient is the one who makes him feel like a Good Therapist.*

Schofield also showed that psychotherapists strongly preferred patients with the "YAVIS syndrome"—young, attractive, verbal, intelligent, successful. Being relatively healthy, YAVIS patients offer therapists a virtually guaranteed success. Almost by definition, insight-oriented psychotherapy works best for patients who are verbal and intelligent.

In former years many psychiatrists assumed that insight-oriented psychotherapy also worked best for younger patients. Psy-

---

dence that psychiatric treatment of any kind cures racism. Third, although as a physician I feel ethically bound to treat his mental disorder, I feel under no ethical obligation to devote the many years it might take to change his deeply racist personality; I'd rather spend the time helping anyone but Jack.

chiatrists widely felt that by the time a person turns forty, he has become so rigid he cannot change through psychotherapy. Few modern psychiatrists would make this claim, and even fewer would make it in public. Nevertheless, psychiatrists still believe that younger patients are more interesting in psychotherapy, and despite any hard evidence, psychiatrists believe that younger patients do better in psychotherapy. Finally, psychiatrists enjoy treating younger patients because they like being a mentor—half teacher, half parent.

Another reason for the YAVIS syndrome is that psychiatrists, like most people, prefer being associated with people they find personally appealing—the "reading class," intellectuals, artists, celebrities, writers, politicians, and the successful. When treating society's powerful and important, the psychiatrist feels that he himself becomes more powerful and important.

Scientific psychiatry has diminished the influence of the YAVIS syndrome. Schofield published his findings during the heyday of psychoanalysis when the only treatment psychiatrists valued was insight-oriented psychotherapy. If a patient was not endowed with the characteristics of being a good psychotherapy case, such as having the YAVIS syndrome, he had far less chance of being liked by his therapist. Today, however, because scientific psychiatrists feel they have many first-rate treatments from which patients get better, psychiatrists like treating many more patients without the YAVIS syndrome. For example, scientific psychiatrists are very gratified by patients, such as the elderly, not psychologically minded lady who recovers from panic attacks with tricyclics, systematic desensitization, and supportive psychotherapy.

Initially, psychiatrists prefer patients with a background and interests similar to their own. They are people the shrink would like as friends. Yet over the long haul, this matters less.

Therapists become fascinated when a patient describes a job, a life-style, an experience, or anything about a world that is foreign to the therapist. Patients charm psychiatrists by making delightful observations that would never occur to the psychiatrist. I recall a thirty-two-year-old woman who, after weighing 275 pounds, had part of her bowel surgically removed; six months later she weighed 140 pounds. Although her dramatic weight loss was ostensibly desirable, she became depressed; she suddenly found it hard to adjust to her new image. For the first time in her life, men were attracted to her, and she felt painfully awkward in dealing with them. In the process of talking aloud during a psychotherapy session, she observed, "Funny thing, losing all that weight: I lost one hundred and thirty-five pounds. That's a *whole person.* I wonder where that person went." It is just because this incidental remark so charmed me that, although more than a decade has passed, I continue to remember this patient vividly. She wasn't trying to endear herself to me, but she did. How? Not by self-consciously saying what she thought might interest me, but rather by talking freely about her own experiences and observations; by doing so, she afforded me a delightfully different way of looking at things.

As the psychiatrist gets to know a patient better, he starts seeing traits he admires within the patient, such as taking himself seriously but not too seriously, seeming authentic, having the courage to risk change, displaying integrity and a sense of humor, exhibiting self-criticism along with self-respect, appreciating arts or current events, and being able to forgive.

As discussed in Chapter 7, psychiatrists like patients who examine issues psychologically and not judgmentally. If a psychiatrist observes, "You seem upset every time I mention your father," he prefers a patient who becomes psychologically curious about his reactions, as opposed to the patient who closes off psychological exploration by moralistic responses, such as "I guess that means I'm bad."

Psychiatrists like patients who work hard in therapy, those who, for example, make it their business to think about therapy between hours and to arrive at sessions prepared to discuss these thoughts. (Some patients actually schedule time to think solely about therapy.) Psychiatrists get annoyed when they ask a patient, "How did you feel about our last meeting?" and the patient replies, "I really hadn't thought about it." The psychiatrist's chief concern is what accounts for the patient's apparent uninvolvement in therapy. Beyond this, however, the psychiatrist may feel put down, believing he has failed to engage the patient sufficiently in psychotherapy.

Therapists respect patients who use their time with the psychiatrist to focus on problems, instead of trying to amuse, impress, or seduce him. Psychiatrists like patients whose approach to therapy is "I can't do much to change others, but I can change myself.'' Therapists much prefer patients who take it upon themselves to raise issues in therapy and not wait for a therapist to lead them by the nose. Regardless of the type of therapy, psychiatrists like patients who take responsibility for their treatment and for themselves.

WHAT PSYCHIATRISTS DISLIKE IN PATIENTS

I'm reluctant to discuss this topic. Repeatedly, I've seen my friends and acquaintances who are in therapy become self-conscious when I start mentioning the traits psychiatrists find objectionable in patients; they wonder if their shrink thinks they have these traits. Although everyone assumes that psychiatrists would not like certain qualities in patients, making this explicit frequently alienates laymen from psychiatrists. When a psychiatrist says patients can be obnoxious, laymen often respond, ''Well, I hope *my* shrink doesn't find *me* obnoxious,'' or ''Who in hell is a psychiatrist to call anyone obnoxious? Psychiatrists should like their patients, not put them down!'' That's reasonable: Nobody wants a therapist who dislikes them.

Nevertheless, this kind of response suggests the layman doesn't understand what a psychiatrist means when he says a patient is ''obnoxious''; moreover, the layman is certainly missing the spirit in which the psychiatrist says this. When therapists dislike particular traits in a patient, that does not mean they dislike the patient. Right now I'm thinking of a patient whose obsessiveness really bugs me, but she has so many other fine qualities, I'm always glad to see her.

More important, when a psychiatrist dislikes something about a patient, the psychiatrist does not think less of the patient; rarely does this thought ever occur to him. Instead, after the psychiatrist makes sure that the problem lies with the patient and not himself, he focuses all his energies on trying to figure out why this trait exists—that is, what psychological, biological, or social factors produced it

The major point that laymen overlook when a psychiatrist finds unlikable traits in a patient is that the shrink views the finding less as a criticism of the patient and more as a mystery to be solved— the mystery being why the patient acts this way. When a psychiatrist responds to information judgmentally and not psychologically, he stops being therapeutic. My feeling that Jack Jonas was a slime was not unprofessional—feelings are feelings and mandating them away doesn't make them disappear. But if I had treated Jack as a slime, that would have been unprofessional.

An extreme situation

It is rare for psychiatrists to be so provoked by a patient that they abandon all their professionalism. Nevertheless, it happened with Harold, a twenty-eight-year-old outpatient with the diagnosis of borderline personality disorder. Patients with this diagnosis habitually worship, then denigrate people, including therapists. Therefore, Harold's psychiatrist, Dr. Sebastian, had grown accustomed to Harold's unrelenting harangues that he was insensitive, dumb, and useless. After two years of outpatient psychotherapy, these harangues turned vicious. At three o'clock every morning Harold would telephone Sebastian and inquire, "Did I wake you? Sorry." At first, Sebastian behaved professionally; he tried to figure out why Harold was escalating his offensiveness. Harold started making twenty calls a day to clog up Sebastian's telephone-answering machine. Soon after Sebastian brought a new oriental rug into his office, Harold "accidentally" spilled coffee on it. Sebastian clung to being professional. A week later, however, Sebastian's father died, and Sebastian told Harold that he would be away for several days. Harold immediately responded by joking about dead fathers, about Sebastian "fucking" his father, wanting him dead, and so on. Sebastian blew his cool. "Enough. You're being a shit, and I don't give a damn why." Harold was startled and began to apologize. Sebastian interrupted, "Don't bother."

In discussing this episode with colleagues, Dr. Sebastian explained, "Harold obviously got under my skin, and however understandable my behavior, it was still unprofessional, and therefore wrong. Sometimes—although far less than on *Marcus Welby*—an outburst such as mine may turn a patient around. But not Harold; he was too impaired. After this episode, therapy degenerated altogether. I hope I never have another outburst, but if a similar situation arose and I found myself about to get vindictive, I'd try to cool myself off, and if I couldn't, I'd end the session before I said something I'd later regret."

The typical dislikes

There's an old psychiatrist's joke in which the shrink is asked by a friend, "How can you stand listening to patients all day?" The psychiatrist replies, "Who listens?" With boring patients, that's what happens: The psychiatrist doesn't listen.

Patients who bore psychiatrists don't realize their ramblings are of absolutely no interest to the psychiatrist. When a psychiatrist asks if he checked the want ads, the bore doesn't just say yes but details all thirty-seven of them. The shrink drifts off as the bore once again explains that her husband married her because "he thought I was the most beautiful girl in the world." For all practical purposes, the bore talks to himself, leading the psychiatrist to feel useless.

The ultimate bore may have been the man whose chart (which I reviewed) read, "Except for a minute each visit, the patient hasn't spoken in fifteen sessions. He claims he has nothing to say, but enjoys coming." A few patients will plop themselves into a chair, say little, and wait for the psychiatrist to fill all silences; constantly trying to extract information, the psychiatrist begins to feel like a dentist. Eventually, the psychiatrist can't figure out what the patient wants him to do, or for that matter, why he's bothering to see a psychiatrist at all. Feeling ineffective and drained, the psychiatrist worries that he's seeing the bore only for the money.

Patients often express concern that they are boring their psychiatrist. "You must have heard this story a thousand times." "I guess I'm not a very interesting case." In my experience, few patients bore their psychiatrist, and certainly far fewer than the number who worry about it. Moreover, patients who fret about being boring aren't boring; the occasional patient who is boring seems oblivious to the fact.

If a patient wonders if he is boring his psychiatrist, he should bring this up during a session. Some therapists might say, "No, not at all." Others might ask, "I wonder why you feel that way?," and if the patient replies, "You keep dozing off," the patient has good reason to be distressed—and to get another psychiatrist. Far more often, discussing this topic uncovers concerns outside of therapy, such as with Mike, a middle-aged actor:

Mike:	I feel like I'm boring you.
Maxmen:	Why?
Mike:	It's just a feeling. Nothing specific.
Maxmen:	This must concern you.
Mike:	Sure does. Always has. As far back as I can remember I've been deathly afraid of being dull. When I was twelve, I desperately wanted to be in our [summer] camp's production of *Oklahoma!,* because I was sure that being an actor made you interesting.

When they are bored by a patient, psychiatrists ask themselves why. It might be because the patient has hit one of the psychiatrist's sore spots, causing the psychiatrist to tune out, feel bored, and initially to attribute this boredom to the patient. On the other hand, when the psychiatrist is reasonably sure it's the patient who is boring, he generates and tests psychological hypotheses to account for this. An example from later in Mike's psychotherapy:

Maxmen:	I was struck that when I asked if you were up for a part, you listed everything you auditioned for during the past year. How come?
Mike:	I thought you'd be interested.
Maxmen:	Come on, Mike. You know better than that! I think you were trying to tell me something.
Mike:	I don't think you realize how frustrating it is to be an actor—to keep going from audition to audition and to keep getting rejected. That hurts!
Maxmen:	I understand your frustration, but I don't understand why, after I ask if you're up for a role, you recite every one of your auditions.
Mike:	Now it's *you* who should know better! I want you to understand all the heartache and effort I put into my career. I want you—
Maxmen	(interrupting):—to approve of you?

Mike: Yes.

Maxmen: But this is not an audition. You don't have to win my approval, you've already got it. Were you aware of this?

Mike: Yes. (pause) I'm not sure. Maybe not. I never feel certain anyone likes me.

Maxmen: So what do you do about it?

Mike   (laughing): I bore you to death by listing two million auditions!

More distressing for the psychiatrist is the patient who continually imposes his view of the world on the psychiatrist, and when the psychiatrist doesn't agree, complains his shrink doesn't understand him. All psychiatrists are familiar with exchanges like the following:

Patient: Do you think my mother caused my depression?

Psychiatrist: She's played a big role in your depression, but I don't think she's the only cause.

Patient: If you can't see she is the cause, then you don't know the first thing about me.

In facing this kind of patient, the psychiatrist feels he's never doing anything right. The patient will arrive fifteen minutes late, and then bitch if the therapist doesn't extend the session. He may spend every visit attacking the psychiatrist's perceptiveness, intelligence, experience, sex, theory, fee, furnishings, or clothes; when the psychiatrist asks why he does this, the patient retorts, "You're being defensive."

Every psychiatrist has his soft spots, and some patients know precisely where they are. When introduced to my very first psychiatric patient, he shook my hand and asked, "When will I leave the hospital?" Having just arrived on the ward, I didn't have the foggiest idea. When I answered, "I don't know, but I could check," he replied, "Don't you know anything?" I felt like an idiot. He was right: I didn't know anything. But then, why should I? He knew I was a beginning med student and that I had just arrived.

With his radar for vulnerability, he sensed I was very insecure about my inexperience and deliberately made me uncomfortable.*

A few patients exasperate psychiatrists by habitually putting them in "no-win" situations. At times, what appears as flattery is just the opposite. A patient insisted that *every* one of my interpretations was "brilliant," thereby demeaning all of them. Another patient did nothing but demean herself. If I sympathized with her, she'd say, "You don't mean it"; if I was silent, she'd reply, "You see, I'm so despicable, even you can't stand me"; if I pointed any of this out to her, she'd confess, "You're right. I'm pathetic." There's the patient who greets every observation by the therapist with "That's so true, you know. In fact, I've already given that a great deal of thought." The shrink restrains himself from saying, "If you've already thought of everything I say, then why are you here?" Some patients will quote the psychiatrist incorrectly or out of context, and then condemn him for what he never said. If the psychiatrist tries to set the record straight, the obnoxious patient attacks the psychiatrist for being "defensive."

Contrary to what many patients believe, most psychiatrists are not angered by patients' asking for a second opinion. (If the doctor is angry, the patient needs a new shrink more than a new opinion.) Like many patients, I too had falsely assumed that my personal physician would resent my getting a second opinion. My doctor's response reassured me: As might any decent psychiatrist and physician, he said, "That's a good idea. If a second opinion will help treatment in any way, I'm all for it." It is precisely for these reasons that psychiatrists will sometimes be quite eager for a patient to obtain a second opinion; even if no new ideas come forth, at least everyone knows that what can be done is being done.

Psychiatrists become annoyed when patients engage in a "pseudotherapy," in which the patient deflects every sensitive issue by endlessly discussing and debating irrelevent intellectualisms. The ones I hear most are drugs versus talk, the right to suicide, biological versus psychological causes of mental illness, and the pros and cons of different therapies. Pseudotherapy often

---

*Whatever his other motives, this patient was testing to see if I would not crumble under his attack. When patients, especially inpatients, get a new psychiatrist, they often do this to find out if their new psychiatrist will be able to endure when things get tough.

begins with "what-if statements": "What if my wife had remained, I bet I'd be happy with life." "What if I were born rich." Mitchell, a middle-aged man, kept skirting any discussion of a job he had lost the day before.

Maxmen: How do you feel about losing your job?

Mitchell: I don't know.

Maxmen: But surely you know what your *feelings* are.

Mitchell: No. But I do wonder about a lot of things. I mean what if I lived under socialism; there, everyone works. If this were a socialist country, I would still have my job. Don't you think socialism is good for mental health?

Maxmen: I don't know.

Mitchell: The problem in America is that bosses run everything, just like my father tried to run me. I have an authority problem.

Maxmen (finding Mitchell's "insight" too pat): But you've *just* lost your job. I realize it might be hard to discuss, but you still haven't said how you feel.

Mitchell: That doesn't matter. What's important is that I get to the root of my problem—my father.

To be sure, Mitchell's relationship to his father had led to authority problems, but at this moment, he was focusing on that relationship as pseudotherapy to avoid discussing his more immediate and painful feelings about the job.

DO PSYCHIATRISTS TAKE A PERSONAL INTEREST IN PATIENTS?

The answer, of course, is yes, but how much and in what way are the real questions; their answers depend in part on the psychiatrist, but also on what the patient means by "personal interest." It could mean being his psychiatrist's favorite patient; or the psychiatrist's worrying about him if he misses an appointment; or the psychiatrist's liking him as a friend; or his case being so fascinating that the therapist discusses it with colleagues or writes about it in a professional journal. Since there are numerous dimensions to whether a psychiatrist takes a personal interest in a patient, when patients do raise the issue, many therapists will reply, "I'll answer your question, but first I'd like to know what you mean by 'taking a personal interest.' If I know that, I can give a better answer."

It's unusual, though not unknown, for patients to confront psychiatrists with this question explicitly, but they will raise it obliquely. For instance, patients will inquire why the psychiatrist is not taking notes during a session on the false assumption that the more notes a psychiatrist takes, the more the psychiatrist cares about the patient.*

When patients wonder if their psychiatrist takes a personal interest in them, some patients want to know if anything they say or do ever shocks the psychiatrist, upsets him, moves him, gets under his skin, or in any way touches him. The answer is again yes, but it's often hard for patients to know this, especially if the psychiatrist is conducting traditional insight-oriented psychotherapy. The psychiatrist will avoid saying how a patient affects him, because doing so undermines a key psychotherapeutic tool—the psychiatrist's being a "blank screen" onto which the patient projects his feelings and fantasies. (See Chapter 7.) But even when the psychiatrist is not being a blank screen, in order to maintain his objectivity he may not divulge that the patient has shocked him.

Psychiatrists are moved, shocked, amazed, disgusted, thrilled, disappointed, enchanted, and everything else by patients. Let me cite a few incidents from my own experience.

A middle-aged woman stabs herself through the heart with a knitting needle; she lies there, still very much alert, and observes, "Maybe I shouldn't knit anymore." A group therapy session of ultra-chic New Yorkers are politely discussing the "changing mores

---

*Whether taken during or after sessions, the psychiatrist's notes range from verbatim recordings to a few sentences about the hour's major themes, medication changes, side effects, or suggestions about what to do during the next meeting. In most situations, psychiatrists make notes to refresh their memories. When they record verbatim, they might well be using the notes for supervision. If patients are concerned about who other than their psychiatrist will see these notes, they should raise this concern. Increasingly, psychiatrists write notes to satisfy bureaucratic requirements and to protect themselves from lawsuits.

of male–female relationships." Quite distinct from the rest, an elderly black man from Harlem remains quiet, but is finally prodded into talking. "The real problem is that women won't blow ya," he says. Stony silence. His frankness enchants me. A young woman, friendless for years except for the animals she hallucinates, announces to me one day, "During the last six months I've made some friends, and so as of this morning, I've stopped hallucinating." That's not how hallucinations stop, but they did, and I'm astounded. After a year of intense work with a very ill young man, I was able to discharge him after fifteen years of state hospitalization. Three hours later he returned. "I can't do it," he said. "The world's too frightening." I don't cry easily, but I did then.

Very often, "taking a personal interest" means viewing the patient as a human being, and not just a bundle of psychopathology. Although psychiatrists vary, by the very nature of their work, most psychiatrists would find it extremely difficult to think of a patient as "just another case," or as just a diagnostic category, or as just a psychodynamic constellation. Don't mistake what I'm saying: Psychiatrists do think about patients as "a borderline" or as "the one with all that castration anxiety," but that is not the *only* way they think about them. If you have a close friend who is a staunch socialist, that doesn't mean it is the only way you know him; the same holds for how a psychiatrist knows a patient. Just by hearing the details of the patient's situation, the psychiatrist can't help but appreciate the uniqueness of the patient's story and personality, and therefore to see and care about him as a distinct individual.

A big pleasure in being a psychiatrist is discovering how each patient is different. I, for one, am always amazed that everyone doesn't see the world exactly as I. I can make this discovery repeatedly, especially because I am a psychiatrist; indeed, the chance to know patients as people is a major reason medical students become psychiatrists. (See Chapter 10.)

How a patient feels about his psychiatrist affects how his psychiatrist feels about him. Psychiatrists care more about patients who seem to care about them. Several times I've been hospitalized medically, and I was surprised by how much I appreciated get-well cards from patients. It's a small thing and I don't believe it influenced how I treated these patients, but for what it's worth, I felt warmer toward them.

All psychiatrists want their patients to like them for particular virtues—intelligence, loyalty, sophistication, attractiveness, warmth, wisdom. No psychiatrist is immune from simple vanity. When a shrink asked his female patient how she felt about seeing a male therapist, she said, "Oh, that makes no difference. You're not a man, you're a doctor." Half-jokingly, the psychiatrist replied, "Thanks a lot!"

Psychiatrists *do* think about their patients between sessions, but in different ways. Sometimes they entertain various psychological, biological, or social explanations to account for the patient's behavior. Sometimes they search for a way to overcome an obstacle in psychotherapy or to find an effective medication. Sometimes they wonder how crucial events between sessions turned out: Did the patient get the job he wanted? Did his long-feared family reunion go all right? Did he reveal his affair to his wife? Sometimes they dwell on a hurtful comment by the patient: "Am I really as rigid as my patient says?" "Is he partly right to accuse me of seeing him only for the money?" Sometimes they contemplate possible parallels between the patient's life and their own: "Is my dislike of my father not unlike the patient's dislike of his father?" Sometimes they reflect on their feelings toward the patient: "Am I sexually attracted to this patient? "Why can't I get this patient off of my mind?" "Am I unnerved by his homosexuality?" Sometimes they think twice about something the patient said: "What did the patient mean when he said, 'Where there's death there's hope'?" Sometimes they fantasize about being the patient's friend, lover, son, or parent. Sometimes they worry about a patient's getting worse: becoming more depressed, returning to heroin, or going psychotic. Sometimes they have the Ultimate Fear: The patient will kill himself or somebody else.

When patients are not improving, on a personal level the therapist feels bad for the patient. On a professional level, his frustration is like that of any other physician whose patient isn't improving—but with one key difference. When most doctors have, let's say, a cancer patient, they know what can and cannot be done, and once they've done everything possible, they no longer worry if they've done enough. But a psychiatrist never knows if he's done enough and can never quite shake the idea that another psychiatrist might do better.

Although psychiatrists are personally invested in their patients, this investment is not unlimited. Therapists like patients to like them, but if they don't, it's not the end of the world; the therapist's self-esteem does not hinge on the patient's approval. The reality is that the psychiatrist plays a greater role in the patient's life than the patient does in the psychiatrist's life. This inequality rubs some patients the wrong way; they insist the psychiatrist feel about them as they feel about the psychiatrist. The patient may call twice a day, or repeatedly slash his wrists, or take mild overdoses, or attend sessions while intoxicated—all in a desperate effort to gain the therapist's attention, engage his concern, possess him completely, and prevent anyone else from having him. Before matters get out of hand, the psychiatrist will try to set limits while making it clear his patience is running out. Otherwise, the therapist goes from being annoyed to being angry to being indifferent.

Psychiatrists get very uncomfortable when they reach this point, since feeling indifferent toward patients is incompatible with doing clinical practice. For any sustained period, psychiatrists cannot fake being interested in their work or in their patients; eventually, patients detect when their psychiatrists don't care. To avoid burnout and to receive any satisfaction from their work, psychiatrists have to be interested in their patients.

ARE PSYCHIATRISTS SEXUALLY ATTRACTED TO PATIENTS?

I can't say for sure, but it seems that psychiatrists are more inclined to *find* patients sexually attractive than to *be* sexually attracted to patients. I myself have never daydreamed about having sex with a patient, but I have imagined going on dates with patients and spending cozy evenings watching TV with them. However dull, my fantasy life is surely not atypical for psychiatrists.

As if on automatic pilot, when most psychiatrists realize they are sexually attracted to a patient, they quickly neutralize these feelings by examining them professionally. They'll start asking themselves, "Is the patient being seductive, or am I, for irrational reasons, misinterpreting the patient's behavior? Have I confused wishing to hug and comfort the patient with being sexually attracted toward the patient?'' No matter how a shrink answers these and similar questions, most have enough ethical, clinical, and common sense not to indulge their sexual feelings.

There are exceptions. Before my psychiatric residency, I felt the moral outrage against having sex with patients hid a legitimate scientific question: Would some patients benefit from sleeping with their therapists? The closed-mindedness over this question seemed like that encountered by Freud when he dared to suggest that children had sexual thoughts. Therefore, when I met my first (and only) psychiatrist who admitted having sex with patients, I matter-of-factly asked him, ''If you did an outcome study, what would the results be?'' In the spirit of scientific objectivity, he matter-of-factly replied, ''I've done it with nine patients. A third got better, a third got worse, and a third stayed the same.''

Many psychiatrists argue that it doesn't matter if sex helps the patient, since it exploits the inherent inequality of the psychotherapeutic relationship. Because especially vulnerable patients feel like helpless children and view psychiatrists as omnipotent father figures, the therapist who has intercourse with a patient commits an act which the patient experiences as incest. In fact, the most common thread in these patients' histories is that their fathers sexually abused them.

Other psychiatrists emphasize that despite any conceivable immediate benefits, in the long run the patient suffers. A California State Psychological Association task force found that according to subsequent therapists, about 90 percent of 559 patients who had had sexual relations with therapists had major problems, including the inability to trust a new therapist or any male, severe depression, drug abuse, and suicide.

According to this task force, about 5.5 percent of male psychologists and 0.6 percent of female psychologists have had intercourse with a patient who was in therapy. An additional 2.6 percent of male therapists and 0.3 percent of females said they had had intercourse with patients within three months after therapy terminated.

Psychiatrists believe their profession is scapegoated whenever any nonpsychiatric mental health professional is discovered to have sex with a patient, since psychiatrists assume that as a profession they exert greater self-restraint than other psychotherapists. Yet the data, however sketchy, don't support this belief: The evidence suggests that psychiatrists are no better or worse than psychologists, but—surprising to me—less likely to take advantage of patients sexually than other physicians. A survey of 460 male physicians published in 1973 revealed that about 5 percent of psychiatrists had sex with their patients, which was less than the 5 to 13 percent usually seen with other doctors, with obstetricians and internists leading the pack. In 1976, none of the 167 female physicians surveyed claimed to have ever had sex with a patient.

Whenever any psychiatrist has sex with a patient, it blemishes the entire profession; psychiatrists would feel like asking the offending psychiatrist, "Dammit, if I can control myself, why can't you?" Many psychiatrists I know were pleased that in 1982 two women received $250,000 in a malpractice suit against a New York psychiatrist, who, according to one plaintiff, was paid $45 an hour for therapy sessions that included sex and an additional $10 to view a videotape of the session.

Psychiatrists feel the reasons therapists give for sleeping with patients are rationalizations. "The patient is seductive." So what? Vancouver psychiatrist Dr. Enid Pine points out that a therapist should no more respond sexually to a seductive patient than he would join a violent patient in smashing windows. "The patient yearned to know that somebody could love her." "She desperately needed a boost to her self-esteem." "She wanted to free herself of frigidity." Psychiatrists reject all of these justifications, noting there are plenty of other effective ways to accomplish these goals without risking the long-term deleterious effects of sexual intercourse.*

Psychiatrists who use patients to satisfy their sexual appetites usually have severe personal problems, most often a rocky marriage. Frequently in their forties, they either seek a boost to their own sexual self-esteem or see themselves as sexual superstars. At other times these "Don Juan therapists" unknowingly turn to sex-

---

*One of these ways is by getting sex therapy, another product of modern scientific psychiatry. Historically, psychoanalytic psychiatrists attributed all sexual problems to neurotic conflicts, and therefore they used their only treatment, insight-oriented psychotherapy, to resolve them. This approach took years and rarely succeeded. In contrast, the work of Masters and Johnson, whatever its flaws, encouraged psychiatrists to apply scientific principles in researching and treating sexual problems. Today, most sex therapy yields excellent results in six to twelve weeks.

ual intercourse to gain relief from what they experience as the un-relenting tediousness of listening to patients.

It's virtually impossible to prevent these therapists from prac-ticing. It's not so much that mental health professionals actively protect sexual abusers (since they are a blight on all therapists), but that they don't want to know about them. They don't want to get involved. When they do know about it, they're apt to view the offender as more pathetic than bad, and to urge him to obtain therapy rather than report him to professional or legal authorities. If he rejects therapy, his peers will report him to a local medical or psychiatric society, most of which have programs for treating abusers while allowing them to maintain confidentiality and to keep their licenses. Depending on the situation, hospitals and clinics may either insist on closer supervision of the psychiatrist or not allow him to practice within their facility. But even when hospital and state medical officials try to stop them from practicing, the courts frequently claim that they don't have the right to deprive a person of his livelihood, or that because intercourse was consensual or physical abuse was minimal, the penalty is too severe. And even when the judge upholds the taking away of a medical license, nothing prevents the defrocked psychiatrist from practicing as a "psychotherapist," since legally anybody can do so.

"IDENTICAL MATCHING" OF PATIENTS AND THERAPISTS

This concern over male therapists' sexual abuse of female pa-tients reinforced a belief advanced by many civil-, women's-, and gay-rights groups that psychiatrists and patients should be "iden-tically matched"—that is, women should treat women, blacks should treat blacks, gays should treat gays, and so on. In the 1970s a common view was: "Male psychologists, psychiatrists and so-cial workers must realize that as scientists they know nothing about women; their expertise, their diagnoses, even their sympathy is damaging and oppressive to women. Male clinicians should stop treating women altogether."

By the 1980s, however, most psychiatrists had abandoned identical matching, asserting that a therapist's *competence* was far more important than whether his or her sex, race, class, and sex-ual orientation matched the patient's. Studies confirm this belief. Moreover, a therapist with virtually the same outlooks as the patient may lack the objectivity and distance needed to conduct effective treatment.

This does not imply that demographic differences between psychiatrist and patient never interfere with treatment. They do. For example, misunderstandings and prejudices may induce psychiatrists to set lower expectations of black patients, and black patients to attribute racism to a psychiatrist's critical remarks. On the other hand, when a black patient is treated by a white psychiatrist (and vice versa), race is not the only difference between them: Differences may also exist in age, social class, education, sex, sexual orientation, marital status, political convictions, psychiatric ideology, and so on. Any one of these may interfere with therapy as much as, if not more than, race. Therefore, any problems in therapy pertaining to race should be discussed, just as those pertaining to any of these differences should be discussed. Therapy falters not because these fundamental differences exist, but because therapy fails to examine them.

Although demographic matching of patients and therapists may not affect outcome, it may influence which issues are discussed. For example, a woman patient may learn more about her fear of men with a male therapist and more about her feminine identity with a female therapist. What issues are discussed also depends on prevailing social norms.

PSYCHIATRISTS AS MIRRORS OF SOCIETY

Psychiatrists always reflect their culture. In 1917, the American *Psychoanalytic Review,* edited by the respected William Alanson White, published the following:

> The Negro . . . appears to be at a much lower cultural level than the Caucasian. It is true that with his talent for mimicry, recalling to us in some measure our jungle cousins, he is able to present a remarkably exact, albeit superficial representation of the white man. . . .
> The precocity of the children, the early onset of puberty, the failure to grasp subjective ideas, the strong sexual and herd instincts with the few inhibitions, the simple dream life, the easy reversion to savagery when deprived of the restraining influence of the whites (as in Haiti and Liberia), the tendency to seek expression in such rhythmic

means as music and dancing, the low resistance to such toxins as syphilis and alcohol, the sway of superstition, all these and many other things betray the savage heart beneath the civilized exterior. Because he wears a Palm Beach suit instead of a string of cowries, carries a gold-headed cane instead of a spear, uses the telephone instead of beating the drum from hill to hill and for the jungle path has substituted the pay-as-you-enter street-car, his psychology is no less that of the African.

Today, psychiatrists are as much products of society as they were then, for psychiatry can never be practiced in isolation from social values. As a result, how psychiatrists view and treat patients does, and always will, mirror society.

For example, the women's movement helped to change conventional psychiatric wisdom during the 1970s. At the beginning of the decade, psychiatrists often blamed overbearing, intrusive "schizophrenogenic" mothers as being the major cause of schizophrenia. Today, nobody says this—at least not in public. For years the psychoanalytic concept of "penis envy"—among women, not men—was viewed as a woman's pathological desire to be a man, whereas now it means that women desire the same rights and opportunities as men, and not that women want to be men.

Overall, psychiatrists believe the women's movement has facilitated their work. Men are more willing to seek help and to express feelings. Because psychotherapy tries to encourage assertiveness, independence, and being responsible for one's actions and circumstances, women's liberation reinforces the goals of psychotherapy. Thus, whereas before women's lib, social pressures worked against the psychiatrist's efforts to help women get control over their own lives, it now affords a social sanction for these efforts.

THE MORAL-EXISTENTIAL PERSPECTIVE

Although they might use different terms, I believe most scientific psychiatrists would agree with Dr. Eugene Abroms's formulation that modern psychiatric treatment evolves in three stages: biological, psychosocial, and moral-existential. The psychiatrist first ensures that the patient has a stable biological platform; if necessary he will prescribe medications to remedy symptoms. Second, he remedies distressing issues with psychosocial therapies.

The third stage, which I have not explored until now, goes beyond symptoms and issues, and, to quote Abroms, "into a realm of pure value, where the ultimate aim is integrity of the person." For this to occur, the therapist-patient relationship involves more than a contract: It is also a covenant, in which "moral qualities of trust and gratitude, of loyalty and devotion, and above all, of respect" are exchanged. In respecting the patient, and in appreciation of the patient's trust to share the intimate details of his life, "the therapist becomes firm in the resolve to stand by the patient, even to tolerate a measure of moral failure." Despite episodically disapproving of each other, eventually there emerges a fiduciary relationship. These loyalties are earned, not ordained. (This moral-existential perspective does not mean that psychiatrists have a greater understanding of morality or of life's meaning and purpose.)

Moral-existential considerations pertain to all psychiatric treatment, not only intensive psychotherapy. For example, take a patient with a straightforward case of major depression whose therapy is primarily tricyclic antidepressants. At the most concrete level, the doctor-patient relationship will affect this treatment, because if the patient does not trust his doctor, he may not take his tricyclics. On a more abstract level, the psychiatrist uses the doctor-patient relationship to convey his sense of loyalty to the patient and to show his respect for him as a human being. He does so less because these are nice things to do and more because they have specific therapeutic intent: When a patient feels that his doctor, a respected authority figure, values him as a person, his ego is boosted and his trust in therapy is bolstered.

How the psychiatrist translates these moral-existential considerations into actual clinical interventions varies according to the psychiatrist, the patient, and the situation. Very often how the psychiatrist does so has less to do with *what* he says than with *how* he says it. If a psychiatrist says to a patient, "I hope you feel better," the patient can usually tell if the shrink means it or is faking it. If the patient believes the psychiatrist's concern is genuine, the patient will be more confident about treatment and about himself.

Ideologues, whether psychological or biological, run the risk of inadvertently ignoring a patient's moral-existential needs. Historically, psychoanalytic psychiatrists viewed patients as "culprits," in the sense that patients were somehow responsible for their own problem. Believing that a patient's mental disorder was a product of the patient's personality, the psychiatrist acted as if the patient *were* the illness. For instance, in discussing a depressed patient with colleagues, a psychoanalytic psychiatrist says, "Unless this guy stops being so rigid, he's always going to be depressed." When the patient doesn't improve, the psychiatrist would claim, "The patient doesn't want to get better; it's part of his masochism." When speaking at a meeting of group therapists, I was describing how patients in a particular group became distraught when one patient started to yell at them. Although I thought it was quite natural for these patients to become distraught—after all, who likes to be yelled at?—my audience strongly disagreed and insisted these patients "had problems dealing with anger." In short, psychological ideologues are prone to view patients as "nothing but an illness."

On the other hand, biological ideologues tend to see patients as "containers," in the sense that they're treating an "illness-that-happens-to-be-in-a-person," instead of a "person-who-happens-to-have-an-illness." To biological ideologues, mental disorders are mental disorders, and if the mental disorder is major depression, it doesn't really matter if the patient is a politician or a drag queen, since the treatment will be the same—tricyclic antidepressants. In a weird way, viewing patients as interchangeable containers of a specific illness leads psychiatrists not only to "forget" they are treating a person, but also to prescribe medications as if they are pouring chemicals into a test tube. When ideologues view patients either as culprits or as containers, they ignore the moral-existential dimension of psychiatric care.

Moral-existential elements of psychiatric treatment also exist, because as therapy evolves, it becomes clear that patients complain of more than symptoms and problems in living; at some point they question whether, after all the psychologizing is done, they are good or bad. Psychiatrists frequently hear patients say, "If you really got to know me, you'd find out how really disgusting I am." Not uncommonly, patients fear that if they reveal the supposed ugliness within them, it would drive away or even destroy their therapist. To admit any of this to anybody, including a psychiatrist, is very painful. In situations like these, the need for moral-existential interventions becomes most apparent. It is here that, in some way or another, the therapist conveys to the patient, "I understand your pain, and no matter how awful you think you are, I value you and want to stick by you."

Dick Cavett, who had hospitalized himself for depression, later revealed how he felt while hosting a Public Broadcasting System talk show in 1981: "I would see myself laughing on the monitor and would think, 'If you [the audience] could see my interior landscape, I would have stepped in front of a car.'. . . Psychiatry saved my life." Many, many patients have shared such feelings, and how a psychiatrist responds to them may influence how a patient values himself.

When I treat patients, I make a special point of discovering the good within them. I don't say very much about this in public; it sounds corny—even to me. Nevertheless, in describing themselves, many patients feel, as one patient expressed it, "underneath madness lies badness." They assume, consciously or not, that the mere existence of their illness or problem is clear proof that they are fundamentally bad, and thus unworthy of another's loyalty. When this psychological dynamic exists, the patient may find that his dislike of others derives largely from his own underlying sense of badness. Widely held, this conviction in one's badness is so basic and powerful that it demands a moral-existential examination.

I do not tell patients, "So what if you slaughtered your mother; nobody's perfect." Instead, I try to help patients identify the genuine virtues within them that they have overlooked. I don't invent virtues, I merely point out what's already there. I try to correct their distorted notions of what's bad. A patient thinks he is bad because he has ambivalent feelings toward his parents; that's not bad, that's human. I try to show patients that given their circumstances, what they think was bad may not have been so bad. Finally, I try to delineate the good from the bad. Then I examine the bad not to flagellate the patient, but to help him learn from it so that in the future, he will rely more on his better instincts.

If I am to develop an authentic bond of loyalty to a patient, then I must eventually find his admirable traits. I don't have to like everything about a patient to feel this bond, any more than the patient has to like everything about me. Yet the very nature of practicing psychiatry makes it easy to discover the virtues in patients. When psychiatrists speak of cherishing their relationships with patients, they are usually referring to these discoveries.

TEN

Becoming a Psychiatrist

Since the new scientific psychiatry is making dramatic progress, one might assume that students flock to become psychiatrists. They don't. In fact, it's just the reverse. From the end of World War II until the late 1960s, 7 to 10 percent of medical students chose psychiatry. Starting in the 1970s, this figure plummeted, and it has remained at roughly 4 percent. This decline is occurring despite a shortage in 1981 of 9,400 psychiatrists in the United States, and by 1990 a projected shortage of 13,000.

The reasons this shortage exists and relatively fewer medical students are becoming psychiatrists reveal a lot about how the revolution from psychoanalytic to scientific psychiatry has affected the profession and the type of people who enter it.

CHOOSING PSYCHIATRY

The most common time for students to choose psychiatry as a career is in medical school. Two percent do so during childhood, 8 percent in high school, 16 percent in college, 44 percent during medical school, 16 percent while training in another specialty, and 14 percent during other periods (e.g., military, Peace Corps). Thus, two groups exist: a smaller group who decide before medical school, and a larger group who decide during medical school.

Although for different reasons, both groups find that medical school does more to discourage than to encourage students to become psychiatrists. Overall, the number of students wishing to become psychiatrists *declines* as medical school proceeds. Among the group that want to be psychiatrists before entering medical school, most are ambivalent about being physicians; they view medical school as a painful distraction they must endure to reach their real goal of becoming psychiatrists. In general, the larger group want to be physicians; their choice of psychiatry was made despite social pressures within medical school against becoming a psychiatrist and despite personal fears that in doing so they would lose their hard-earned medical identity. In short, medical schools turn students off to psychiatry.

Why student-doctors don't become psychiatrists

Anybody who becomes a psychiatrist does so in the face of all the reasons his fellow students give not to enter the field. The main reason medical students don't wish to specialize in psychiatry is that they believe it lacks scientific rigor, therapeutic effectiveness, and a clearly delineated role. Typical student comments are: "There's too much dogma and not enough science," "There's little tangible result per time spent," "Psychiatry interests me, but it's not like being a 'real' doctor," "Psychiatrists know very little medicine and are alienated from other doctors," "Current therapies are inadequate," "I can do all the psychiatry I want as an internist," "Psychiatry seems to be all theory, and none of it very useful," "Psychiatrists are glorified social workers." When asked what they liked best about their psychiatric clerkship, the kindest thing several students could think of was "infrequent night call"; one added pointedly, "playing Ping-Pong with patients."

Medical students generally view psychiatrists as nice guys who are clinically inept, fuzzy thinkers, thin-skinned, too concerned with being liked, screwy or nuts, and with crazy kids to boot! This picture, though drawn from society's, derives primarily from medical school professors and house staff.

Quite naturally, medical students want to please their teachers, but those selecting psychiatry must often buck their professors. When as a medical student I told our chairman of urology that I was going into psychiatry, he scoffed, "I deal with the *real* thing!'' Never again did he acknowledge my existence. Why bother teaching urology to a nonphysician?

Psychiatrists feel they're getting a bum rap. They'll argue that although many psychiatric patients aren't completely cured, neither are most medical patients. Internists don't cure heart disease, strokes, cancer, or diabetes any better than psychiatrists cure schizophrenia; physicians, including psychiatrists, only cure acute episodes. Psychiatry might not be sufficiently scientific, but it's getting there. The rest of medicine is practiced far more subjectively than most physicians let on. Psychiatrists do forget a lot of general medicine, but so do neurologists, surgeons, obstetricians, and every other specialist who doesn't routinely use it. Although psychiatrists may lean toward nonconformity, it's highly doubtful they are any screwier than anyone else.

Medical school discourages students from becoming psychiatrists in other ways. Some students cite poor teaching, especially during the first two (preclinical) years. During the final two years, in which they do full-time clinical work, some students find psychiatry boring, but most feel emotionally drained by it. One student explains, "During college I was interested in psychiatry, but when I came face to face with real patients, including two who committed suicide, I found it too demoralizing. Since my patients weren't getting any better and I kept overempathizing with them, every night I came home depressed." Another said, "I'm still considering psychiatry, but worry about the personal risks of alcoholism, job frustration, and suicide."

Psychiatrists frequently claim that students avoid psychiatry because it is the third-lowest-paid of all medical specialities. Yet this disincentive can't be all that compelling, because only a third of students know that psychiatrists make less, two thirds claim that financial concerns don't influence their choice of specialty, and students who do become psychiatrists are more aware of the economic disadvantage than those who don't.

The growth of family practice may be taking students away from psychiatry. Over the past thirty-five years, roughly a tenth of all medical students have been continually at odds with medicine's increasing specialization and "dehumanization." To escape these trends, students once turned to psychiatry, but now they choose family practice, which has regained respectability. On the other hand, the low percentage of students who become psychiatrists may reflect psychiatry's success and not its failure, since a large infusion of psychiatric concepts helped family practice to regain its respectability in the first place.

I too have a theory. Historically, those medical students with antiestablishment, "poetic" streaks were specifically attracted to *psychoanalytic* psychiatry, just because it seemed subjective, intellectual, abstract, artistic, and humanistic. Therefore, as scientific psychiatry emerged, what drew these students to psychiatry was gone. Not only did psychiatry appear to lose its poetry, but as a science, it seemed unable to measure up to the rest of medicine. Perceiving modern psychiatry as neither good art nor good science, some potential psychiatrists have turned elsewhere. However, as students and their mentors become acclimated to the new psychiatry that uses art to supplement science (and not vice versa), I suspect more students will enter the profession.

Why students do become psychiatrists

"Everybody" knows people become psychiatrists to solve their own problems. Yet in truth, although this motivation might exert more influence on other mental health professionals, I've rarely heard a psychiatrist say he entered the field to feel happier," or "to stop being anxious," or "to get along better with people." About a quarter of psychiatrists believe they were attracted to the field because they were curious about their own psychology or because they were helped by psychiatry, but that's different from selecting a specialty for therapeutic reasons.

When interviewing applicants to psychiatric residencies, psychiatrists will encounter students who want psychiatry for all the wrong reasons: the applicant who's oblivious to the psychological significance of his choosing psychiatry when his mother had a "nervous breakdown," or the applicant who says, "I feel more at home with psychiatric patients than with normal people." These red flags induce psychiatrists to reject the student's residency application, and sometimes to suggest he examine his motivations in therapy and think twice about entering the profession. Psychiatrists don't mind applicants who are in therapy, but they do mind applicants who want their residency to be therapy.

In a 1983 survey, 531 psychiatrists were allowed to indicate as many motivations for their choice of career as they deemed important. Table 10-1 shows their responses:

A Columbia student anticipating a career in psychiatry mentions some frequently heard themes: "I find it much more interesting to talk about real life problems with patients than to discuss their liver. Each person's story is unique, but their spleens are all the same. . . . I'm a good listener, and I think I'm pretty good at helping people."

His classmate observed, "When [psychiatric] patients tell me their stories, I often wonder what I'd do if I had their illness or was stuck with their situation. On the other hand, these questions

TABLE 10-1*
WHY MEDICAL STUDENTS BECOME PSYCHIATRISTS

REASON	RATING OF IMPORTANT/ VERY IMPORTANT
Knowledge within the field	45%
Experience with ill patients	36%
Challenge of the field	35%
Opportunity to add to the field	34%
Medical school teaching	31%
Own problems and/or treatment	25%
Identification with teacher	21%
Apparent ease of the profession	20%
Identification with relative (who's in a related field)	15%
Illness in family or friends	14%
Exhaustion and desire to try another specialty	7%

*Taintor Z, Morphy M, Seiden A, and Val E (1983) Psychiatric residency training: relationships and value development. *American Journal of Psychiatry*, 140: 778–780.

never occur to me in medicine. In fact, in medicine *nothing* occurs to me. Medicine is 'psychic numbing.' Psych patients have showed me that you can be a doctor and still feel. In medicine you're always suppressing your feelings, but in psychiatry you're always using them. That's exciting. I don't want to go through life as a split-brain preparation."

Students often view their choice of psychiatry as an alternative to the nitty-gritty of medicine. A psychiatrist from Los Angeles recalls: "The sights and feel of medicine were all wrong for me. I hated sticking people to draw blood or putting in IVs; all that poking around till you find a vein, and then you miss the vein and have to stick the patient again. Jabbing patients with needles is necessary, and I got good at it, but I was always bothered by it. Blood cakes under your fingernails; there's too much saliva and vomit. . . . I don't like touching sick people; their skin decays, they're usually unwashed, and it's unappetizing to keep poking your finger next to their scrotums and into their rectums. Doing pelvics is a gushy mess.

"Having patients die was the worst part. It happens so routinely in medicine that after a while, doctors become desensitized to it, as if a dead person was a broken machine headed for the scrap heap. I understand the necessity for this attitude, but I didn't want to become that way. . . . Death scares me, and a big reason I chose psychiatry was to avoid it. Too often I was hurt by getting to know a person well and then watching him die."

Some psychiatrists enter the profession because they're fascinated with the mind and brain, how each affects the other, and how environment influences both.* They see psychiatry as medicine's last frontier, a field ripe for innovation and professional advancement.

Others are attracted to psychiatry because they had a good experience in psychotherapy. A child psychiatrist said, "What

---

*A psychiatric resident says, "During medical school I was reading how normally Parkinson's patients walk no faster than a snail. But then, almost as an afterthought, the text noted that if there is a fire in a theater, these patients will run out of the theater as fast as everyone else. Now here are patients with genuine destruction of brain tissue, and yet how they behave is a product of the brain interacting with the environment. This insight so intrigued me, I figured, why not make a career pursuing it?"

clinched my choice of psychiatry was my year in therapy during medical school. It turned my life around. In part, I wanted to emulate my shrink. More important, although I was intrigued by psychiatry, I always had grave doubts about its working, until my own treatment convinced me it did.''

Like many others, I chose psychiatry to rectify, as my diary reads, "the cerebral ossification of medical school." By the final year, medical school had become quicksand, snatching me away forever from everything I loved, such as politics, theater, Japanese studies, and history. Choosing psychiatry was the only snap decision I've ever made, and I recall the precise moment. I was lamenting my intellectual stagnation and growing isolation from "interesting" (i.e., nonmedical) friends, when I started to wonder if specializing in psychiatry might be the answer. I picked up my unused psychiatric textbook and on page 1 it read: ". . . psychiatry is a generality and not a specialty." This line confirmed my hope and changed my life.

Only years later did I discover that I might have a talent for psychiatry and that I enjoyed helping people; these came as delightful surprises. Yet initially, I chose psychiatry for selfish reasons. Psychiatry was to be my costume, an identification badge indicating how I wanted others to see me. The people I respected were emotionally indifferent about physicians, but they always felt strongly about psychiatrists. Not viewing myself as particularly interesting, I figured that if my profession was, then by osmosis, I would be too. Becoming a psychiatrist was my way of discovering, and later fulfilling, an idealized self-image. In this, I'm hardly unique.

What kind of students become psychiatrists?

As far as I'm concerned, the more interesting ones. Granted, I'm biased. Yet having spent fifteen years teaching medical students and running their training programs, I've known thousands of medical students, and in general, those entering psychiatry stand out. They're more concerned with people than things. Ideas intrigue them. For most students, medicine is their life; for future psychiatrists, medicine is only part of it. Their interests are more diverse: They're more inclined to paint, to write poetry, to act politically. They're more open-minded, more comfortable with uncertainty, more willing to experiment with drugs, alternative life-styles, or Eastern religions, or to travel to exotic lands. Studies confirm my impressions.

In comparison to their peers, medical students who become psychiatrists are more likely to be single and from large cities. In general, their parents are wealthier and exert less influence over their choice of a career, a mate, or a marital status. More often they are agnostic or nonreligious, but if neither, they're likely to be Jews and Catholics more than Protestants.

The percent of women becoming psychiatrists is rising faster than the percent of women becoming medical students. From 1974 to 1982 the proportion of women entering psychiatric residencies climbed from 22 to 38 percent, while in medical school it increased from 15 to 24 percent.

Personality profiles of future psychiatrists show they are better able to tolerate unstructured, ambiguous situations. Psychological tests show that in comparison to other medical students, they are less willing to control other people's behavior, but more willing to influence their moral standards. They score higher on measures of nurturance, intimacy, and autonomy. They show less concern for power and status. They are closer to their mothers and tend to identify with them. They are more open about feelings and dissatisfactions; their self-esteems are lower. They are more cynical, generally anxious, and relatively worried about death.

They're brighter and more verbal, according to their general scholastic aptitude scores on the Medical College Admission Test (MCAT). On the other hand, their academic records in college and medical school are mediocre, and their class rankings in medical school are usually below the norm. In fact, future psychiatrists are the only student-physicians whose MCAT scores and academic ranks don't correlate.

They are more likely to major in the humanities and social sciences than in the natural sciences. Drawn to the abstract instead of the practical, they are more concerned with the psychological, philosophical, aesthetic, and humanistic. They are less racist and lean to the political left.

These people are not like most medical students—dependable "grinds," who are conventional, conservative, and conformist. Feeling they'd be out of place in medical school, many psychiatrically inclined college students avoid medical school altogether;

they become psychologists. They consider premed a rat race with cutthroat competition, and for what? Medical school, which they view as dull and irrelevant, if not harmful, to becoming a good psychotherapist.

Those undergraduates who feel it's worth becoming a physician enter medical school holding their noses. Eight to ten years later, when they'll finally become full-fledged psychiatrists, they'll usually say they made the right choice and that things turned out as expected. Of more interest is what they didn't expect. For beyond the predictable advantages of being a physician—e.g., greater income, more status, ability to prescribe drugs—a medical education changes them in more fundamental, crucial, and enduring ways.

MEDICAL SCHOOL AND INTERNSHIP

From day one, students discover that medical school is as rumored: a marathon of memorizing facts. Only scientific facts count. Despite every medical school's brochure insisting that faculty value a "broad liberal arts education," that's all a lie, and every medical student knows it. Creativity, cleverness, and intelligence don't facilitate a medical education; they only distract from amassing facts. Every vein, artery, nerve, bone (all 206 of them), fiber, muscle, joint, cartilage, gland, and lymph node must be found and named. Even empty spaces get names. Students will name their ("Abra") cadaver, but there's one name they rarely learn—their cadaver's real name. (After nine months of gross anatomy, I was shaken to discover I'd been dissecting one Faye Ryan.) In medical school, the importance of a course is in direct proportion to the number of facts students should be able to regurgitate on exams.

In psychiatry, there were no facts—or so I as a student in 1964 was led to believe. With no facts, there was no need to study psychiatry, and therefore nobody did. I exaggerate. There was one fact. A huge sign sprawled across a shrink's office read, "Adolescence is not a disease." During my first two years of medical school, that was all the psychiatry I learned. Today's psychiatry does have facts, but most students assume it's devoid of facts—a hodgepodge of theories, opinions, and common sense.

Students come to freshman psychiatry with so many diverse

and enormous expectations that inevitably they are disappointed. They want freshman psychiatry to be an oasis amid a desert of data, the only "humanistic," "intellectual," and "civilizing" course during the first two years of school. Those who'd considered careers in psychology want freshman psychiatry to be what they fantasize psychology grad school would have been: a scholarly study of Freud, Jung, Skinner, etc. Other students want psychiatry to be those dearly missed late-night bull sessions which, because of medical school, are no more. Some students expect psychiatry to provide analyses of society, blueprints for political action, guides for ethical practice, techniques (or tricks) for talking with patients, and encounter groups for self-actualization. Many hopes ride on this course, but after several lectures, most of these hopes are dashed.

Students have these bloated expectations of psychiatry because, like most laymen, they assume that psychoanalytic psychiatry still reigns and that psychiatric expertise is boundless. Yet, as discussed in Chapter 1, psychiatry is not about anything which involves thinking, feeling, perceiving, and behaving—in other words, everything. Instead, medical students discover that where psychiatric expertise genuinely rests is with the study, diagnosis, and treatment of patients with mental disorders.

Psychiatry is the only *clinical* discipline taught during medical school's first two years; all other courses are devoted to medicine's basic sciences. Talking about clinical work holds little meaning for medical students unless they're also doing it. After I lectured to first-year students about patients' getting angry at doctors, a student asked, with complete sincerity, "But if you treat patients properly, why would they ever be angry at you?" It's not until their third year when they become directly involved in treating patients that they can answer this question for themselves, and understand what psychiatry does.

In their first two years, students receive about fifty lectures on subjects such as human development, psychoanalytic theory, psychiatric diagnosis, psychobiology, psychopharmacology, human sexuality, doctor-patient relationships, and psychiatry in general medicine. During their junior year, students take a five or six week clerkship, usually on psychiatric inpatient services, where they accompany and assist a resident. Under supervision, they interview new patients, make diagnoses, write histories, suggest treatments, conduct psychotherapy, talk to families, and help arrange for the patient's discharge.

This third year of medical school might well be the most important in any physician's career. At the start of the year, he thinks of himself as a layman, and by its end, as a doctor. This is the first time he spends his days (and nights) directly caring for patients. After years of *preparing* to be a physician, the student is finally *performing* as a physician. Now he learns primarily from patients instead of books.

During this third year, all medical students take clerkships in surgery, internal medicine, pediatrics, obstetrics and gynecology, neurology, and psychiatry. Although the future psychiatrist doesn't realize it at the time, his identity as a physician begins with these clerkships. This medical identity distinguishes him from all other mental health professionals. Without minimizing the importance of having more pay, status, power, responsibility, clinical tools, and biological knowledge, being a physician influences one's entire career in far more profound ways.

Medical training enmeshes one in people's births, deaths, and many agonizing traumas in between. As a physician, the psychiatrist has seen the splattered remains of auto victims, the bleeding chests of gunshot wounds, and the ravings of madmen. He's observed abortions and delivered newborns. He's treated the stabbed, the mauled, the crushed, the deformed, and the amputated. He's known the blind and the demented. He's touched every organ, fingered every orifice. He's accustomed to people under great stress and suffering. Since he must rectify diseases and devastations, a medical education trains him to take charge, to exercise authority, to assume ultimate responsibility, and to act calmly in crises. It acclimates him to being idolized and vilified by patients. It teaches him that his making a fatal mistake is not a possibility, but an inevitability.

By the end of his internship, these experiences, insights, and attributes have become second nature. So when he starts to train specifically as a psychiatrist, unlike other mental health professionals, he's already had at least three years of caring for patients, touching them, seeing their pain, knowing their intimacies, letting them down, harming them, but with luck, not yet killing anybody. These experiences, ingrained for life, are what psychiatrists feel is special about being a physician.

Although professional chauvinism and romanticism surely lead psychiatrists to overvalue their medical training, there's evidence to support their belief. From 1970 to 1975, when psychoanalytic psychiatry had so detached itself from medicine, internships were no longer required of psychiatrists. Because internship is the most intensive medical training in a physician's entire career, comparing psychiatrists who interned with those who didn't could show if medical training was all that useful. It was. Those with internships related better to staff, spoke more easily with patients, and were more adept at handling emergencies. Psychiatric supervisors found the internship group displayed superior clinical judgment, carried larger caseloads, and had fewer patients drop out of treatment.

Though medical experience trains psychiatrists to assume responsibility, especially in a crisis, it does not necessarily better prepare them to conduct other psychiatric skills. For instance, in one study psychology trainees outperformed psychiatric residents in assessing suicide.

There's a down side to this medical identity. It's a natural setup to breed arrogance, condescension, and callousness. Some argue it encourages psychiatrists to treat patients as things, to overemphasize biology, and to underestimate psychology and sociology. Surely this occurs, but I haven't seen any solid evidence for it.

During the fourth year, medical students may take four to eight weeks of psychiatric electives, which often help them decide about becoming psychiatrists. Yet for many tangled administrative reasons, medical students seeking top-notch psychiatric residencies must apply during their third year. This means that since most psychiatrists choose their specialty during their junior and senior years of medical school, a majority of students are selecting psychiatry *before* they've taken an elective, and sometimes before they've even had a clerkship. Thus, psychiatrists-to-be make career plans having had little, if any, opportunity to see what psychiatrists do.

PSYCHIATRIC RESIDENCY

Following internship, doctors train in a specialty during their residencies. If they study adult psychiatry, the residency takes three years. If they want to be child psychiatrists, they'll spend two years in a basic adult psychiatric residency followed by a two-year residency in child psychiatry. Whereas all psychiatrists receive some training in child psychiatry, roughly 10 percent go on to do a residency in it.

Although less so today, what a residency emphasizes significantly influences how a psychiatrist will practice. During the psychoanalytic era in which psychology and biology were markedly polarized, when a student selected a residency, he was in effect deciding his lifelong professional orientation. In today's scientific psychiatry, however, all modern residency programs stress psychology *and* biology, and so most younger graduates are adept at both. Still, each program focuses a bit more on certain aspects of psychiatry, and thus, so will its graduates. At the same time, although psychiatrists reflect their residencies, their choice of a residency reflects them.

Choosing residencies

Given the national shortage of psychiatrists, students have no problem getting a residency; their problem is to get one they want. Since top-notch residency programs receive about twenty applications for each position, most students who apply to these programs don't get their first choice. Many of these students are stunned and hurt, since it may be the first time they've been rejected by a program. On the other hand, there are so many excellent psychiatric residencies throughout the country that most American-trained medical students can obtain good psychiatric training.

The selection of residents is, in fact, highly arbitrary. Although one would like the choices to be made objectively, there's no reasonable way to accomplish this. Residency training directors start by getting from the applicant's medical school a "Dean's letter," three letters of recommendation (from psychiatric or nonpsychiatric faculty), and grades. These letters all sound alike: "Mr. Applicant is honest, trustworthy, hard-working, diligent, concerned with patients, well liked by peers and teachers, eager to learn, and psychologically sensitive." Few faculty have the guts to write critical letters, and now with the Buckley Amendment allowing students to see everything that's written about them, teachers are more reluctant than ever to write anything critical about students; moreover, writing critical letters doesn't encourage students to become psychiatrists. Grades don't help, since some schools have eliminated them, while others have adopted an "honors, pass, fail" system, which is equally uninformative because, depending on the school, 2 to 30 percent of the students will receive "honors."

All this paper isn't totally useless. Over the years faculty and program directors have evolved a language of code words and practices to communicate when a student is particularly gifted. At the bottom of a typed letter, a teacher may write in longhand, "This student's *really* good!" All letters are favorable; only a few are ecstatic. Yet given that the value of these letters lies more in the realm of inference than information, they're not a very sound basis for selecting residents.

Consequently, a major determinant of who gets accepted into a residency is how the student performs during his three or four forty-five-minute interviews at each program. The candidate typically spends one interview with a resident to get the "real scoop" on the program. Another interview is often with the training director or department chairman, both to find out about the program and to massage the applicant's ego. To see how a program treats women, female applicants usually talk to a woman resident or staff member; blacks and Hispanics meet with someone from those minorities.*

Interviewers usually ask about the student's reasons for becoming a psychiatrist, his future career plans (e.g., community psychiatry, private practice, research), his upbringing, his family, and if he's had psychological problems and psychotherapy. Whether the applicant has had such problems and received psychotherapy

---

*Not so for gays. Fearing discrimination, roughly half don't mention their homosexuality. Although homosexuality hasn't officially been a mental disorder since 1973, a large minority of psychiatrists still believe that it is psychopathological and object to having gay residents. The only hard data that are even related to this subject come from a survey of third-year psychiatric residents, in which 45 percent of males and 53 percent of females believed psychiatrists "should be heterosexuals." (Some psychiatrists maintain that homosexuality is a mental disorder, but will argue just as strongly that this does not justify any discrimination against gay applicants.) In reality, most residency programs accept gay applicants, but with some reluctance. I suspect this reluctance has less to do with the usual "homophobia" than with psychiatrists' feeling inept and uncomfortable when supervising gay residents on their feelings toward patients of the same sex.

doesn't work against him, and sometimes it's even a plus, a sign he's sufficiently in tune with himself to know he needs help. Interviewers are less concerned with the applicant's knowledge of psychiatry than with his eagerness to learn.

During the interview, all the successful applicant must do is appear intelligent, intuitive, understanding, empathetic, psychologically minded, verbal, friendly, flexible, cooperative, tolerant, sincere, responsible, warm, extraverted, mature, fairly sane, independent without being hostile to authority, and physically attractive. He should display leadership abilities and nonmedical interests.

Applicants usually find these interviews to be stressful, since beyond feeling that their entire careers hinge on how well they convey all these attributes, they correctly feel their character is being judged, their minds probed, and their sanity tested. To a question such as "Could you tell me something about your family?" all an applicant for most positions has to say is something like "My mom's a teacher and my dad's a pharmacist." Yet if an applicant for a psychiatric residency says nothing but this, he's considered shallow. The applicant must prove he is psychologically self-aware by describing his family's problems, conflicts, and passions. Although I have qualms about using a job interview as a psychotherapy session, some exploration of the applicant's psychological awareness pays off. I recall asking an applicant, "Does having parents who are both psychiatrists ever pose any problems for you?" With complete sincerity, he replied, "No." He then looked at me with genuine bewilderment and asked, "Why would you ever think it would?" If he has to ask, I have to wonder if he belongs in psychiatry.

Among the profession's most inglorious traditions is the "stress interview." Although used far less often today, it's still employed to see how applicants function under stress, the idea being that good psychiatrists are cool under fire. Most applicants don't know stress interviews exist until they've been through one. One famous stess-interview technique is matter-of-factly asking the applicant to open a window, which unbeknownst to him is nailed shut. The applicant tries, looks like a klutz, stumbles over apologies, and feels like a jerk. Another script has the applicant entering the interviewer's room only to find the psychiatrist on the floor looking for a nonexistent contact lens. The interviewer doesn't explain himself or even acknowledge the applicant's presence. The flustered candidate wonders what he should do. Should he help the poor prof by getting down on the floor, or would he look silly (and mess up his only suit) crawling around down there?

I was unaware of the stress interview when I first encountered it. Sure that my utter sincerity would charm my interviewer (since I had nothing else going for me), I began this interview by confessing I knew far less about psychiatry than most students. But my oh-so-refreshing candor did not refresh my interviewer; he became angry and grilled me for thirty minutes. He'd name a book on psychiatry, ask if I'd read it (knowing I hadn't), and then attack me for not reading it. He did this with four different books. The sadist moved on to drugs and dreams and defense mechanisms, and over and over again I pleaded deficient. What seemed to anger him most was that it was I who volunteered my ignorance, rather than he who discovered it.

Since the Grand Inquisitor wasn't impressed with me, I hoped he'd be impressed with my wife.* I mentioned I was on my honeymoon. He couldn't care less. "But she's a costume designer." His ears perked up. "What does she design for?" he growled. Finally I knew an answer: "The theater." But that angered him more. "Why doesn't she design for movies?" he demanded. "I don't know. She likes theater." He became infuriated. "What do you mean, you don't know? Don't you talk to your wife? What kind of crummy marriage do you have? Can't you do *anything* right?" I was devastated. I left the office, and vomited.

A psychiatrist later told me I'd been subjected to a stress interview, and that I should be ready for them. I was.

At the next program, the interviewer asked me to pass an ashtray. I tried, but it wouldn't move. "It must be glued to the table," I said. The interviewer belly-laughed; he liked being caught.

At another program I was interviewed in the office of a Park Avenue psychoanalyst. Her third question was "How often do you masturbate?" "Thirty-two times a day," I replied. She told me I was hostile. I agreed.

I mention these incidents because they're part of the profes-

---

*I've long believed the best way to learn about an applicant is to meet his spouse. Who better demonstrates what a candidate likes and values than the person he lives with?

sion's folklore. All psychiatrists have similar stories, and all love talking about them.

Ostensibly, interviews are to find out about the applicant. Yet candidates who receive the highest ratings are usually those who allow the interviewer to do most of the talking.

Faculty prefer applicants who've *done* something, especially things that psychiatrists value. The applicant may have played the violin, organized a poverty program, served in the Peace Corps, published a scientific paper, helped crippled children, written a novel. Selection committees attribute great importance to such accomplishments, because they are among the few concrete bits of data which they can use to choose one candidate over another. That's why they are far more likely to accept applicants whose clinical work they have directly observed during a clerkship or an elective.

Above all else, faculty don't want hassles. They don't want residents who are mental cases or troublemakers. For instance, they don't want an applicant who refuses to do ECT; he'd cause constant disputes and inconvenience the faculty, who would have to give ECT to his patients who need it. Faculty don't relish applicants who are adamantly against anything, fearing they'll be unpleasant, argumentative, and dogmatic. The only dogmatic residents faculty accept are those whose dogma is within the profession's mainstream.

Faculty members pick residents who share their general ideology and personality. Psychiatrists teach to convey tradition, to maintain academic immortality. Psychiatrists speak of their teachers as others speak of their family trees. "My mentor was a student of Ernest Jones, who was a student of Freud." Because the faculty know they will have to spend three long years teaching a resident, they want to make sure they will like him, be able to influence him, and effectively teach him. In the final analysis, the Good Applicant makes the psychiatrist feel like a Good Teacher.

The first year

After waiting for years to be a psychiatrist, the first day of residency is a dream fulfilled, a "Now I'm finally doing what I really want to do." Yet it doesn't take long for the new resident to feel like an absolute idiot. My case is typical.

As I entered the inpatient service on the first day of my residency, Jon, the ebullient chief resident, whisked me into group therapy while telling me I was to lead it. Jon introduced me to the group's eight patients. Perhaps I was paranoid, but they seemed annoyed at having to break in yet another new psychiatrist. So they ignored me—thank God!—and in silent awe I sat amazed at how skillfully they discussed their problems. After ten minutes, Jon intervened. "How come your new doctor has yet to speak? I bet you're wondering if he knows anything." I hid my fury. Why was this prick making a fool of me in front of my patients? Jon wouldn't relent. He turned to me and said, "The patients are worried that you're incompetent and don't know how to take care of them. But instead of reassuring them, you make matters worse by staying mute." With eighteen eyes riveted on me, I had to say something, and fast. But what? So like a jerk I mumbled, "I'm looking forward to knowing all of you." Jon said to the group, "See what I mean? How many of you found what Dr. Maxmen said comforting?" No hands were raised. I was ready to kill. Instead, I kept quiet.

After the group, as Jon and I went to his office, I was looking for a place to dispose of his body. Jon, who was in great spirits and was pretending to be unaware of my rage, feigned astonishment: "You don't look pleased. Did I say something wrong?"

"Yeh! You made me look like an idiot before my own patients!"

"Hey! Stop being so serious," Jon replied. "I assume you're objecting to what everybody already knew—the truth. The fact is that you *didn't* say anything. The patients are no fools; they have good reason to worry whether their new doctor knows what to do, especially since he's a near-mute the first time they meet him. I mean, it's true isn't it?—you don't know anything. That's okay; that's why you take a residency."

Jon was right. Like me, most psychiatric residents spend their first year on an inpatient service, mainly because they don't know very much. On an inpatient unit there are plenty of staff around to correct a beginner's blunders, thereby instructing residents and protecting patients.

After growing accustomed to being a competent physician, the new resident finds it both strange and stimulating to be unknowledgeable and unskilled once again; but this time, it's as a psychiatrist. For most psychiatrists, the first eight months of residency are wonderful: They're doing and learning psychiatry all day long and rapidly becoming competent at it. It's like a ballplayer who gets to the major leagues, an astronaut at his first launch, a kid at Christmas. Every day the novice psychiatrist goes home and talks to his mate nonstop. Each day provides a new insight, a new discovery, a new experience, a new role model, a new problem, a new pain.

"The first-year blues"

At around eight months, however, for many residents the bottom drops out. "The first-year blues" set in, because after the initial rush of knowledge and skills, novelty wears off, the rate of learning slows down, and new disappointments arise. Because residents know more, they recognize more psychopathology in their patients. Those patients who initially seemed well now appear clingy, demanding, and nasty. When residents discover they feel this hostility toward patients, especially when it's so intense and new to them, they often become angry at themselves, demoralized, or depressed. Residents find that their "profound" insights are neither profound nor insightful, and certainly not effective. Carefully made plans for patients don't work out. For example, after six months of supporting a thirty-year-old's living away from her family, the resident feels like a total failure when she ends up back home. Eight months is enough time for the resident to have at least one patient elope from the hospital while his one and only outpatient drops out of treatment. Two or three others whom the resident discharged from the hospital in good condition have now been readmitted.

Residents feel useless, and once again incompetent. As one resident observed, "I'm not really helping patients. I just *manage* them." Referring to his ward chief, he said, "Gary's therapy is ingenious. When *he* talks, patients listen. When *I* talk, nothing happens. Maybe I should change fields." Another resident said, "I used to love going to work. Now I avoid it. Every time I walk down the corridor [on the inpatient unit], all seven of my patients line up to see me, each claiming a dire emergency. For some, it's always a dire emergency; they're a pain in the ass. But others really do have emergencies, and I feel terrible for them, since I don't have the time nor the energy to give them what they need. Sometimes I'm so discouraged, I hide in my office."

Yet nothing, and I mean nothing, devastates the beginning resident as much as having his first patient commit suicide. Since suicide inflicts enormous pain on the living, the therapist included, the resident gets angry at the deceased, but then feels guilty for feeling so angry. He feels guilty for the mistakes he did, and did not, make. Although every physician feels guilty over committing technical errors, only the psychiatrist feels additional guilt about his own feelings and motivations. The psychiatric resident will ruminate about whether he unconsciously wanted his patient to die, something that would never occur to a resident in any other specialty. The resident will flagellate himself by wondering if he may have been acting out his negative feelings toward the patient by not paying sufficient attention to the patient's suicidal hints.

To help the resident deal with these feelings, and more important, to prevent future deaths from suicide, faculty members will hold a teaching exercise every time a patient commits or seriously attempts suicide; this exercise is called a "psychological autopsy." The entire inpatient staff, usually fifteen to twenty mental health professionals from various disciplines, will review the case to identify what, if anything, could have been done better. This review is the overt agenda of the meeting; its covert agenda is to offer psychological support to the deceased patient's resident. Faculty will stress that although most people don't think about it this way, mental illness can be as fatal as physical illness, and that all psychiatrists, regardless of their ability, have had patients who commit suicide. Every psychiatrist attending the psychological autopsy feels that "but there for the grace of God go I"—that is, it could have just as well been his own patient who killed himself. Not infrequently, the psychological autopsy's overt and covert agendas clash: Having conducted many of these psychological autopsies, I have found that in the staff's eagerness not to compound the resident's already enormous guilt, they may avoid clearly specifying, before all assembled, where the resident blew it.

It usually takes weeks, and sometimes months, for the resident to get over this trauma. The resident finds that his colleagues are very sympathetic and go out of their way not to rub salt into his wounds. Yet whether or not his fears are justified, the resident usually cannot shake the feeling that his colleagues are questioning his ability and judgment. Having a patient commit suicide has led some residents to leave psychiatry.

At some point in their training, about 10 percent of psychiatric residents change specialties. Another 4 percent switch to another psychiatric residency. The first-year blues prompts many of these changes, and induces many residents to obtain personal psychotherapy.

When the first-year blues stem from boredom, they are easily remedied: Come July, when residents shift services and start treating outpatients, they feel revitalized.

The T-group

Before the first year ends, another way residents deal with the first-year blues is by confiding in each other in a T-group—an institution in 80 percent of all psychiatrists' training. In retrospect, some psychiatrists believe their T-group was the most rewarding experience of their entire education; others consider it their weirdest.

Imagine a dozen psychiatrists in a room with no specified agenda, and then imagine what they might do. One might expect them to psychoanalyze one another. They don't, and what's more, they are very self-conscious about playing shrink all the time. Nor do they run around naked, although I guess they could. Psychiatric residents aren't the type, especially on the East Coast.

Although T-groups have many different formats, the ones at Columbia, which I know best, are typical. Starting in their first year, each residency class has its own T-group. Participation is voluntary. Residents select their own T-group "leader," a psychiatrist who has no administrative authority over their careers; this allows residents to speak more freely within the group.

The T stands for "training," not "therapy," even though these groups may be therapeutic (see Chapter 5). At the outset, the "leader" announces, "This T-group will meet for ninety minutes a week, for the next fifty-two weeks. The goal of a T-group—some call it a 'process group'—is to study how groups, all kinds of groups, function. The method of study will be experiential; you'll learn by direct involvement. I won't give lectures, nor will I lead the group. I will, however, try to facilitate your learning by being a 'consultant.' " At this point, the consultant stops talking.

The residents get restless. They don't know what to do. This is the first time they've not been told what to do. Unclear on what the consultant meant by the group's purpose, the residents scramble to find one. Residents who frequently bitch about tyrannical authorities are now insisting on their own agenda; others look to the consultant for leadership, and when they don't get it, they're surprised at how dependent they've become on authorities. Group members will try to be the "smartest," the "funniest," the "sexiest," the "most insightful." Residents discover they're more competitive than they'd imagined. Finding it safer, they'll vent their spleens about lousy teachers, incompetent nurses, and frustrating patients.

One might expect that it would be relatively easy for psychiatrists to talk about their personal feelings and concerns. Not true. They find it hard to open up, less because of their initial reason— "We all have to work together"—than because, like most people, they feel that sharing intimacies exposes one's deficiencies and vulnerabilities. These fears are compounded by the not unrealistic concern that everything they say will be "analyzed" by their peers. To avoid opening up, they'll fret that secrets will leak from the group. But more compellingly, residents are fully aware that if members speak their mind, personal dislikes of one another will eventually emerge. They don't want this to happen, and many a resident has said, "If my feelings are to be devastated, I much prefer it be done in private with my analyst than in public with my peers." Indeed, some residents so dread the possibility of being hurt by others' insensitivity or criticism that many T-groups have an unspoken rule never to criticize a member.

The residents' fear that opening up before their colleagues will render them dangerously vulnerable gives rise to a paradox. On the one hand, I have heard many a resident, myself included, say in a T-group, "I'm always meeting everyone else's emotional needs, but I wish that sometimes somebody would spend a few moments to take care of *my* emotional needs." Yet, when this opportunity presents itself as it does in a T-group, residents, like most psychiatrists, prefer to offer, and not to receive, emotional support. It is almost as if by asking for such support, the resident would turn into a patient, or at the very least, an emotional weakling—hardly the stern stuff of the "stable" psychiatrist.

Eventually, as trust develops within the group, residents do open up, but far more about professional than about personal concerns. Most of the discussion is shoptalk: how they're treated by faculty; how they wish to gain the approval of certain professors; how they're overworked; how they are treated differently by friends just because they are now psychiatrists; how they worry about not doing enough for their patients; how some patients drive them crazy; and how, on rare occasions, a resident fears that a patient, whom he may or may not know, is threatening to kill him.

Meanwhile, the consultant helps the residents see what's going on in the group. He frequently does so by the classic "T-group comment," a deliberately enigmatic statement which suggests something without being clear about it. In response to a dominant occurrence in the group that nobody will acknowledge or talk about, such as a subtle flirtation between members, the consultant may remark, "Sweat's running down my thigh." This type of comment, which usually amuses and infuriates residents, is designed to be suggestive enough to give them a clue that something sexual is going on in the group, but vague enough to make them see it and bring it up for themselves.

In learning how all groups function, in the T-group residents directly observe people's ambivalence toward authority. Residents see how competitive they become with the consultant, attacking him for being too "domineering," "self-centered," "ineffective," "withholding," "hypocritical," and "insensitive." At other times, they worship the consultant, praising him for having incredible depth, wisdom, sensitivity, and insight.

Residents never forget their T-group. It's the only time during a resident's training that he's both a subject and an object of investigation. For the 50 percent of psychiatric residents who are not receiving personal therapy, the T-group is often their closest experience to being in psychotherapy. A middle-aged psychiatrist, who had never obtained personal psychotherapy, looked back on his T-group and said, "I was such a stiff person before I joined; it really opened me up." Even those residents who are in therapy acknowledge the T-group's effect on them. "I hadn't realized until the group how viciously competitive I get." Although every psychiatrist remembers his T-group, not all remember it favorably. "I hated my T-group. I felt under constant pressure to discuss my feelings, and I simply didn't want to. The more I refused, the more people got on my case. One day I got so fed up, I simply left the room and never returned." Many psychiatrists believe their T-group deepened their understanding of how patients experience group therapy. "When you have *ten* people all telling you that you're full of shit, that's awesome! I saw how groups, whether for good or ill, can be frighteningly powerful. It clued me in to how patients must feel in a group.''

That most psychiatrists reflect positively on their T-groups is clear; that they learn how groups function—its main purpose—is not. Maybe that's not so important; there are other ways to learn about groups. Yet because residents work in psychologically charged environments, T-groups afford them a good opportunity to unwind, to support one another, and to realize they are not alone in facing the stresses of becoming a psychiatrist.

Curriculum

When psychiatric educators were asked which of over 900 topics should be taught to residents, every one agreed on the following: (a) the evaluation and basic treatment of mental disorders as described in *DSM–III,* (b) the evaluation and treatment of psychiatric emergencies, (c) the clinical assessment of brain disease, (d) the hypothesized causes of psychoses, (e) a psychodynamic understanding of psychotherapeutic relationships, and (f) basic psychotherapeutic skills.* These six areas constitute the core curriculum in all psychiatric training, and thus the basic expertise of all psychiatrists. Most residents feel they've acquired this basic expertise by the end of their second year of training.

Because the psychiatrist's expertise is the diagnosis and treatment of mental disorders and serious problems in living, many subjects which the public assumes psychiatrists know about are rarely taught. Residents receive little or no training in transactional analysis, Jungian therapy, Adlerian therapy, sociology, psychodrama, Rolfing, ESP, mental health, psychosurgery, or the psychology of social and cultural phenomena (e.g., drama, art, computers, politics, racism).

During a typical week, a resident spends ten hours in lectures or seminars, six hours receiving supervision on his cases, and thirty to thirty-five hours treating patients. Although objectively resi-

---

*"Basic psychotherapeutic skills" normally include conducting supportive, insight-oriented, couples, family, and group psychotherapy, as well as using medication and ECT. Although psychoanalysis receives considerable attention, the ability to perform it is not considered an essential psychiatric skill. Training in behavior therapy and child psychiatry vary a lot depending on the program.

dents know they learn from all these experiences, subjectively they feel that treating patients is "service" and not training. This perception leads to the residents' most frequent gripe: "Our service commitments are so excessive, we're not getting enough teaching." Faculty respond, "You're not just students; you're being paid sixteen to twenty thousand dollars a year to provide service." Then, after acknowledging the importance of training, faculty zing residents with their two favorite cliches: "Service *is* training," and *"All* patients are interesting." Although true, these lines never assuage residents. On the other hand, good supervision does.

Supervision of patient care

Although in theory residents are supervised on all their cases, in practice they usually receive careful supervision on roughly half of them. This instruction normally consists of one resident discussing one patient with one supervisor. Other formats may be employed, such as five to ten residents intensively exploring one case with a supervisor.

Faculty members are assigned to supervise specific aspects of a resident's work. For example, Columbia's second year residents each have seven different supervisors for an hour a week. One teacher is for group therapy, another for family therapy. Two instructors supervise "patient management," which covers initial evaluations of new patients' diagnoses and psychodynamics, deciding and implementing treatment plans for new patients, monitoring medications, providing brief psychotherapy, and handling "practical" problems during the course of treatment (e.g., "Should I hospitalize a suicidal patient?" "Should I allow an extremely depressed patient to attend his mother's funeral?" "Should I have a session with Mr. Schwarz if he comes intoxicated?") Two teachers supervise the resident's long-term, intensive, insight-oriented psychotherapy, while another monitors the resident's psychopharmacologic treatment.

To learn how to use medication, residents must treat hundreds of patients, but to learn the basics of psychotherapy, residents need excellent supervision on just a few patients; from them, one hopes, residents will extrapolate to others.

In general, a resident will discuss a patient in supervision without his teacher's ever seeing the patient and without the patient's ever knowing his case is being supervised. If a patient wonders if his case is being supervised, he should ask his therapist.* At times, a supervisor may directly observe the resident's interview of a patient; he might even interview the patient himself. (Psychiatrists speak of "interviewing" patients, not "talking with" them.) Supervisors occasionally use audiotaped or videotaped recordings of psychotherapy sessions,† but in most situations their advice is based on what the residents tell them.

A more structured, but less used, approach is for the supervisor to hear the resident's "process notes"—transcripts of psychotherapy sessions recorded by the resident, as verbatim as possible, right after the hour. Supervisors comment on what the resident recorded and on what he "may have accidentally" left out. The supervisor might ask, "Why did you focus on your patient's anger toward her mother, but avoid her obvious anger toward you?" Or "Why is it that according to your notes, all the women in the group talk, while all the men are speechless? Does this reflect the men or *your feelings* about the men?" or "Do you believe your patient's incessant ramblings about his boss have oedipal overtones?" Taking process notes is an arduous, time-consuming task, but it teaches residents how to remember the details of a psychotherapy session.

In most jobs, when a novice errs, inexperience or a lack of knowledge is blamed. Not so in psychiatry. When a resident makes a mistake, he would rather attribute it to countertransference than to inexperience. Psychiatric residents take great pride in their intelligence, and so when anything goes awry in treatment, they are loath to admit it was because they don't know something. On the other hand, they are quite willing to fault their own psychology, since by attributing all errors to a neurotic countertransference, they can show off their psychological sophistication. For example, I was supervising a first-year resident on his evaluation of a

---

*Residents are not the only psychiatrists who receive supervision. After their residencies, many psychiatrists pay for supervision to sharpen their skills, and thereby, help their patients.

†Patients, who must consent to being taped, can turn off the machine whenever they wish. The tape recorder is placed where the patient can see it, but outside his immediate line of vision. Typically, after five minutes of tape recording, both patient and therapist are no longer fazed by it. Some patients feel they get far more out of a session by listening to a tape recording of it at home.

new and elderly patient. The resident made a beginner's mistake: He failed to inquire if his patient abused alcohol. The resident automatically ascribed his oversight to "ambivalent feelings I have toward my father." But so what? Even assuming the resident has mixed feelings about his father—who doesn't?—inexperience is still the most likely cause of the error. If the resident were to make the same mistake *repeatedly,* then, and only then, would counter-transference be the chief culprit. Every resident sees his emotions adversely affect treatment, but in most cases, the experience he acquires during training shows him how to avoid repeating such mistakes. During my residency, this fact became embarrassingly apparent.

Under the best of circumstances, children and I do not get along. Thus, when we began to learn how to conduct play therapy with children, I was the first in my class to volunteer; I figured I would be inept anyway, so why not get it over with? So having never evaluated or treated a child, I was to assess Carl, an eight-year-old bed wetter. This evaluation took place in a room loaded with toys and decorated with a one-way mirror; observing us from behind this mirror were my fellow residents. (Carl knew he was being observed.)

At our first meeting, although I had no idea of what to do, Carl rescued me by suggesting we play Go to the Head of the Class, a board game. Carl explained the rules to me—something about rolling dice, picking cards, answering questions, and moving Alfred E. Neuman–like tokens. We start playing, and very soon, I'm having a great time, and so is my new playmate. In fact, I am so absorbed in the game, I forget that I'm being observed and that my whole purpose for being there is to evaluate this child. As the game draws to an end, it's nip and tuck: We both have three spaces to go before reaching the head of the class. By this time, my competitiveness has taken over. No eight-year-old bed wetter is going to beat me! Victory hinges on the next question. I pick a card, and read the question to Carl. "How do you spell the word 'speech'?" (I may have no ability with children, but I have even less ability at spelling.) Very carefully, Carl replies, "s-p-e-e-c-h." I'm ecstatic: The bed wetter has blown it! "Wrong!" I proclaim. "It's s-p-e-*a*-c-h." I pounce my token three spaces ahead and declare myself the winner. Hoots, yelps, and guffaws are heard from the adjacent room. Laughing hysterically, my dear classmates are even pounding the one-way mirror. Little Carl is bewildered. I'm baffled: Why all the commotion? It was only after the session that I realized my spelling blunder, but more important, I saw how much my competitiveness ran amok and interfered with therapy. Since then, I have tried to keep this competitiveness in check.

In supervision, residents learn more than psychological complexities and clinical techniques; they learn fundamental ways of behaving with patients. Simple things, but things that can greatly influence psychotherapy. Residents enter training with society's stereotypes about how psychiatrists are *supposed* to behave, and during a residency these are unlearned. For instance, because psychotherapy is a serious enterprise, I assumed it was highly unprofessional to crack a joke. This sounds naive, but at the time, that's what I believed. Mind you, I told jokes anyway, but fearing my supervisors' disapproval, I hid this from them. Finally, I confessed to a supervisor, who not only told me that telling a joke was okay, but more significantly, how to employ humor to advance psychotherapy. Like most good supervisors, he was showing me how to avoid being a psychiatric robot and to use my personal style toward professional ends.*

The second year

The chief pleasure for the second-year resident is that he spends at least half his time performing insight-oriented psychotherapy with outpatients. The remainder of his time is typically split between doing outpatient evaluations, medication maintenance, emergency-room psychiatry (see Chapter 8), and child psychiatry.

During the second or third year, the resident also provides consultation to house staff on the psychiatric problems of medical and surgical patients. These consultations are usually requested on hospitalized patients who are confused, suicidal, and, most often, uncooperative with treatment, tearing out IVs or refusing therapy.

Because a major reason students become psychiatrists is to get

---

*Early in my residency, I proudly told a supervisor that I "did not give in to the manipulations of a sobbing hysteric by passing her a Kleenex." The supervisor told me, "Stop being a schmuck! Be a *mensch* and give her a Kleenex. If you're being manipulated, discuss it later in treatment. Meanwhile, all therapists, even you, should use good manners in treatment." I felt like a jerk: My supervisor was absolutely right. Yet like most residents, I needed to correct the many stereotypes I had about how shrinks are supposed to behave.

away from medicine, when residents start performing consultations and working alongside other physicians, they are "coming home." During the era of psychoanalytic psychiatry, this was usually an unhappy reunion, since psychoanalytic insights were of little practical use to the doctors requesting the consultation; moreover, psychiatrists' downplaying their medical identity did little to endear residents to their medical peers. With scientific psychiatry's "remedicalization" of the profession, psychiatric residents feel more at home with other physicians and can be of greater practical help to them and to their patients. According to recent surveys, doctors implement 80 percent of all psychiatric recommendations.*

When I was a resident, the surgeons asked my supervisor, Dr. Pat McKegney, and me to consult on an older man who had a half-dozen thick six-inch nails lodged in his lower intestine. The surgeons felt the guy was, as they wrote in the chart, "mentally unglued," and they wanted us to evaluate him. The patient, a street vagrant, looked drained, tired, and worn. Speaking in a monotone, he rambled half-coherently about insects, Lyndon Johnson, poetry, and "pandas in heat." The man was a chronic schizophrenic, but his behavior was no odder than the surgeons'. Nails in the bowel constitute a surgical emergency; at any moment they can perforate the intestine, causing peritonitis and death. Since surgeons live to cut, their failure to operate was hard to fathom. But after talking with the surgeons, it became clear they were so put off by this patient's weird behavior that they ignored him. Our job was to get the surgeons to stop being distracted by the man's peculiarities and to pay serious attention to his surgical needs. But how?

The patient, with his apparently hearty appetite, had swallowed more than nails. Pat showed him an X ray revealing what anybody could tell were five fishhooks attached to his esophagus. After the patient calmly examined the X ray, with complete seriousness Pat asked him, "How do you think those fishhooks got there?" Genuinely puzzled, the patient replied, "That's odd. I don't fish."

We told the surgeons of this exchange, and their amusement started to get them invested in the patient. We then calmed their

---

*How often the recommendations of other specialists are accepted is unknown.

unwarranted fears that operating on this patient might exacerbate his schizophrenia.

As in this case, when psychiatrists provide consultations, they address not only the patient's difficulties, but also the psychological obstacles that interfere with the physician's providing good care. Their training in consultation psychiatry teaches residents to give such advice without sounding as if they were psychoanalyzing the physician. While learning this technical skill, the resident is also "rejoining" the medical profession and completing his identity as a physician.

By the start of the third year, residents feel they've learned psychiatry's fundamentals and need far less supervision. Consequently, their final year of training is primarily elective, and depending on his interests, a third-year resident conducts research, administers an inpatient unit or an outpatient clinic, teaches medical students, treats drug addicts, sharpens psychotherapeutic skills, works at a student-health service, or becomes a chief resident. Which of these, and many other, opportunities a resident pursues depends not only on what he wants to learn, but more important, on what he hopes to do when he leaves academia and plops into the "real" world.

ELEVEN

Private Lives

All psychiatrists-in-training ride "the big track"—twenty-four years of nonstop education, which finally terminates at the end of residency.* The track's course is determined by the necessities of training, and the psychiatrist's choice to remain aboard is reinforced by the expectations of teachers. A trainee who takes a detour—like spending a year bumming around Europe or writing a novel—risks having mentors and colleagues question his dedication, seriousness, dependability, and stability. (Academic psychiatrists transmit a mixed message to trainees: They overtly encourage residents to embark on these detours, but covertly discourage them from doing anything that interferes with training.) Many residents daydream about taking a year off "to do what *I* want to do before my career and kids straitjacket me into adulthood." Nevertheless, out of habit, necessity, or desire, most psychiatrists stay on track till the end.

When training is finally over, the psychiatrist suddenly faces the novel situation that *he,* and not academia, must run his life. Ironically, after all these years, the psychiatrist has to do what he

---

*After completing what one resident called "the twenty-fourth grade," many psychiatrists choose to obtain further training, most often in child psychiatry, research, and psychoanalysis.

has been counseling his patients to do—take charge of his own life. For residents, leaving the big track feels similar to leaving home; it's a time to "grow up," to decide for themselves what type of psychiatry to practice and what type of life to live.

LAUNCHING A CAREER

The stress of launching a career outside a university's shrink tank is compounded by faculty, who generally act as though anything other than an academic career is second-rate. So when residents don't follow in their teachers' footsteps, they feel as if they were displeasing their parents. Referring to his favorite faculty member, a near-to-graduating resident confessed, "If I go into private practice instead of joining his research team, I'm afraid he will lose all interest in me." He was exaggerating, but not by much.

Few residencies provide any formal teaching on "How to Conduct a Private Practice" or "How to Make a Living as a Psychiatrist"; informal guidance in these matters is just as rare. Although 90 percent of psychiatrists will eventually do some private practice, their teachers feel it is uncouth to discuss establishing a practice, and worse yet, making money. Since the "good" psychiatrist seeks truth, not dollars, why waste time discussing irrelevancies?

Another reason most instructors avoid discussing how to launch a private practice is that they don't know how. University faculty *automatically* receive their own offices, monthly salaries, insurance, billing systems, answering services, secretaries, and patients. Since many teachers have never arranged for these, not only can't they advise, but some pretend the problems don't even exist. When Harvard psychiatrist Dr. Jonathan Borus conducted a seminar called "Transition to Practice," the residents called it "Reality Rounds."

The first two years following residency are highly stressful. In a survey of 263 psychiatrists completing their residencies, 73 percent complained of moderate anxiety and depression, while 58 percent of the total claimed they were incapacitated by these symptoms. The events that recent graduates cited as stressful, from the most to the least frequently occurring, were: board examinations (66 percent), difficulties with patients (47 percent), marital problems (45 percent), changes in friends (40 percent), moving (39 percent), sexual problems (28 percent), concerns over health (26 percent), sleep disturbances (24 percent), weight changes (23 percent), and separation and divorce (14 percent).

In this study, the single best predictor of which psychiatrists successfully leave the big track is the degree of support they receive from a spouse or loved one. Apparently, this occurs less because more emotionally mature students get married than because marriage itself exerts a "protective" influence. Married medical students experience less stress than nonmarried ones, but only *after* they get married. What's more, being "connected" to others, be it through play, recreation, or professional contacts, is helpful. Residents who best master transition also come from programs with a diverse orientation. In contrast, having personal psychotherapy had no apparent effect, positive or negative, on how well psychiatrists handle this transition.

On the verge of leaving the academic womb, fledgling psychiatrists are suddenly faced by an onslaught of totally unfamiliar questions: "How can I get a salaried part-time job to pay the rent until my practice builds up?" "How do you find an office, and what do you look for?" "Should I go into partnership?" "What do I charge?" "What should I do about patients who don't pay?" "Do I charge for missed sessions?" "How do I get referrals?" "Can I afford to turn down a patient even though he's going to drive me buggy?" "Since they only pay fifteen dollars a session, should I accept Medicare patients?" After years of believing it déclassé to mention money, the psychiatrist who's about to launch a practice finds himself thinking of little else.

Fees, income, and expenses

> . . . money matters are treated by civilized people in the same way as sexual matters—with the same inconsistency, prudishness, and hypocrisy.
> —Sigmund Freud (1913)

When psychiatrists first see private patients, they feel guilty about charging them.* More experienced colleagues, perhaps cor-

---

*Dr. Richard Druss, a Columbia University psychoanalyst, tells the tale of an analyst, who on leaving his car in Manhattan's fashionable Upper East Side is

rectly, label these concerns "neurotic," but the typical new psychiatrist keeps asking himself, "Am I worth seventy dollars an hour? How can I charge just for talking? Since anybody can do what I do, why should I be paid for it? For years I saw patients who paid in the clinic, so why is this bothering me *now*?" The big difference is that now he is getting paid *directly*.

Receiving payment from a patient heightens the psychiatrist's sense of responsibility for that patient. The novice psychiatrist finds himself being a bit more cautious about making aggressive interpretations, since if they lead to the loss of but one patient, his income can drop by 10 to 20 percent. Yet the chief concern of the beginning psychiatrist is whether he deserves his fee. This might be the first time the psychiatrist has ever placed a monetary value on his services and, in his mind, on himself.

When starting a private practice, psychiatrists also worry that by charging a fee, they are harming their patients. For example, soon after a patient agrees to a fee of $90 an hour, he laments that he cannot afford the bicycle his son Steve wants for Christmas. The psychiatrist thinks that by simply waiving the $90 cost of this one session, little Stevie could get his bike. In just one year, many novice psychiatrists have run up thousands of dollars in unpaid bills.

When the rent's due, common sense overcomes guilt and the psychiatrist ends up charging whatever the market will bear.* Most psychiatrists set a basic fee, and will lower it, depending on how busy they are and on the patient's income.

Psychiatrists usually decide to charge for missed sessions depending on whether the patient was absent primarily because of

---

suddenly confronted by a thief who demands, "Give me all your money and drugs!" The analyst empties his wallet and explains, "I don't have any drugs—really." The skeptical thief replies, "You've got MD plates, so you must be a doctor." The analyst interjects, "But I'm the kind of doctor who doesn't use drugs: I'm a psychoanalyst. I *talk* to patients about their problems." Becoming curious, the robber says, "What do you charge for this?" "Eighty dollars an hour." The thief is stunned. "Hot damn! You give no drugs; you just talk. And for that you get *eighty bucks*. And you call *me* a thief!"

*Perhaps only New Yorkers could appreciate the best guideline for setting fees: the cost of a pizza slice. A patient suggested that when a slice goes for 60 cents, charge $60 a session; when a slice is 80 cents, charge $80, and so on. Is there a better barometer of inflation than a pizza slice?

"resistance" or "reality." Because the typical general practitioner sees a new patient every fifteen minutes, if a patient doesn't show up, the doctor can see another patient. Not so with a psychiatrist: If a patient doesn't arrive, there won't be another patient in his office for at least an hour. Thus, if a psychiatrist knows several days in advance of a cancellation, he's less apt to charge for a missed session, since he can schedule another patient.

Psychiatrists are now the third-lowest-paid medical specialists (see Table 11-1). Before taxes, the average physician annually nets $99,500, whereas the average psychiatrist nets $76,500 (in 1982). The reasons for this are many. Whereas psychiatrists can charge only for seeing patients, other physicians can also charge for procedures, such as X rays, operating, and anesthesia. (However, 10 to 15 percent of psychiatrists give shock treatment, and can charge for it.) The time restraints of the standard fifty-minute hour and the emotional intensity of psychotherapy limit the number of patients a psychiatrist can see a day. Psychiatrists work fewer hours and must compete with other mental health providers. When the

TABLE 11-1
ANNUAL NET INCOMES OF
PHYSICIANS

SPECIALTY	NET INCOME*
Radiology	$136,800
Anesthesiology	131,400
Surgery	130,500
Obstetrics/gynecology	115,800
Other†	94,900
Internal medicine	86,800
Psychiatry	76,500
General/family practice	71,900
Pediatrics	70,300

*Average, pretax net income in 1982; i.e., Net Income = Gross Income − Expenses (Table 11-2).
†Includes pathologists, neurologists.

economy is depressed, more patients are hospitalized and enter the public sector; thus, fewer are seen privately. When money is tight, patients are more inclined to dispense with psychiatric than with medical care. Health insurance covers less (if anything) for psychiatric care.

On the other hand, the psychiatrist's expenses are much lower than those of any other medical specialist (see Table 11-2). Little if any medical equipment is needed. Neither are nurses and secretaries; a phone-answering machine suffices. Psychiatrists aren't plagued by mountains of insurance forms and complicated billing systems. For less money, psychiatrists have less hassle. But, if a psychiatrist really hustles in private practice, he can readily net $90,000 from outpatients or $100,000 to $120,000 from inpatients.

Remember that the table of expenses doesn't include the roughly $18,000 a year he may be paying for his own analysis, nor does it include payments on the $20,000 to $40,000 in debt that most residents incur by the end of medical school.

Compared to all other physicians who treat patients, psychiatrists are sued the least and pay the least in malpractice premi-

TABLE 11-2
ANNUAL EXPENSES OF PHYSICIANS

SPECIALTY	EXPENSES*
Obstetrics/gynecology	$109,000
Surgery	105,000
Internal medicine	75,800
General/family practice	75,700
Radiology	68,100
Other†	67,600
Pediatrics	66,700
Anesthesiology	52,300
Psychiatry	37,200

*Average practice expenses for self-employed physicians in 1982.
†Includes pathologists, neurologists.

ums. From 1978 to 1983, the number of psychiatrists filing malpractice claims climbed from one out of fifty to one out of twenty-five. Despite this rise, it is nowhere near the average for other physicians: Each year one out of four files malpractice claims. Malpractice suits stem more from poor doctor-patient relationships than from poor treatment, and psychiatrists are probably sued less because they have better relationships with their patients. When they are sued, 27 percent of suits are about "improper treatment," with a majority of these involving sex between psychiatrist and patient; 18 percent are over "drug reactions," including side effects and failure of medications to work as promised; and another 18 percent are about failures to prevent suicides. A mere 1 percent were related to ECT. During the past five years, malpractice insurance has doubled for psychiatrists, so that in 1983, its yearly cost in New York City was $1,784, and in California, $1,920.

Like most professionals, psychiatrists prefer to live in large cities or college towns with good schools and good cultural and recreational facilities, but the single greatest consideration for psychiatrists is the extent to which the area's health insurance plans cover psychiatric services. From 1970 to 1979, communities that provided extensive insurance for psychiatric care increased their psychiatrist-population ratios by 100 percent, whereas those that didn't increased their ratios by only 25 percent.

Boards

Nothing stresses new psychiatrists more than having to take the "boards," officially called the American Board of Psychiatry and Neurology (ABPN). Since their inception in 1934, the boards' format has continually changed, but there are usually two parts. Part I is an all-day written exam, consisting largely of multiple-choice questions, one third on neurology and two thirds on psychiatry. Although psychiatrists can take Part II, "the orals," within nine years of passing Part I, most do so within a year. In Part II the psychiatrist observes two psychiatric patients, one for twenty minutes on videotape, and the other for thirty minutes "live." After each, for the remainder of the hour, two examiners ask the board candidate about the patient's assessment, diagnosis, psychology, and treatment.

Whereas physicians, including psychiatrists, are *licensed* to practice legally by states, psychiatrists and neurologists are *certified* by the ABPN, which means they have demonstrated not excellence, but *basic competence*. Because a "board-certified" psychiatrist is likely to be a "safe" psychiatrist, patients seeking a good psychiatrist should definitely ask if the psychiatrist is board-certified. For psychiatrists, at most board certification may raise their annual salary by $1,000; otherwise, it is without legal status and not having it rarely disqualifies a psychiatrist from a job.

Even though boards have little practical meaning, psychiatrists get very nervous taking these exams. There are countless stories about keys being lost, pipes crunched, and glasses broken. Realizing that 40 percent of candidates fail Part II, even highly knowledgeable psychiatrists will devote three to six months preparing for each part of the exam; many will spend $500 to $1,500 taking courses that are specifically designed to prepare them for boards. On the day of the oral exam they sit stiffly in rows, as if awaiting execution. When they finally meet the patient, many normally calm, courteous, and sensitive psychiatrists suddenly forget to introduce themselves; they'll fumble for words, not hear the patient, ask questions out of sync, and forget major parts of the interview, such as the patient's family history.

Since boards are the profession's chief standard of clinical competence, if a psychiatrist fails them, does that mean he is incompetent? Perhaps; it varies with the person. It doesn't help that boards present a "no-win" situation: Everybody assumes the psychiatrist will pass, so when he does it's no big deal; if he fails, everybody politely says the boards "don't matter," but the flunked shrink is sure they're wondering about his professional ability and why he screwed up. This concern is not imaginary; 71 percent of younger psychiatrists believe all psychiatrists should be board-certified.

But more important than what colleagues think is what the psychiatrist himself thinks. In failing the exam, he not only questions his professional competence but wonders if his failure reflects some "unconscious masochism" or "need to fail." After failing boards, psychiatrists have been known to endure three to eighteen or more months of demoralization, agitation, nightmares, sulkiness, and despair. Even when boards are passed without difficulty, taking them is always traumatic.

After twenty-four years of school, once boards are completed, most psychiatrists may never take another exam. With boards behind him, the psychiatrist has entered professional adulthood and can get on with his personal life.

SOCIAL LIFE

Outside the office, when a psychiatrist lets his profession be known, people respond in ways all too familiar to every psychiatrist. If the psychiatrist wants to get involved giving serious answers, he might well reply:

Layman: Can you read people's minds?

Psychiatrist: No.

Layman: Still, I'd better watch what I say. Are you going to analyze me?

Psychiatrist: Not in the sense that you mean it. Whether or not they are psychiatrists, most sophisticated people "analyze" or size up other people's psychology. I'm not analyzing your psychology any more than you're analyzing mine. "Analyzing people" is something we do for a living, not something we do socially. At first, during my residency, I found it hard to stop analyzing people, but now the novelty of being a psychiatrist has worn off and I automatically shut off all that psychologizing.

Layman: Do you diagnose people you meet?

Psychiatrist: Not really. First off, I don't have nearly enough information to make a diagnosis; to get that, I'd have to do a clinical interview. Even if I thought you might be depressed, I wouldn't ask you about your sleep, appetite, or bowel habits in a social situation. Second, although sometimes I can't help but wonder if somebody has a mental illness, so does everyone else. Third, when my wife and I meet somebody, I might suspect the person has a borderline personality disorder while my wife thinks he's a bum. Our labels differ, but being a psychiatrist doesn't make

287

me any better at dealing with that person *socially* than my wife; *clinically* I could, but that's different.

Layman: How can you stand listening to people all day?

Psychiatrist: Because we do more than listen: We help people. We're not passively absorbing information, but actively trying to use what we hear to advance treatment. Even when psychiatrists are silent, they are constantly formulating and testing hypotheses, and trying to figure out what to say next.

Layman: Isn't it frustrating to be a psychiatrist?

Psychiatrist: Sometimes. But then, I would assume that sometimes you also find your work frustrating.

Layman: What kind of psychiatrist are you?

Psychiatrist: A good one.

Layman: What I mean, smart-ass, is if you are a Freudian or a Jungian. Do you use drugs or psychotherapy?

Psychiatrist: Most psychiatrists today, myself included, use both biological and psychological treatments. We don't view them as antagonistic, but complementary; each does something different. Many basic psychoanalytic concepts, such as defense mechanisms and the unconscious, are taken for granted by psychiatrists, no matter what kind of practice they have. Sure, some psychiatrists are more interested in psychobiology and others in psychoanalysis, but most contemporary psychiatrists draw from both; they view the debates, such as drugs versus talk or Freud versus Jung, as passé.

Layman: Do you think psychiatry works?

Psychiatrist: Yes, although it depends on what you mean by "work."

Layman: Well, you can't cure people.

Psychiatrist: By and large, that's true. But then, most doctors don't cure their patients; physicians don't cure di-

	abetes, heart disease, cancer, strokes, hypertension, arthritis, or the majority of illnesses they treat. They can help a lot, but so can we.
Layman:	The reason I'm asking is that I'm thinking about seeing a psychiatrist, but what holds me back is that I'm not sure I have faith in psychiatry.
Psychiatrist:	Faith has nothing to do with it. After you give treatment a reasonable chance to work, you can determine for yourself whether it is, or is not, helpful. What matters is not faith, but results.
Layman:	But a friend of mine has been in therapy for three years, and he says he really doesn't know if it's helped. His shrink tells him that he's made a lot of progress, but my friend isn't so sure. So it's still a question of faith: Does he have faith in his own judgment or his shrink's?
Psychiatrist:	I don't know your friend's situation, but it seems to me the issue is not about having faith in therapy or even if therapy works: The issue here is that your friend doesn't trust his own judgment.

In general, psychiatrists are glad to supply friends with the names of therapists or tell them what to look for in getting a therapist. Psychiatrists don't mind discussing psychiatric issues as long as the discussion isn't an excuse for a patient to seek advice on his treatment. Not only doesn't the psychiatrist have enough clinical information to make an informed judgment, but he worries that whatever he says may undermine the person's therapy. On social occasions, most psychiatrists prefer not to debate psychiatric ideologies, make diagnoses, interpret dreams, judge the quality of a person's treatment, or perform therapy.

A psychiatrist's attributes outside his office have no bearing on his abilities inside his office. Psychiatric expertise is limited to clinical situations; psychiatric training neither improves personality nor bestows social grace. Thus, when first meeting a psychiatrist socially, don't be surprised if he is interpersonally inept, psychologically obtuse, or devoid of self-awareness. In social settings, shrinks usually talk about children, cars, home furnishings,

August vacations in Cape Cod,* the high cost of living, and their most frequent ailment—backaches. In my experience, psychiatrists are generally no more, or less, interesting or profound than others with similar backgrounds.

When psychiatrists engage in shop talk at parties, they are more likely to gossip about the politics and personalities of a training institution, hospital, or psychiatric society than to discuss their patients. They avoid talking about patients partly because, after seeing them all day long, they are eager to talk about *anything* but patients. Moreover, psychiatrists take confidentiality seriously. Nevertheless, they are prone to name-drop: "I was treating this well-known Republican who was close to Nixon, and he described Nixon as . . ."

When psychiatrists and patients meet socially, if anyone feels awkward, it is usually the patient. The chief concern of the psychiatrist is that the patient's seeing him might undermine the patient's confidence. The psychiatrist might be drunk, gallivanting with another woman or with a homosexual partner; he might be in swim trunks that reveal an unflattering belly. As a result, most therapists will go to some, although not a great, extent to avoid seeing a patient socially.

Psychiatrists often feel they are treated differently just because they are psychiatrists. An unmarried psychiatrist ran into a woman with whom he'd once had an affair: "I was aghast! After several drinks she says, 'I'd recharge our relationship, but I could never do that with a shrink.' " Newer psychiatrists complain that long-standing close friends now avoid sharing intimacies, claiming they're afraid of "being psychoanalyzed." As one psychiatric resident complained, "I feel cheated. Being a psychiatrist, I'm suddenly disqualified from having heart-to-heart conversations." Once the psychiatrist's friends realize that he's not analyzing them, they treat the psychiatrist normally. On the other hand, casual acquaintances may not. At a party when a psychiatrist simply says somebody's "crazy," listeners often take this as a virtual diagnosis; if anybody else says the same thing it's no big deal.

Like most psychiatrists, I often feel pressured, either by oth-

---

*All mental illness disappears in August, except in Cape Cod, where 31,000 American psychiatrists congregate to wear Bermuda shorts, lie on the beach, and read John Updike.

ers or by myself, to behave therapeutically. When an acquaintance tells a layman, "My marriage is on the rocks," the layman can merely say, "That's too bad," without feeling obligated to help in resolving the person's problem. Not so with a psychiatrist. If I were to respond, "That's too bad," it would seem vapid, unworthy of a psychiatrist. Correctly or not, psychiatrists usually assume the acquaintance expects them to say something more profound or therapeutic.

FAMILY LIFE

In essence, the psychiatrist's family life is the same as anyone's of similar socioeconomic standing. Where exceptions exist, they stem more from how outsiders view psychiatrists than from how psychiatrists or their families behave.

Children bear the brunt of belonging to a psychiatrist's family. Classmates will tease them, saying that they or their psychiatrist-parent is crazy, a loony, or a mental case. Kids always tease each other, but what's different for a psychiatrist's child is that he has to prove his sanity, and that when he does anything odd, others will "explain" it by saying, "Everybody knows that psychiatrists raise the screwiest kids." After hearing this enough, some children of psychiatrists start worrying about their sanity. Since they are repeatedly asked, "Does your father (or mother) analyze you?" most psychiatrists' children go through a period when they view everything their parent says about their behavior as a psychiatric interpretation instead of a normal parental comment.

As happens with most spouses of psychiatrists, my wife encounters two typical reactions: "How great to have a live-in shrink who solves all your problems" and "Isn't it awful to have somebody analyzing you all the time?" Although a costume designer, my wife is constantly being asked for her "expert" advice on medical, and to a lesser degree psychiatric, matters. Doctors—not normal people but doctors—assume that because I am a physician, she's a nurse. This book's editor, Nick Bakalar, is married to a psychiatrist, and thus is condemned to a lifetime of being called "doc" by tollbooth operators and gas-station attendants who spot the MD license plates on his car.

Like most psychiatrists, I don't tell my wife anything about my patients. First, she's not interested. Second, she feels information about patients is none of her business—and I agree. Third, although I'm not concerned she will gossip, something can always slip out by accident; if I tell her nothing, this can't happen.

Psychiatrists have the same rate of bad marriage and divorce as other physicians (47 percent), and this rate is not much higher than that of similar socioeconomic groups (32 percent). In comparison to other mental health professionals, psychiatrists have the lowest rate of separation and divorce: For psychiatrists it is 6.1 percent, for psychologists 10.5 percent, for psychiatric social workers 13.3 percent, for psychiatric nurses 16 percent, and for other mental health workers 14.3 percent.

When troubles do arise in a psychiatrist's marriage, studies show the most frequently heard complaint, from about half of all psychiatrists' wives, is that their husbands use interpretations and jargon in addressing ordinary domestic problems. One wife says, "I have been called a dentate vagina and paranoid, and have had explained to me that my behavior results from parental suppression." Another wife observes, "I find that what I say is interpreted to mean the exact opposite of what I intended." Other complaints include "My husband's psychiatry has contributed to my lack of confidence" and "With the experience gained in his career, he developed a superior attitude. He became extremely skillful in rationalizing situations to suit himself. . . . I felt intimidated and put down."

When marital problems occur when one member is an attorney, spouses complain of being treated like a jury; when one is a teacher, spouses complain of being treated like a student. I've heard a man bitch to his actress wife, "I'm not one of your fans!" Just as being an attorney, teacher, or actress is not the *cause* of marital problems but the way they're *conceptualized,* so too with being a psychiatrist.

Generally speaking, spouses of psychiatrists will express certain sentiments much *less* than laymen might expect. It is unusual for a spouse to complain that her psychiatrist mate "cares more about his patients than about me," or that "he takes his frustrations with patients out on me." Partly because psychiatrists try to leave their patients' problems at the office, if anything, their spouses complain their mates don't talk enough about their frustrations with patients, even in the most general of terms. (Psychiatrists are much more likely to discuss professional frustrations unrelated to patients.)

THE IMPAIRED PSYCHIATRIST

This subject is taboo. Patients avoid it because they don't want their psychiatrist to be too ill or too crazy to help them; psychiatrists avoid it because they don't want to be patients. So what if eventually *all* doctors become patients? Patients get ill, not doctors; patients go mad, not doctors; patients die, but never physicians.

In July 1972, a forty-seven-year-old psychiatrist in a private group practice died unexpectedly. Within forty-eight hours, his partners contacted his patients and offered supportive counseling, which most patients appreciated. (In response to a similar offer when another psychiatrist died, a patient responded, "You couldn't even wait until the body was cold before recruiting patients for yourself!") Patients grieved, cried, expressed fears of being alone; many responded with increased somatic complaints, others with stoicism and especially denial.

Some patients and even a few psychiatrists tried to maintain contact with the deceased. One patient was consoled by clipping and cataloguing articles from psychiatric journals in the dead man's office. Another patient wanted (and received) a trinket from the psychiatrist's bookshelf. Months later at a Broadway play, one of his partners was transfixed, momentarily convinced a man sitting in the orchestra was the deceased returned to life.

Without ever explicitly asking about suicide, many patients wanted to know if there was an autopsy, what it revealed, whether the coffin would be open (it wasn't, thereby increasing denial), when the funeral would be, and the location of the grave.

Everybody reacted personally. A twenty-nine-year-old female patient proclaimed, "God is dead . . . He was my only Jesus. . . . I know this is selfish, but what's going to happen to me?" A thirty-year-old man who'd regarded the psychiatrist as a shield from his castrating mother stated his situation succinctly: "My mother has won."

As months passed, the initial grief and denial were superseded by feelings of abandonment, rejection, and finally anger. Some patients attacked their new therapists for not being as good as their old therapist, while others (including the patients' friends and relatives) continually berated the dead therapist for "overworking himself," being "accident-prone," and virtually causing his own death. Some patients had resurrection fantasies, such as one who said, "I know he's alive in the grave; he almost died before."

Physical illness

Living with Crohn's disease, a chronic bowel disorder that usually bothers and sometimes hospitalizes me, I've found that my psychological reactions to physical illness are quite similar to those of other psychiatrists, including the widely respected psychoanalyst Dr. Paul Dewald. After being hospitalized for six weeks from a serious stroke which caused him to be unconscious and amnesic, he recovered at home for another four weeks before gradually returning to practice.

When our illnesses became worse, and in Dewald's case life-threatening, we both became masters at denial.* At first, we put off informing patients we were ill. Then, after being hospitalized and riddled with tubes, we told our patients we'd see them next week. Dewald said his denial was "rationalized by me as protecting the patients from undue anxiety associated with learning I was seriously ill."

Once I became self-absorbed with my illness, I tried to avoid patients who would telephone, even if only to wish me well. Dewald and I worried that whatever information we gave patients about our illnesses would someday complicate psychotherapy. Although this was a valid concern, at the time I was more concerned with being left alone, freed from any burden (real or imagined) to care for patients, and with avoiding being in a "one-down" position with my patients.

When I began to improve physically, I became increasingly eager to speak with patients, and if possible, to advise them clini-

---

*Another psychiatrist told me that on the very night of the day he started his own psychoanalysis, he awoke with severe back pain. Never had the power of psychoanalysis loomed so impressively—until three hours later when he passed a kidney stone.

cally. I enjoyed having the company and being helpful. If I could help others, I was no longer sick.

Dewald and I started to fret that colleagues would displace us and patients would leave us. He calls this "neurotic," but I'm not totally sure: If I were a patient, no matter how much I liked my therapist, if he wasn't available, what good would he be? We not only worried about losing income and craft, but as friends and family encouraged us to "take it easy," we feared becoming "addicted" to the regression we'd secretly come to enjoy.

Gradually returning to work, we had to decide which patients to see first. I felt conflicted between wanting to see healthier, and therefore less demanding, patients first, as opposed to initially seeing more disturbed patients who, although needing more help, would be a far greater strain on me. Both Dewald and I started to worry about how the patients would interpret our choices. Would the earlier-seen patients think they were sicker, needier, nicer, or our "favorites"?

Once back at work, instead of feeling relieved, the residual effects of illness disrupted our concentration. Trying extra hard to be in top form, we privately grumbled that our patients weren't appreciating all our efforts. We'd rationalize our anger at patients for not suffering as we had by thinking, "The patients must be angry at us for being ill and leaving them."

When psychiatrists are physically ill, they spin endless mental gyrations deciding if their symptoms are physical or mental. Do I feel lethargic because I'm depressed or because of my Crohn's disease? Am I sleepy because I'm tired or because I want to avoid work? For psychiatrists, these ruminations are the norm, not the exception.

Suicide

People often feel guilty when a person they know commits suicide. Yet when a psychiatrist kills himself, his colleagues will experience additional guilt, believing that just because they are psychiatrists, they should have, and could have, prevented the psychiatrist's death. So when a psychiatrist does commit suicide, an unspoken thought in the minds of many psychiatrists is: "The guy might still be alive if the psychiatrists working with him were paying enough attention to him." Psychiatrists realize this sentiment is unfair, since any psychiatrist sufficiently determined to kill himself knows how to hide his intention from colleagues.

On the other hand, there are times when psychiatrists consciously or unconsciously avoid recognizing a potentially suicidal colleague. Psychiatrists might not want to "get involved." They might feel so drained by patients they lack the energy to recognize, and to deal with, a suicidal colleague. They might not wish to see a colleague's despair, fearing that if he can get suicidal, so can they. For all these reasons, whenever a psychiatrist commits suicide, the psychiatrists who knew him may well have a reason to feel some guilt.

Despite some disagreement among experts, it appears that psychiatrists commit suicide at a rate twice that of other physicians, and that physicians do so at a rate similar to other age-matched professionals. It's unknown whether psychiatrists kill themselves more often because of their profession, their personalities, or something else. Psychiatrists tend to be less religious, and less religious people more often kill themselves. In comparison to most families, those of psychiatrists are more likely to admit to a suicide. Psychiatrists are better able to commit suicide than laymen because they know what's required to avoid botching the job.

Since 50 to 70 percent of suicides occur during a major depression, could it be that doctors prone to depression choose psychiatry, or that psychiatric work prompts depression and suicide? Nobody knows. Could it be that the stress of treating patients induces a major depression that leads to suicide, or does the psychiatrist first develop a major depression, which then, as he is en route to committing suicide, makes him feel that work is more stressful? Once again, nobody really knows. Unscrambling this chicken-and-egg problem is difficult, but psychiatrists are more inclined to believe the severe depression came first, and that the stress of treating patients and the eventual suicide are the result, not the cause, of the depressive illness.

Figures suggest that women psychiatrists, like other female professionals, seem to commit suicide four times as often as age-matched American white females. Women in the general population commit suicide three to four times less often than men, and this higher suicide rate among female psychiatrists brings them up to the rate of their male colleagues.* Surveys show that women psychiatrists are less satisfied with their training and their careers, and even if one controls for their shorter work week and smaller chance of being board-certified, they still earn less. But whether any of these factors account for why women psychiatrists commit suicide more than women in general remains unknown.

Burnout

Whereas depression and not work is the main cause of psychiatrists' suicides, depression is only one of many causes which lead psychiatrists to burn out. Although frustrations at work play a major role whenever a psychiatrist burns out, the fantasy of many patients that their not getting better caused their shrink to burn out is grandiose. All psychiatrists are frustrated by patients; only a few burn out.

Feeling indispensable is the dominant trait of psychiatrists who burn out. Concerned with losing face or revealing professional inadequacies, they're reluctant to refer patients. Being excessively fussy and perfectionistic, they waste time on unimportant details, work endlessly, and avoid vacations and recreation. They need to be needed.

Earlier in their careers, burned-out psychiatrists were often idealistic, hardworking overachievers; now they're martyrs. Instead of writing their usual half-page note in a patient's chart, they now fill two to four, and sometimes ten or more, pages. They make sure everyone sees they are swamped with work and dedicated to patients. Despite all these efforts, little gets accomplished. They fret about falling behind professionally, but read few technical journals and attend few educational meetings. In their hurried existence, working, sleeping, and eating schedules become chaotic. To maintain their energy or to calm their nerves, the burned-out psychiatrist is rarely drug-free, abusing narcotics the most.

When patients detect a burned-out psychiatrist, they see a therapist who is disheveled and frazzled, is increasingly late for appointments, and often misses them altogether. For session after session, he talks far more than usual and frequently off the point;

---

*Statistically, this rate of 40.7 per 100,000 differs little from the 35.7 per 100,000 seen with male physicians.

at other times, he's virtually mute. His concentration wavers. He's not as sharp. His sense of humor is gone. Patients begin to feel that his well-being hinges on their own well-being. Although usually minor, his prescription errors become frequent and his handwriting is shakier.

Every psychiatrist has his off days. Every psychiatrist goes through periods when the craziness of his patients gets to him. Every psychiatrist becomes overwhelmed by the miseries and futilities of his patients. Every psychiatrist has days, if not weeks, of feeling he is of absolutely no help to his patients. When such difficulties persist, and the psychiatrist begins to sense the specter of burnout, most psychiatrists will do something about it. They may seek therapy. They may take courses, join professional discussion groups, talk things over with trusted colleagues, or switch jobs. Because psychiatry is such an emotionally charged profession, the risk of burnout is high, yet burnout is avoidable.

While nobody would dispute the wisdom of "Physician, heal thyself," many traits of the good psychiatrist conflict with the traits of a good family member and of a sane human being. Psychiatrists control feelings, healthy people express them. Good psychiatrists work long hours, good family members don't. Good therapists respond to every emergency; healthy therapists take the phone off the hook.

Speaking as a patient, I want the best for my doctor. Yet for this to happen, when I'm ill on weekends and unable to reach him, I must settle for his partner, who knows little of my case. If we want saner doctors, we should expect to see less of them. Similarly, burned-out psychiatrists do nobody any good, but to prevent burnout from happening, each psychiatrist knows that he will be less than fully dedicated to his patients.

PERSONAL THERAPY

Half of my first-year residency class trained at the West Haven V.A. Hospital while my half trained at the Yale–New Haven Medical Center. At West Haven a resident was assumed "crazy" if he did *not* receive a personal analysis; at Yale–New Haven, he was "crazy" if he *did* receive an analysis. These convictions revealed less about analysis than about those who held them. They also reflect a split within the profession. For contrary to myth, only half of all psychiatrists receive individual psychotherapy or psychoanalysis (which I'm lumping together and calling "personal therapy").*

The value psychiatrists have placed on obtaining personal therapy has changed over time. In 1912, when Freud became convinced that all analysts should be analyzed, he wrote that it wasn't enough for the analyst to "be an approximately normal person . . .[he should also] have undergone a psychoanalytic purification. . . ." From the 1930s through the 1950s, Freud's belief was generally accepted by American psychiatrists. They were convinced that completing a personal analysis (not therapy) provided a "necessary insurance against persistent character defects," as if bestowing an "official endorsement of normalcy." Today, such expectations are considered grandiose, even by psychiatrists who staunchly believe that every psychotherapist should have his own psychoanalysis or personal therapy.

There are two basic rationales for obtaining personal therapy. First, there are its *therapeutic* functions, which entail resolving or "curing" a psychiatrist's conflicts, impairments, mental illness, or problems in living which might interfere with conducting therapy. Second, there are its *training* purposes, which include learning by direct experience what it's like to be a patient, how the unconscious functions, and how a more experienced therapist works. Most psychiatrists who enter personal therapy do so for both reasons.†

Whether personal therapy benefits psychiatrists depends on its purpose. When used strictly for treatment, it probably helps as much (or as little) as it does with anyone else. Studies have shown that personal therapy does not help psychiatrists adjust to problems in living, nor alleviate the stress of moving from a residency

*The American Psychiatric Association asserts that psychiatrists needn't have personal therapy. In contrast, all psychoanalysts must receive a personal analysis.
†The official reasons a psychiatrist gives for obtaining personal therapy often conflict depending on economic considerations. In 1981, the U.S. Tax Court ruled that a psychiatric resident could deduct personal therapy as an *educational* expense, which for many is over $18,000 a year. However, if personal therapy is an educational expense, it is not a *medical* expense; it should not be covered by health insurance, even though insurance often reimburses psychiatrists for up to 50 to 100 percent of it. Thus, therapy is treatment for insurance companies, but education for the IRS.

into practice. Personal therapy does, however, alter how a psychiatrist conducts treatment. Analyzed therapists are more active with more disturbed patients and quieter with healthier patients. The psychiatrist who's been through intensive personal therapy is more likely to treat patients as his therapist has treated him and to hold more closely to what standard textbooks suggest.

Whether a psychiatrist receiving personal therapy benefits his patients depends substantially on how long he has been practicing. Studies reveal that in contrast to their nonanalyzed peers, the analyzed psychiatrists who are relatively experienced are more helpful to patients and display greater empathy, whereas newer therapists are relatively cold, unempathetic, distant, and ineffective. They might, for example, be so in awe of their analyst that they redeploy one of their analyst's "brilliant" interpretations onto their own patients, who sit there confused, unable to figure out what this interpretation has to do with them.

Most psychiatrists still feel that receiving a personal therapy is valuable, but mainly for psychiatrists who primarily conduct insight-oriented psychotherapy. Yet, with the shift from psychoanalytic to scientific psychiatry, relatively fewer psychiatrists have practices limited to performing intensive psychotherapy, and therefore, from a strictly professional (rather than personal) standpoint, fewer psychiatrists feel a need to obtain personal therapy.

ALL THINGS CONSIDERED

Although many people leave professions to become psychiatrists, the reverse is rarely the case. Psychiatrists change jobs, but almost always inside, and not outside, the field. As a whole, psychiatrists seem glad to be psychiatrists.

The profession's rewards are obvious. When surveyed, psychiatrists claimed that what they liked most about their profession was (in order) helping patients, feeling socially useful, having a good income, financial security, favorable working conditions, status, opportunities for professional advancement, and intellectual stimulation and excitement.

Of these psychiatrists, 35 percent could not name any career dissatisfactions; 13 percent complained they lacked status, especially among other physicians; 11 percent didn't like their working conditions; and 9 percent griped about a low income. Other concerns were "long office hours," "constant tension of practice," "the loneliness of office practice," "endless paperwork," and "isolation from the rest of the community." A few psychiatrists worried that they weren't "sufficiently effective."

Like most of my colleagues, when I became a psychiatrist I assumed certain benefits woud accrue which, to my surprise, never did. Although being a psychiatrist has taught me something about living sensibly, it has never resolved any of my own psychological concerns. Being a psychiatrist has not made me a better (or worse) husband, friend, or person, and if I had kids, I'd still be the same type of father. Although I can spout many psychiatric terms and explanations, being a psychiatrist *per se* has neither helped nor hindered my understanding of people or of the world. I am no wiser, but no more foolish; no happier, yet no sadder.

Being a psychiatrist allows me to know people in ways that few other professions make possible—but I anticipated this. There are days when nothing is going right for any of my patients, and when these days occur, I retreat to bed three hours earlier than usual and remain awake all night long; I also anticipated this. I expected to learn from my patients, and I have.

On the other hand, when I chose to become a psychiatrist in 1966 I never anticipated that within fifteen years my profession would undergo the most profound change since the Freudian revolution. During the past decade, my ability to help patients has expanded enormously, not because of me, but because of this revolution. My diagnoses illuminate prognoses and suggest treatments. I have many new and different drugs to offer my patients; so too with the many types of family, couples, group, behavioral, and cognitive, as well as traditional, psychotherapies.

Let my confession be clear. When I entered psychiatry, I expected to learn about patients, but in all honesty, not to *help* them. I expected to learn about ids and egos, but not to make symptoms go away. I expected the biological, psychosocial, and moral-existential aspects of treatment to be in conflict, but not to be synthesized. I expected to be a philosopher, but not a doctor. I expected to be an artist, but not a scientist.

I am glad the new scientific psychiatry has proved me wrong.

Source Notes

(In these notes the *American Journal of Psychiatry* will be abbreviated as "Am J Psy" and *Archives of General Psychiatry* as "Arch Gen Psy.")

Chapter 1 THE SECOND REVOLUTION

PAGE

15   "Since recently most . . .": Strauss GD, Yager J, Strauss GE (1984): The cutting edge in psychiatry. Am J Psy, 141: 38–43

15   "Although constituting less . . .": Gross ML (1978): The Psychological Society. Random House: NY; Gruel L (1980): Psychiatric Manpower for the 80's. American Psychiatric Association: Washington, DC; Light D (1980): Becoming Psychiatrists. Norton: NY; American Psychiatric Association (1983): Economic Fact Book for Psychiatry. American Psychiatric Press: Washington, DC; English JT, Kritzler ZA, Scherl DJ (1984): Historical trends in the financing of psychiatric services. Psychiatric Annals, 14: 321–331

17   "Of the 31,000 . . .": Gruel; American Psychiatric Association; Henry WE, Sims JH, Spray SL (1973): Public and Private Lives of Psychotherapists. Jossey-Bass: San Francisco; Blum JD, Redlich F (1980): Mental health practitioners: old stereotypes and new realities. Arch Gen Psy, 37: 1247–1253; Goldstein MZ, Bromet EJ, Hanusa BH, Lasell RL (1981): Psychiatrists' life and work patterns: a statewide comparison of women and men. Am J Psy, 138: 919–924; Fenton WS, Leaf PJ, Moran NL, Tischler GL (1984): Trends in psychiatric practice, 1965–1980. Am J Psy, 141: 346–351

17   "Since 1965, psychiatrists . . .": Fenton

17   "Roughly a quarter . . .": Morrow JS (1983): Personal correspondence from American Psychiatric Association, May 22; Werner R (1984): Personal correspondence from American Medical Association, May 3

17n   "Although the American . . .": Werner; Maxmen JS (1970): On joining the AMA. Medical Opinion and Review, 6: 50–57

23   ". . . in 1964 *Fact* . . .": Rogow AA (1970): The Psychiatrists. G. P. Putnam's Sons: NY

23n   "With clear political . . .": Ibid

23   "Theoretically psychiatrists can . . .": Menninger W (1967/1947): The

world today. In A Psychiatrist for a Troubled World: Selected Papers of William C. Menninger, M.D., 2: 570–573

25 ". . . it appears in . . .": Jaspers K (1972/1923): General Psychopathology. University of Chicago Press: Chicago, pp 301–303

29 "There can be . . .": Alexander FG, Selesnick ST (1966): The History of Psychiatry. Basic Books: NY, pp 290–291

30 "In treating patients, . . .": Abroms EM (1983): Beyond eclecticism. Am J Psy, 140: 740–745

31*n* "As with this explanation . . .": Unger RM (1982): A program for late twentieth-century psychiatry. Am J Psy, 139: 155–164

Chapter 2 *HOW PSYCHIATRISTS DIAGNOSE*

PAGE
35 *"The Diagnostic and . . .":* The Diagnostic and Statistical Manual of Mental Disorders, Third Edition (DSM-III) (1980). American Psychiatric Association: Washington, DC

36 "The concept of . . .": Szasz T (1979): The lying truths about psychiatry, in The Encyclopedia of Delusions. Edited by Duncan R, Weston-Smith M. Wallaby: NY, p 123

40 "What once in . . .": Alexander FG, Selesnick ST (1966): The History of Psychiatry. Harper & Row: NY, p 164

41 ". . . US/UK Study . . .": Cooper JE, Kendell RE, Gurland BJ, Sharpe L, Copeland JRM, Simon R (1972): Psychiatric Diagnosis in New York and London. Oxford Univ Press: NY

41 "Indeed, just one . . .": Kendell RE, Cooper JE, Gourlay AJ, Copeland JRM, Sharpe L, Gurland BJ (1971): Diagnostic criteria of American and British psychiatrists. Arch Gen Psy, 25: 123–130

42 "That's why the . . .": Srole L, Langner TS, Michael ST, Opler MK, Rennie TAC (1962): Mental Health in the Metropolis: The Midtown Manhattan Study. Volume 1. McGraw-Hill: NY

42*n* "When clearly defined . . .": Freedman DX (1984): Psychiatric epidemiology counts. Arch Gen Psy, 41: 931–933; Robins LN, Helzer JE, Weissman MM, Orvaschel H, Gruenberg E, Burke JD, Regier DA (1984): Lifetime prevalence of specific psychiatric disorders in three sites. Arch Gen Psy, 41: 949–958

42 "For example, in 1975 . . .": Woodruff RA, Clayton PJ, Guze SB (1975): Is everyone depressed? Am J Psy, 132: 627–628

43   "The excessive diagnosis . . .": North C, Cadoret R (1981): Diagnostic discrepancy in personal accounts of patients with 'schizophrenia.' Arch Gen Psy, 38: 133–137

45   "For instance, studies . . .": Simon RJ, Fleiss JL, Gurland BJ, Stiller PR, Sharpe L (1973): Depression and schizophrenia in hospitalized black and white mental patients. Arch Gen Psy, 28: 509–512; Raskin A, Crook TH, Herman KD (1975): Psychiatric history and symptom differences in black and white depressed inpatients. Journal of Consulting Clinical Psychology, 43: 73–80; Adebimpe VR (1981): Overview: white norms and psychiatric diagnosis of black patients. Am J Psy, 138: 279–285

46   "Because these criteria . . .": Feighner JP, Robins E, Guze SB, Woodruff RA, Winokur G, Munoz R (1972): Diagnostic criteria for use in psychiatric research. Arch Gen Psy, 26: 57–63

47   "DSM-II: DEPRESSIVE NEUROSIS . . .": The Diagnostic and Statistical Manual of Mental Disorders, Second Edition (DSM-II) (1968). American Psychiatric Association: Washington, DC, p 40

47   "DSM-III: DIAGNOSTIC CRITERIA . . .": DSM-III, pp 222–223

51   "Psychiatrists are far . . .": Spitzer RL, Endicott J, Robins E (1975): Clinical criteria for psychiatric diagnosis and *DSM-III*. Am J Psy, 132: 1187–1192; Andreasen NC, McDonald-Scott P, Grove WM, Keller MB, Shapiro RW, Hirschfeld RMA (1982): Assessment of reliability in multicenter collaborative research with a videotape approach. Am J Psy, 139: 876–882

51   "The types of . . .": Spitzer; Klein DF (1967): Importance of psychiatric diagnosis in prediction of clinical drug effects. Arch Gen Psy, 16: 118–126

53   ". . . *DSM-III* is reductionistic . . .": Vaillant GE (1984): The disadvantages of *DSM-III* outweigh its advantages. Am J Psy, 141: 542–545

55   *"DSM-III* points out . . .": DSM-III, p 6

55   ". . . a mental disorder . . .": Ibid

56   "This expansion of . . .": Light D (1980): Becoming Psychiatrists. Norton: NY, p 19

58   "Every textbook of . . .": Klerman GL (1984): The advantages of *DSM-III*. Am J Psy, 141: 539–542

Chapter 3 *MENTAL DISORDERS*

PAGE
61   "In one of . . .": Rosenhan DL (1973): On being sane in insane places. Science, 179: 250–258

61   "Much can be . . .": Spitzer RL (1976): More on pseudoscience in science and the case for psychiatric diagnosis. Arch Gen Psy, 33: 459–470

63   "The either/or concept . . .": Marcus RL (1984): Mentally ill criminals: 'as culpable as anyone.' Letter, New York Times, March 15, p A30

67*n*   "Only 20 percent . . .": Shapiro S, Skinner EA, Kessler LG, Von Korff M, German PS, Tischler GL, Leaf PJ, Benham L, Cottler L, Regier DA (1984): Utilization of health and mental health services. Arch Gen Psy, 411: 971–982

67*n*   "In 1980, according . . .": American Psychiatric Association (1983): Economic Fact Book for Psychiatry. American Psychiatric Press: Washington, DC

68*n*   "Using *DSM-III* diagnostic . . .": Regier DA, Myers JK, Kramer M, Robins LN, Blazer DG, Hough RL, Eaton WW, Locke BZ (1984): The NIMH Epidemiologic Catchment Area Program. Arch Gen Psy, 41: 934–941; Myers JK, Weissman MM, Tischler GL, Holzer CE, Leaf PJ, Orvaschel H, Anthony JC, Boyd JH, Burke JD, Kramer M, Stoltzman R (1984): Six-month prevalence of psychiatric disorders in three communities. Arch Gen Psy, 41:959–970

72   "Each year, about . . .": Minkoff K (1978): A map of the chronic mental patient, in The Chronic Mental Patient. Edited by Talbott J. American Psychiatric Association: Washington, DC, pp 11–38

72   "The annual cost . . .": Gunderson JG, Mosher LR (1975): The cost of schizophrenia. Am J Psy, 132: 901–906

72   "Schizophrenics occupy roughly . . .": Berger P, Hamburg B, Hamburg D (1977): Mental health: progress and problems. Daedalus, 106: 261–276

75   "About a quarter . . .": Ludwig AM (1980): Principles of Clinical Psychiatry. Free Press : NY

76   "Fifty to 70 . . .": Goodwin DW, Guze SB (1984): Psychiatric Diagnosis. Oxford University Press: NY

76   ". . . virtually all suicides . . .": Markham M (1981): Suicide without depression. Psychiatric News, 16(20): 8, 24–25, October 16

76   "Because suicide is . . .": Pokorney AD (1983): Prediction of suicide in psychiatric patients. Arch Gen Psy, 40: 249–257; Tefft BM, Pederson AM, Babigian HM, Haroutin M (1977): Patterns of death among suicide attempters, a psychiatric population, and a general population. Arch Gen Psy, 34: 1155–1161; Spitzer RL, Endicott J, Woodruff RA, Andreasen N (1977): Classification of mood disorders, in Depression: Clinical, Biological and Psychological Perspectives. Edited by Usdin G. Brunner/Mazel: NY, pp 73–103

79 "In one study, . . .": Targum SD, Dibble ED, Davenport YD, Gershon ES (1981): The family attitudes questionnaire: patients' and spouses' views of bipolar illness. Arch Gen Psy, 38: 562–568

81 "While these patients . . .": Wender PH, Klein DF (1981): Mind, Mood & Medicine: A Guide to the New Biopsychiatry. New American Library: NY

82 "Many psychiatrists claim . . .": Wender; Shader RI, Goodman M, Gever J (1982): Panic disorders: current perspectives. Journal of Clinical Psychopharmacology, 2: 2S–10S

82 "The most popular . . .": Ewalt JR (1967): Other psychiatric emergencies, in Comprehensive Textbook of Psychiatry. Edited by Freedman AM, Kaplan HI. Williams and Wilkins: Baltimore, pp 1179–1187

Chapter 4 HOW PSYCHIATRISTS EVALUATE PATIENTS

PAGE

104n "Frame-by-frame analysis . . .": Sloman L, Berridge M, Homatidis S, Hunter D, Duck T (1982): Gait patterns of depressed patients and normal subjects. Am J Psy, 139: 94–97

107 "For example, a . . .": Hamilton M (1960): A rating scale for depression. Journal of Neurology, Neurosurgery, and Psychiatry, 23: 56–62

108n "In the near . . .": Maxmen, JS (1976): The Post-Physician Era: Medicine in the 21st Century. Wiley: NY

109 "Unfortunately, the DST . . .": Goodwin FK, Paul SM (1983): The uses and misuses of biological tests in psychiatry. Current Comments, May, pp 5–7

109 "According to one . . .": Muecke LN, Krueger DW (1981): Physical findings in a psychiatric outpatient clinic. Am J Psy, 138: 1241–1242

109 "Although psychiatrists debate . . .": Patterson CW (1978): Psychiatrists and physical examinations: a survey. Am J Psy, 135: 967–968

Chapter 5 HOW PSYCHIATRISTS DETERMINE TREATMENT

PAGE

111 "The future may . . .": Freud S (1938/1964): An Outline of Psychoanalysis, in Complete Psychological Works, standard ed, vol 23: 141–207. Translated and edited by Strachey J. Hogarth Press: London, p 182

112 "Dr. Robert Michels . . .": Michels R (1981): The psychoanalytic par-

adigm, in Models of Clinical Psychopathology. Edited by Eisdorfer C, Cohen D, Kleinman A, et al. Spectrum: NY, pp. 5–12

112   "Similarly, for modern . . .": Karasu TB (1982): Psychotherapy and pharmacotherapy: toward an integrative model. Am J Psy, 139: 1102–1113

113   "When today's psychiatrists . . .": Abroms EM (1983): Beyond eclecticism. Am J Psy, 140: 740–745

116   "In 1973, the . . .": Donnelly J (1978): The incidence of psychosurgery in the United States, 1971–1973. Am J Psy, 135: 1476–1480; Fink M (1981): Book review of The Psychosurgery Debate: Scientific, Legal, and Ethical Perspectives. Am J Psy, 138: 408–409.

117   "Despite numerous anecdotal . . .": Pauling L (1974): On the orthomolecular environment of the mind: orthomolecular theory. Am J Psy, 131: 1251–1257

117   ". . . there are no . . .": Comments on Dr. Pauling's article by Drs. Wyatt RF, Klein DF, and Lipton MA. Am J Psy, 131: 1258–1267; Winick M (1980): Nutrition in Health and Disease. Wiley: NY

117   "Conversely, taking high . . .": Winick

120   "Patients claim that . . .": Yalom ID (1970): The Theory and Practice of Group Psychotherapy. Basic Books: NY; Maxmen JS (1973): Group therapy as viewed by hospitalized patients. Arch Gen Psy, 28: 404–408; Schaffer JB, Dreyer SF (1982): Staff and inpatient perceptions of change mechanisms in group psychotherapy. Am J Psy, 139: 127–128

122   "American psychiatrists have . . .": Gruel L (1980): Psychiatric Manpower for the 80's. American Psychiatric Association: Washington DC, Tables 6.1, 6.2

123   "Numerous studies confirm . . .": Ochitill H, Kellner R (1982): Somatoform disorders, in Treatment of Mental Disorders. Edited by Greist JH, Jefferson JW, Spitzer RL. Oxford: NY, pp 266–308

125   "It is much . . .": Flinn DE, Leon RL, McKinley RL (1981): Psychotherapy: the treatment of choice for all. Psychiatric Annals 11: 335–344, p 337

125   "Studies do reveal . . .": Rounsaville BJ, Klerman GL, Weissman MM (1981): Do psychotherapy and pharmacotherapy for depression conflict?: empirical evidence from a clinical trial. Arch Gen Psy, 38: 24–29

128   "When actually tested . . .": Wilkins W (1973): Expectancy of therapeutic gain: an empirical and conceptual critique. Journal of Consulting Clinical Psychology, 40: 69–77; Bloch S, Bond G, Qualls B, Yalom I, Zimmerman E (1976): Patients' expectations of therapeutic improvement and their outcomes. Am J Psy, 133: 1457–1460

130*n*   "Even if offering . . .": McGlashan TH (1984): The Chestnut Lodge follow-up study, II. Arch Gen Psy, 41: 586–601

131   "Research shows that . . .": Vaughan CE, Leff JD (1976): The influence of family and social factors on the course of psychiatric illness. British Journal of Psychiatry, 129: 125–137; Anderson CM, Hogarty GE, Reiss DJ (1980): Family treatment of adult schizophrenic patients: a psycho-educational approach. Schizophrenia Bulletin, 6: 490–505

134   "There is, however, . . .": Frances A, Clarkin JF (1981): No treatment as the prescription of choice. Arch Gen Psy, 38: 542–545

137   *"Cognitive therapy. In . . .":* Beck AT (1976): Cognitive Therapy and the Emotional Disorders. International Universities Press: NY; Silverman JS, Silverman JA, Eardley DA (1984): Do maladaptive attitudes cause depression? Arch Gen Psy, 41: 28–30; Murphy GE, Simons AD, Wetzel RD, Lustman PJ (1984): Cognitive therapy and pharmacotherapy: singly and together in the treatment of depression. Arch Gen Psy, 41: 33–41

Chapter 6 THE BIOTHERAPIES

PAGE
145   "Light, natural and . . .": Rosenthal NE, Sack DA, Gillin C, Lewy AJ, Goodwin FK, Davenport Y, Mueller PS, Newsome DA, Wehr TA (1984): Seasonal affective disorder. Arch Gen Psy, 41: 72–80

145   "Dr. Eric Kandel . . .": Kandel ER (1983): From metapsychology to molecular biology: explorations into the nature of anxiety. Am J Psy, 140: 1277–1293; The neurosciences and behavior: an emerging biology of the mind (1982): P&S, The Journal of the College of Physicians and Surgeons of Columbia University, 2(2): 19–22

147   "It now appears . . .": Crowe RR, Noyes R, Pauls DL, Slymen D (1983): A family study of panic disorder. Arch Gen Psy, 40: 1065–1069; Torgersen S (1983): Genetic factors in anxiety disorders. Arch Gen Psy, 40: 1085–1089

147   "For example, the concordance . . .": Kendler KS, Robinette CD (1983): Schizophrenia in the National Academy of Sciences–National Research Council Twin Registry: a 16-year update. Am J Psy, 140: 1551–1563

148   ". . . psychiatrists Seymour Kety . . .": Kety SS (1983): Mental illness in the biological and adoptive relatives of schizophrenic adoptees: findings relevant to genetic and environmental factors in etiology. Am J Psy, 140: 720–727

149   "The schizophrenic spectrum includes . . .": Kety; Kendler KS, Gruenberg AM (1984): An independent analysis of the Danish Adoption Study of Schizophrenia. Arch Gen Psy, 41: 555–564

149*n*   "An example of . . .": Torgersen S (1984): Genetic and nosological aspects of schizotypal and borderline personality disorders: a twin study. Arch Gen Psy, 41: 546–554

149   ". . . cluster with alcoholism . . .": Weissman MM, Gershon ES, Kidd KK, Prusoff BA, Leckman JF, Dibble E, Hamovit J, Thompson D, Pauls DL, Guroff JJ (1984): Psychiatric disorders in the relatives of probands with affective disorders. Arch Gen Psy, 41: 13–21; Knorring AL, Cloninger R, Bohman M, Sigvardsson S (1983): An adoption study of depressive disorders and substance abuse. Arch Gen Psy, 40: 943–950; Leckman JF, Weissman MM, Merikangas KR, Pauls DL, Prusoff BA (1983): Panic disorder and major depression: increased risk of depression, alcoholism, panic, and phobic disorders in families of depressed probands with panic disorder. Arch Gen Psy, 40: 1055–1060

149   "In other studies . . .": Winokur G (1979): Unipolar depression: is it divisible into autonomous subtypes? Arch Gen Psy, 36: 47–52

151   "The patient, on . . .": Henderson D, Gillespie RD (1952): A Textbook of Psychiatry for Students and Practitioners, Seventh Edition. Oxford University Press: London, p 337

154   "The single most . . .": Caton CLM (1984): Management of Chronic Schizophrenia. Oxford: NY

155*n*   "Depending on the . . .": Caton; Crane GE (1971): Persistence of neurological symptoms due to neuroleptic drugs. Am J Psy, 127: 1407–1410; Asnis GM, Leopold MA, Duvoisin RC, Schwartz AH (1977): A survey of tardive dyskinesia in psychiatric outpatients. Am J Psy, 134: 1367–1370; Chouinard G, Annable L, Ross-Chouinard A, Nestoros JN (1979): Factors related to tardive dyskinesia. Am J Psy 136: 79–83

156   "Depressive disorders are . . .": American Psychiatric Association (1983): Economic Fact Book for Psychiatry. American Psychiatric Press: Washington, DC

160   "In the article . . .": Friedberg J (1975): Electroshock therapy: let's stop blasting the brain. Psychology Today, 9(3): 18–23, August

161   "In the newsletter . . .": Pribram K (1974): Interview. APA Monitor, Sept–Oct, pp 9–10

161   ". . . the actual use . . .": Mills MJ, Pearsall DT, Yesavage JA, Salzman C (1984): Electroconvulsive therapy in Massachusetts. Am J Psy, 141: 534–538

161   "Nonetheless, more than . . .": Klein DF, Gittelman R, Quitkin F, Rifkin A (1980): Diagnosis and Drug Treatment of Psychiatric Disorders: Adults and Children, Second Edition. Williams & Wilkins: Baltimore

161   "Studies reveal that . . .": Hurwitz TD (1974): Electroconvulsive therapy: a review. Comprehensive Psychiatry, 15: 303–314

161   "Of the seven . . .": Klein et al

162   "A recent survey . . .": Guze SB (1980): Electroconvulsive therapy. Psychiatric Capsule & Comment, 2(12): 1–2

162   "The most dangerous . . .": Scarf M (1979): Shocking the depressed back to life. New York Times Magazine, June 17, pp 32–36, 42

162   "In a report of 259,000 . . .": Hurwitz

163   "Nevertheless, over the . . .": Guze

163   "Research comparing patient's . . .": Squire LR (1975): Memory functions six to nine months after electroconvulsive therapy. Arch Gen Psy, 32: 1557–1564

163   "Despite the verg . . .": Fink M (1977): Myths of "shock therapy." Am J Psy, 134: 991–996

166   "During the past . . .": Beigel A (1981): Proposals to stimulate competition in the financing and delivery of health care. Presentation before the Subcommittee on Health, House Ways and Means Committee, October 2

167   "Tolerance to their . . .": Maxmen JS (1981): A Good Night's Sleep: A Step-by-Step Program for Overcoming Insomnia and Other Sleep Problems. Contemporary Books: Chicago

167   "From 1971 to 1977 . . .": Maxmen

167   "From 1973 to 1981 . . .": Baum C, Kennedy DL, Forbes MB, Jones JK (1982): Drug Utilization in the U.S.—1981. Third Annual Review. Department of Health and Human Services: Washington, DC, December

168   "For example, a . . .": Keller MB, Klerman GL, Lavori PW, Fawcett JA, Coryell W, Endicott J (1982): Treatment received by depressed patients. Journal of the American Medical Association, 248: 1848–1855

168   "Although the proper . . .": Jick H, Dinan BJ, Hunter JR, et al. (1983): Tricyclic antidepressants and convulsions. Journal of Clinical Psychopharmacology, 3: 182–185

168   ". . . according to one . . .": Orne MT (1983): Perspectives on the VII World Congress of Psychiatry, Volume 2. Wyeth Laboratories: Philadelphia, pp 13–14

Source Notes

Chapter 7 PSYCHOTHERAPY

PAGE

172   "Research comparing individual . . .": Pilkonis PA, Imber SD, Lewis P, Rubinsky P (1984): A comparative outcome study of individual, group, and conjoint psychotherapy. Arch Gen Psy, 41: 431–437

173   "Indeed, when a . . .": Malcolm J (1981): Psychoanalysis: The Impossible Profession. Alfred A. Knopf: NY

178n   "Dr. Roy Schafer . . .": Schafer R (1974): Talking to patients in psychotherapy. Bulletin of the Menninger Clinic, 38: 503–515, p 514

187   ". . . to paraphrase H. L. Mencken . . .": Mencken HL (1916/1955): Theodore Dreiser, in The Vintage Mencken. Gathered by Alistair Cooke. Vintage: NY, pp 35–56

190   "Dr. Jay Haley . . .": Haley J (1969): The art of being a failure as a therapist, in The Power Tactics of Jesus Christ and Other Essays. Grossman: NY, pp 53–61

190   "Dr. Hans Strupp . . .": Strupp HH, Hadley SW, Gomes-Schwartz B (1977): Psychotherapy for Better or Worse: The Problem of Negative Effects. Jason Aronson: NY

190   "When supervisors at . . .": Buckley P, Karasu TB, Charles E (1979): Common mistakes in psychotherapy. Am J Psy, 136: 1578–1580

190   "Professionals even find . . .": DeWitt KN, Kaltreider NB, Weiss DS, Horowitz MJ (1983): Judging change in psychotherapy: reliability of clinical formulations. Arch Gen Psy, 40: 1121–1128; Chevron ES, Rounsaville BJ (1983): Evaluating the clinical skills of psychotherapists: a comparison of techniques. Arch Gen Psy, 40: 1129–1132

194   "Strolling through Leyden . . .": Jones E (1955/1970): The Life and Work of Sigmund Freud, Volume 2. Basic Books: NY

195   "For example, Manhattan . . .": Levinson P, McMurray L, Podell P, Weiner H (1978): Causes for the premature interruption of psychotherapy by private practice patients. Am J Psy, 135: 826–830

198   "A study of . . .": Harty M, Horowitz L (1976): Therapeutic outcome as rated by patients, therapists, and judges. Arch Gen Psy, 33: 957–961

198n   "Psychotherapy research also . . .": Mosher LR, Keith SJ (1979): Research on the psychosocial treatment of schizophrenia: a summary report. Am J Psy, 136: 623–631

199   ". . . Abraham Kardiner when . . .": Kardiner A (1977): My Analysis with Freud. Norton: NY, pp 69–70

199   "In the most . . .": Weissman MM, Prusoff BA, DiMascio A, Neu C, Goklaney M, Klerman GL (1979): The efficacy of drugs and psychotherapy in the treatment of acute depressive episodes. Am J Psy, 136: 555–558; DiMascio A, Weissman MM, Prusoff BA, Neu C, Zwilling M, Klerman GL (1979): Differential symptom reduction by drugs and psychotherapy in acute depression. Arch Gen Psy, 36: 1450–1456

Chapter 8 PUBLIC PSYCHIATRY

PAGE
201   "In truth, a majority . . .": American Psychiatric Association (1983): Economic Fact Book for Psychiatry. American Psychiatric Press: Washington, DC

201   "Therefore, during a . . .": Gruel L (1980): Psychiatric Manpower for the '80s. American Psychiatric Association: Washington, DC

202   "Roughly a third . . .": Ibid

206   "Over the past . . .": American Psychiatric Association

210   "The average occupancy . . .": Ibid

210   ". . . in Manhattan in . . .": Netzer D (1983): The report of the subcommittee on the New York City psychiatric bed crisis. Governor's Select Commission on the Future of the State-Local Mental Health System, December

211   "In 1979, the . . .": American Psychiatric Association

214   "For patients having . . .": Ibid

214   "Research conducted during . . .": Glick ID, Hargreaves WA, Drues J, Showstack JA, Katzow (1977): Short vs long hospitalization: a prospective controlled study. Arch Gen Psy, 34: 314–317; Herz MI, Endicott J, Spitzer RL (1977): Brief hospitalization: a two-year follow-up. Am J Psy, 134: 502–507

219   "In 1981 a . . .": Who Are the Homeless? (1982). New York State Office of Mental Health: NY, May

220   "Studies throughout the . . .": Caton CLM (1984): Management of Chronic Schizophrenia. Oxford: NY

220   "For example, in New York . . .": Hoffman SP, Rosenfeld R, Wenger D, Shimono J (1984): The homeless mentally ill: what went wrong? Paper presented at the annual meeting of the American Orthopsychiatric Association, Toronto, April

221 "Unfortunately, much of . . .": Maxmen JS (1984): Hospital treatment, in Management of Chronic Schizophrenia. Edited by Caton CLM. Oxford: NY, pp 55–74

Chapter 9 *HOW PSYCHIATRISTS FEEL ABOUT PATIENTS*

PAGE
226 "Psychologist Dr. William . . .": Schofield W (1964): Psychotherapy: The Purchase of Friendship. Prentice Hall: Englewood Cliffs, NJ

226 "In other words, . . .": Ames E (1980): What your shrink really thinks of you. Reflections, 15(4): 19–31

240 "A California State . . .": Nelson B (1982): Efforts widen to curb sexual abuse in therapy. New York Times, November 11, p C1, 3

240 "According to this . . .": Ibid

241 "A survey of 460 . . .": Kardener S, Fuller M, Mensh I (1973): A survey of physicians' attitudes and practices regarding erotic and non-erotic contact with patients. Am J Psy, 130: 1077–1081; Perry JA (1976): Physicians' erotic and nonerotic physical involvement with patients. Am J Psy, 133: 838–840

242 "But even when . . .": New York Post (1983): "N.Y.'s mental hospitals can't let this ruling stand." Editorial. January 5, p 32; Psychiatric News (1981): MD condemns sex with patients, urges widespread education. 16(21): 30, 34, November 6

242 "Male psychologists, psychiatrists, . . .": Chesler P (1971): Women as psychiatric and psychotherapeutic patients. Journal of Marriage and the Family, 33: 746–759

242 "Studies confirm this . . .": Mogul KM (1982): Overview: The sex of the therapist. Am J Psy, 139: 1–11

242 "Moreover, a therapist . . .": Shapiro ET, Pinsker H (1973): Shared ethnic scotoma. Am J Psy, 130: 1338–1341

243 "The Negro . . . appears . . .": Lind JE (1917): Phylogenetic elements in the psychoses of the Negro. The Psychoanalytic Review, 4: 303–332, pp 303–304

244 "THE MORAL-EXISTENTIAL . . .": Abroms EM (1983): Beyond eclecticism. Am J Psy, 140: 740–745

247 "Dick Cavett, who . . .": Dick Cavett says thanks (1983). Psychiatric News, 18(21): 38, November 4

Chapter 10 BECOMING A PSYCHIATRIST

PAGE

249   "From the end . . .": Nielsen AC III, Eaton JS (1981): Medical students' attitudes about psychiatry: implications for psychiatric recruitment. Arch Gen Psy, 38: 1144–1154

249   "This decline is . . .": Freedman DX (1976): The alma mater is smoking—this is dangerous to your health! Arch Gen Psy, 33: 407–410; Why don't medical students want to be psychiatrists? (1981). Roche Reports, 12(11): 12–13

249   "The most common . . .": Taintor Z, Morphy M, Seiden A, Val E (1983): Psychiatric residency training: relationships and value development. Am J Psy, 140: 778–780

250   "Overall, the number . . .": Eagle PF, Marcos LR (1980): Factors in medical students' choice of psychiatry. Am J Psy, 137: 423–427

250   "The main reason . . .": Nielsen

250   "This picture, though . . .": Ibid; Eagle; Yager J, Scheiber SC (1981): The career choice of psychiatry: a national conference on recruitment into psychiatry. Journal of Psychiatric Education, 5: 258–268; Sierles F (1982): Medical school factors and career choice of psychiatry. Am J Psy, 139: 1040–1042

251   "Yet this disincentive . . .": Nielsen

252   "About a quarter . . .": Taintor

255   " '. . . psychiatry is a generality . . .' ": This remark is attributed to Alan Gregg in Redlich FC and Freedman DX (1966): The Theory and Practice of Psychiatry. Basic Books: NY, p 1

256   "In comparison to . . .": Eagle

256   "The percent of . . .": American Psychiatric Association (1980): Selected data from APA census of psychiatric residents. Unpublished; Datagram (1974): Journal of Medical Education, 49: 305; Datagram (1982): Journal of Medical Education, 57: 498

256   "Personality profiles of . . .": Light D (1980): Becoming Psychiatrists. Norton: NY

256   "They are less racist . . .": Light

260   "Those with internships . . .": Karasu TB, Stein SP, Charles ES (1976): A preliminary study of the elimination of the internship. Arch Gen Psy, 31: 269–272

260 "Psychiatric supervisors found . . .": Karasu TB, Stein SP, Charles ES (1978): A three-year follow-up study of the elimination of the internship. Arch Gen Psy, 35: 1024–1026

260 "For instance, in one . . .": Burstein AG, Adams RL, Giffen MB (1973): Assessment of suicidal risk by psychology and psychiatry trainees. Arch Gen Psy, 29: 792–793

262*n* "The only hard . . .": Taintor

267 "At around eight months . . .": Skodal AE, Maxmen JS (1981): Role satisfaction among psychiatric residents. Comprehensive Psychiatry, 22: 174–178

269 ". . . an institution in 80 . . .": Pinney EL Jr, Wells SH, Fisher B (1978): Group therapy training in psychiatric residency programs: a national survey. Am J Psy, 135: 1505–1508

272 "When psychiatric educators . . .": Bowden CL, Humphrey FJ, Thompson MGG (1980): Priorities in psychiatric residency training. Am J Psy, 137: 1243–1246

272 "Most residents feel . . .": Skodal

277 "According to recent . . .": Popkin MK, Mackenzie TB, Hall RCW, Garrard J (1979): Physicians' concordance with consultants' recommendations for psychotropic medication. Arch Gen Psy, 36: 386–389; Kramer BA, Spikes J, Strain JJ (1980): Compliance with psychiatric consultant's recommendations. Letter to the editor. Arch Gen Psy, 37: 1082

Chapter 11 PRIVATE LIVES

PAGE
280 "The first two . . .": Looney JG, Harding RK, Blotcky MJ, Barnhart FD (1980): Psychiatrists' transition from training to career: stress and mastery. Am J Psy, 137: 32–36

281 "Married medical students . . .": Coombs RH, Fawzy FI (1982): The effect of marital status on stress in medical school. Am J Psy, 139: 1490–1493

281 "What's more, being . . .": Looney

281 ". . . money matters are . . .": Freud S (1913/1958): On beginning the treatment (further recommendations on the technique of psycho-analysis. I), in Complete Psychological Works, standard ed, vol 12: 121–144. Translated and edited by Strachey J. Hogarth Press: London, p 131

282   "In just one . . .": Roche Reports (1982): How to make a living while taking care of patients. February 1, pp 5–6, 14

283   "Psychiatrists are now . . .": American Medical Association (1983): Socioeconomic monitoring system, 2(4), July

283   Tables 11-1 and 11-2, Ibid

283   "The reasons for . . .": Sharfstein SS, Clark HW (1980): Why psychiatry is a low-paid medical specialty. Am J Psy, 137: 831–833

284   ". . . nor does it include . . .": M. S. (1981): Moonlighting, financial astronomy for residents. Association for Academic Psychiatry Newsletter, 8(3): 2, Fall edition; Winslow R (1981): A nation of doctors in debt? New York Times Magazine, November 8, pp 132–141

285   "From 1978 to 1983 . . .": APA Malpractice claim types constant, but frequency, costs have doubled (1983). Psychiatric News, 18(21): 3, November 4

285   ". . . the single greatest consideration . . .": Koran LM (1981): Psychiatrists' distribution across the 50 states, 1978. Arch Gen Psy, 38: 1155–1159

285   "Nothing stresses new . . .": Looney

286   "Realizing that 40 . . .": Rudy LH (1982): 1981 Annual report of the American Board of Psychiatry and Neurology, Inc. Am J Psy, 139: 1403–1404

286   "This concern is . . .": Taintor Z, Morphy M, Seiden A, Val E (1983): Psychiatric residency training: relationships and value development. Am J Psy, 140: 778–780

286   "After failing boards, . . .": Maleson FG, Fink PJ, Field HL (1980): Board certification anxiety. Am J Psy, 137: 837–840

292   "Psychiatrists have the . . .": Goldney R, Czechowicz M, Dibden S, Govan J, Miller M, Tottman J (1979): The psychiatrist's family—a comparative study. Australian and New Zealand Journal of Psychiatry, 13: 341–347; Pearson MM (1982): Psychiatric treatment of 250 physicians. Psychiatric Annals, 12: 194–206; Vaillant GE, Sobowale NC, Mc Arthur C (1975): Some psychologic vulnerabilities of physicians. New England Journal of Medicine, 287: 372–375

292   "In comparison to . . .": Blum JD, Redlich F (1980): Mental health practitioners: old stereotypes and new realities. Arch Gen Psy, 37: 1247–1253

292   "When troubles do . . .": Goldney

293   "In July 1972 . . .": Shwed HJ (1980): When a psychiatrist dies. Journal of Nervous and Mental Disease, 168: 275–278

294   "Living with Crohn's . . .": Maxmen J (1972): The doctor as patient, in Patient-Centered Medicine. Edited by Hopkins P. The Balint Society: London, pp 157–162

294   ". . . Dr. Paul Dewald. . . .": When the analyst is seriously ill ((1981). Roche Reports, 11(4): 12–13, March 15

296   "Despite some disagreement . . .": Rich CL, Pitts FN (1980): Suicide by psychiatrists: a study of medical specialists among 18,730 consecutive physician deaths during a five-year period, 1967–72. Journal of Clinical Psychiatry, 41: 261–263; Preven DW (1983): Physician suicide: the psychiatrist's role, in The Impaired Physician. Edited by Scheiber SC, Doyle B. Plenum: NY, pp 39–47

296   "Since 50 to 70 . . .": Goodwin DW, Guze SB (1984): Psychiatric Diagnosis. Oxford University Press: NY

296   "Figures suggest that . . .": Rich

297n   "Statistically, this rate . . .": Rich

297   "Surveys show that women . . .": Goldstein MZ, Bromet EJ, Hanusa BH, Lasell RL (1981): Psychiatrists' life and work patterns: a statewide comparison of women and men. Am J Psy, 138: 919–924

297   "Feeling indispensable is . . .": Pearson

298   "For contrary to myth . . .": Greenberg RP, Staller J (1981): Personal therapy for therapists. Am J Psy, 138: 1467–1471

299   "In 1912, when . . .": Freud S (1912/1958): Recommendations to physicians practising psycho-analysis, in Complete Psychological Works, standard ed, vol 12: 111–122. Translated and edited by Strachey J. Hogarth Press: London, p 116

299   "From the 1930s . . .": Marmor J (1979): Psychoanalytic training: problems and perspectives. Arch Gen Psy, 36: 486–489, p 488

299   "Studies have shown . . .": Greenberg; Looney

299n   "In 1981, the . . .": Tax court says MD can deduct treatment costs (1982). Psychiatric News, 17(3): 17, February 5

300   "Whether a psychiatrist . . .": Greenberg

300   "When surveyed, psychiatrists . . .": Rogow AA (1970): The Psychiatrists. G. P. Putnam's Sons: NY

Index